Handbook of
Stroke Prevention in Clinical Practice

CURRENT CLINICAL NEUROLOGY

Daniel Tarsy, MD, SERIES EDITOR

Seizures in Critical Care: *A Guide to Diagnosis and Therapeutics,* edited by ***Panayiotis N. Varelas,*** *2005*

Handbook of Stroke Prevention in Clinical Practice, edited by ***Karen L. Furie and Peter J. Kelly,*** *2004*

Handbook of Neurocritical Care, edited by ***Anish Bhardwaj, Marek A. Mirski, and John A. Ulatowski,*** *2004*

Vascular Dementia: *Cerebrovascular Mechanisms and Clinical Management,* edited by ***Robert H. Paul, Ronald Cohen, Brian R. Ott, Stephen Salloway,*** *2004*

Atypical Parkinsonian Disorders, edited by ***Irene Litvan,*** *2004*

Clinical Handbook of Insomnia, edited by ***Hrayr P. Attarian,*** *2004*

Critical Care Neurology and Neurosurgery, edited by ***Jose I. Suarez,*** *2004*

Alzheimer's Disease: *A Physician's Guide to Practical Management,* edited by ***Ralph W. Richter and Brigitte Zoeller Richter,*** *2004*

Field of Vision: *A Manual and Atlas of Perimetry,* edited by ***Jason J. S. Barton and Michael Benatar,*** *2003*

Surgical Treatment of Parkinson's Disease and Other Movement Disorders, edited by ***Daniel Tarsy, Jerrold L. Vitek, and Andres M. Lozano,*** *2003*

Myasthenia Gravis and Related Disorders, edited by ***Henry J. Kaminski,*** *2003*

Seizures: *Medical Causes and Management,* edited by ***Norman Delanty,*** *2002*

Clinical Evaluation and Management of Spasticity, edited by ***David A. Gelber and Douglas R. Jeffery,*** *2002*

Early Diagnosis of Alzheimer's Disease, edited by ***Leonard F. M. Scinto and Kirk R. Daffner,*** *2000*

Sexual and Reproductive Neurorehabilitation, edited by ***Mindy Aisen,*** *1997*

Handbook of
Stroke Prevention in Clinical Practice

Edited by

Karen L. Furie, *MD, MPH*
Massachusetts General Hospital and Harvard Medical School, Boston, MA

and

Peter J. Kelly, *MD, MS, MRCPI*
Mater Misericordiae University Hospital and University College, Dublin, Ireland and Massachusetts General Hospital, Boston, MA

HUMANA PRESS TOTOWA, NEW JERSEY

999 Riverview Drive, Suite 208
Totowa, New Jersey 07512

humanapress.com

This publication is printed on acid-free paper. ∞
ANSI Z39.48-1984 (American Standards Institute) Permanence of Paper for Printed Library Materials.

Production Editor: Robin B. Weisberg.

Cover illustration: Hand-painted interpretation of a stroke event. Cover illustration by Dr. Pei-Chen Ning.

Cover design by Patricia F. Cleary.

For additional copies, pricing for bulk purchases, and/or information about other Humana titles, contact Humana at the above address or at any of the following numbers: Tel.: 973-256-1699; Fax: 973-256-8341; E-mail: humana@humanapr.com, or visit our Website: www.humanapress.com

Printed in the United States of America. 10 9 8 7 6 5 4 3 2 1

E-ISBN 1-59259-769-6

Library of Congress Cataloging-in-Publication Data

Handbook of stroke prevention in clinical practice / edited by Karen L.
Furie, Peter J. Kelly.
p. ; cm. -- (Current clinical neurology)
Includes bibliographical references and index.
ISBN 1-58829-158-8 (alk. paper)
1. Cerebrovascular disease--Prevention--Handbooks, manuals, etc.
[DNLM: 1. Cerebrovascular Accident--prevention & control--Handbooks.
WL 39 H2368 2004] I. Furie, Karen L. II. Kelly, Peter J., MB. III.
Series.
RC388.5.H345 2004
616.8'1--dc22

2003020644

Series Editor's Introduction

Despite major advances in the understanding of stroke mechanisms that have occurred over the past quarter century, stroke continues to rank among the leading causes of death and disability worldwide. Although currently it may be difficult to believe, early doubts were expressed as to whether interventions in risk factors for either coronary disease or stroke would actually lead to a reduction in the incidence of these disorders. However, large clinical trials in hypertension, carotid disease, atrial fibrillation, and antithrombotic and antiplatelet therapies have effectively demonstrated the efficacy of these targeted interventions in reducing stroke incidence. More recently, after earlier uncertainty regarding the role of elevated lipids as a risk factor for stroke, clinical trials of the statins have also demonstrated a significant reduction in the incidence of ischemic stroke. However, as emphasized in *Handbook of Stroke Prevention in Clinical Practice*, despite these gains and the initial decline in stroke incidence that did occur in the 1960s and 1970s, the incidence of stroke disappointingly has failed to show a further significant decline since that time.

The editors of *Handbook of Stroke Prevention in Clinical Practice* raise the very important question of whether recognized strategies for stroke prevention have been widely or effectively implemented. They correctly emphasize the critical importance of identifying the mechanism of stroke in each patient so as to properly direct prevention and treatment. As Dr. Louis Caplan so eloquently stated, the essential question in management of patients with cerebrovascular disease is to first ask and answer the question, "What is wrong with Mr. Jones?" *(1)*. That is, exactly why has this patient had transient ischemic attack? It then becomes clearer what should be done about it. Early stroke prevention and treatment studies considered ischemic stroke collectively without clearly identifying the mechanism of stroke in enrolled patients. Undoubtedly, the same can often be said of stroke management as it routinely takes place in the community. The chapters on vascular, cardiac, embolic, uncommon, and cryptogenic causes of stroke in this volume usefully serve to emphasize the very wide variety of circumstances that can result in ischemic stroke.

The editors have also further updated the list of risk factors for stroke including tobacco and alcohol, obesity and physical activity, hormonal status, serum biomarkers, and genetic factors, all of which will require further study to determine their importance as risk factors and the impact of intervention in these areas. Useful tables and definitive summary statements concerning the current state of the art concerning risk factors and available interventions will hopefully serve to improve the prospects for patients at risk for stroke. The CD-ROM that is included can be downloaded into a computer or PDA and should maximize the value of this information to the practicing clinician.

REFERENCE

1. Caplan LR. TIAs: We need to return to the question, "What is wrong with Mr. Jones?" Neurology 1988;38:791–793.

Daniel Tarsy, MD
Movement Disorders Center,
Beth Israel Deaconess Medical Center,
Harvard Medical School, Boston, MA

Preface

Stroke is a major cause of death and disability worldwide. In the United States, it is the third leading cause of death, after heart disease and cancer. There are approximately 600,000 ischemic strokes each year and up to one-third of these individuals remain permanently disabled. Globally, stroke is projected to be the fourth most common cause of premature death and disability by the year 2020. Since the 1970s, several large international cohort studies have provided a wealth of information about stroke risk factors, many of which may be modified by lifestyle changes or medical therapies. During the same epoch, large clinical trials have established targeted interventions for preventing stroke associated with specific high-risk conditions, such as carotid disease and atrial fibrillation. Yet, even with the risks defined and the prevention strategies proven, the incidence of stroke has not decreased significantly in recent years. Although scientifically validated and widely accepted, these strategies for stroke prevention are often not effectively implemented.

The failure to identify and treat risk factors for stroke contributes to the high rates of recurrent stroke and vascular death seen in patients with cerebrovascular disease. Although issues related to vascular protection are not unique to the cerebrovascular circulation, the failure to modify such risk factors as hypertension, hyperlipidemia, smoking, and obesity contributes to the burden of stroke. Neurologists evaluating an individual at high risk of recurrent stroke following transient ischemic attack or minor stroke are sometimes ill-prepared to assume responsibility for managing such risk factors as hypertension. In contrast, non-neurologists may feel uncomfortable localizing neurological symptoms and determining the pathophysiology for the event, which may lead to a failure to implement a mechanism-based prevention strategy tailored to that individual.

Our purpose in writing the *Handbook of Stroke Prevention in Clinical Practice* was to focus on the practical aspects of managing patients at high risk of stroke and to provide the resources that a practicing clinician might find valuable in assessing and treating these individuals. The summary statements, tables, and graphs were intended to leave sharp impressions that could be woven into the clinical discourse and shared with patients and their families. We sought to include the tools and references we use on a regular basis in our practice and to consolidate them in one text. Our intention was to provide a practical guide, rather than an exhaustive compendium of stroke epidemiology and clinical trial results. We made a determined effort to include the most up-to-date targets and interventions, recognizing that these will likely evolve over time.

Our approach is based on the pathophysiology of cerebral ischemia and infarction. The primary goal of the initial assessment of a symptomatic patient should be to determine the mechanism of ischemia. The classification schemes currently employed are useful, but not optimal, given that an individual might have multiple risk factors and potentially more than one mechanism of disease. Identifying a single cause of symptoms, be it atrial fibrillation or surgically remediable carotid stenosis, should not absolve the physician from identifying and modifying other risk factors. There is increasing evidence that conventional and novel risk factors contribute to stroke through effects on inflammation, endothelial injury, and activation of the hemostatic system. For these reasons, although we address specific mechanisms throughout the text, we chose to structure the book based primarily on states conferring increased stroke risk.

We wish to express our sincere appreciation for the valuable assistance of the clinicians and researchers who contributed their time and expertise to this work. We are grateful to Brenda Thornell and Susan Santilli who provided invaluable assistance in preparing the text. Additionally, we wish to acknowledge Dr. J. Philip Kistler and Dr. C. Miller Fisher of the Massachusetts General Hospital Stroke Service, whose pathophysiologic approach to stroke diagnosis and management has profoundly influenced generations of neurologists.

Karen L. Furie, *MD, MPH*
Peter J. Kelly, *MD, MS, MRCPI*

Contents

Contributors

CENK AYATA, MD • Departments of Radiology and Neurology, Massachusetts General Hospital and Harvard Medical School, Boston, MA

FERDINANDO S. BUONANNO, MD • Department of Neurology, Massachusetts General Hospital and Harvard Medical School, Boston, MA

RACHEL FARRELL, MB, MRCPI • Department of Neurology, Mater Misericordiae University Hospital and University College, Dublin, Ireland

KAREN L. FURIE, MD, MPH • Department of Neurology, Massachusetts General Hospital and Harvard Medical School, Boston, MA

DAVID M. GREER, MD • Department of Neurology, Massachusetts General Hospital, Brigham & Women's Hospital, and Harvard Medical School, Boston, MA

PETER J. KELLY, MD, MS, MRCPI • Mater Misericordiae University Hospital and University College, Dublin, Ireland; and Department of Neurology Massachusetts General Hospital, Boston, MA

J. PHILIP KISTLER, MD • Department of Neurology, Massachusetts General Hospital and Harvard Medical School, Boston, MA

WALTER J. KOROSHETZ, MD • Neurology and Stroke Services, Massachusetts General Hospital and Harvard Medical School, Boston, MA

DONALD M. LLOYD-JONES, MD, ScM • Department of Medicine, Massachusetts General Hospital and Harvard Medical School, Boston, MA

DOMINICK J. H. MCCABE, MB, MRCPI • Institute of Neurology, National Hospital for Neurology and Neurosurgery, London, England

MINGMING NING, MD • Department of Neurology, Massachusetts General Hospital and Harvard Medical School, Boston, MA

RAUL G. NOGUEIRA, MD • Department of Neurology, Massachusetts General Hospital and Harvard Medical School, Boston, MA

CHRISTOPHER J. O'DONNELL, MD, MPH • Cardiology Division, Massachusetts General Hospital and Harvard Medical School, Boston, MA; and NHLBI, Framingham Heart Study, Framingham, MA

GUY RORDORF, MD • Department of Neurology, Massachusetts General Hospital and Harvard Medical School, Boston, MA

JAN L. SHIFREN, MD • Vincent Ob/Gyn Service, Massachusetts General Hospital and Harvard Medical School, Boston, MA

JOHN SIMS, MD • Department of Neurology, Massachusetts General Hospital and Harvard Medical School, Boston, MA

ANEESH B. SINGHAL, MD • Department of Neurology, Massachusetts General Hospital and Harvard Medical School, Boston, MA

STELIOS M. SMIRNAKIS, MD, PhD • Department of Neurology, Massachusetts General Hospital and Harvard Medical School, Boston, MA; and Max Planck Institute for Biological Cybernetics, Tubingen, Germany

ERIC E. SMITH, MD • Department of Neurology, Massachusetts General Hospital and Harvard Medical School, Boston, MA

MEHMET AKIF TOPCOUGLU, MD • Department of Neurology, Massachusetts General Hospital, Boston and Harvard Medical School, MA

MARIA WORMACK, MD • Stroke Service, Department of Neurology, Massachusetts General Hospital, Boston, MA

Value-Added eBook/PDA

This book is accompanied by a value-added CD-ROM that contains an Adobe eBook version of the volume you have just purchased. This eBook can be viewed on your computer, and you can synchronize it to your PDA for viewing on your handheld device. The eBook enables you to view this volume on only one computer and PDA. Once the eBook is installed on your computer, you cannot download, install, or e-mail it to another computer; it resides solely with the computer to which it is installed. The license provided is for only one computer. The eBook can only be read using Adobe® Reader® 6.0 software, which is available free from Adobe Systems Incorporated at www.Adobe.com. You may also view the eBook on your PDA using the Adobe® PDA Reader® software that is also available free from Adobe.com.

You must follow a simple procedure when you install the eBook/PDA that will require you to connect to the Humana Press website in order to receive your license. Please read and follow the instructions below:

1. Download and install Adobe® Reader® 6.0 software
   You can obtain a free copy of Adobe® Reader® 6.0 software at www.adobe.com
   **Note: If you already have Adobe® Reader® 6.0 software, you do not need to reinstall it.*
2. Launch Adobe® Reader® 6.0 software
3. Install eBook: Insert your eBook CD into your CD-ROM drive
   PC: Click on the "Start" button, then click on "Run"
   At the prompt, type "d:\ebookinstall.pdf" and click "OK"
   **Note: If your CD-ROM drive letter is something other than d: change the above command accordingly.*
   MAC: Double click on the "eBook CD" that you will see mounted on your desktop.
   Double click "ebookinstall.pdf"
4. Adobe® Reader® 6.0 software will open and you will receive the message
   "This document is protected by Adobe DRM" Click "OK"
   **Note: If you have not already activated Adobe® Reader® 6.0 software, you will be prompted to do so. Simply follow the directions to activate and continue installation.*
   Your web browser will open and you will be taken to the Humana Press eBook registration page. Follow the instructions on that page to complete installation. You will need the serial number located on the sticker sealing the envelope containing the CD-ROM.

If you require assistance during the installation, or you would like more information regarding your eBook and PDA installation, please refer to the eBookManual.pdf located on your CD. If you need further assistance, contact Humana Press eBook Support by e-mail at ebooksupport@humanapr.com or by phone at 973-256-1699.

1
Epidemiology of Stroke

Eric E. Smith and Walter J. Koroshetz

INTRODUCTION

Stroke is a major burden on public health worldwide. In the United States, it is the third leading cause of death after heart disease and cancer and the leading cause of chronic disability in adults. Despite the recent introduction of new therapies for acute stroke, effective prevention remains the major strategy for decreasing the mortality and morbidity of stroke. This chapter reviews epidemiological methods and risk factors for stroke.

OVERVIEW OF EPIDEMIOLOGICAL METHODS

Measures of Disease Frequency

Measurement of the impact of stroke requires an understanding of its frequency in the population *(1)*. The frequency of a disease is usually described in terms of *incidence* and *prevalence (2)*. *Cumulative incidence* refers to the number of new cases occurring in a defined population in a specified period. However, all individuals in the population under study may not have been observed for the same period of time because some individuals enter the study later than others or some leave the study earlier. In this case, the *incidence rate* is usually calculated as the measure of disease occurrence. As for cumulative incidence, the numerator remains the number of new disease cases. However, the denominator is the product of the number of individuals observed and the total observation time free of disease (Box 1).

In contrast to incidence, which measures new disease occurrence, *prevalence* refers to the proportion of a defined population that has the disease at a given time (Box 1). The prevalence is dependent on the duration of the disease and the incidence. For example, diseases with a high incidence and a long duration (e.g., diabetes) will have a high prevalence compared to diseases of lower incidence or shorter duration (e.g., lung cancer).

From: *Current Clinical Neurology: Handbook of Stroke Prevention in Clinical Practice*
Edited by: K. L. Furie and P. J. Kelly © Humana Press Inc., Totowa, NJ

Box 1
Measures of Disease Frequency

$$\text{Cumulative incidence} = \frac{\text{Number of new cases of disease during a specified time}}{\text{Population at risk}}$$

$$\text{Incidence rate} = \frac{\text{Number of new cases of disease}}{\text{(Population at risk)} \times \text{(Time period of observation)}}$$

$$\text{Prevalence} = \frac{\text{Number of cases of disease at a specified time}}{\text{Total population at risk}}$$

$$\text{Mortality rate} = \frac{\text{Number of deaths due to disease during a specified time}}{\text{Total population at risk}}$$

$$\text{Case fatality rate} = \frac{\text{Number of deaths due to disease}}{\text{Number of persons with the disease}}$$

Design of Epidemiological Studies

Different study designs afford different advantages in cost, effort, and types of data analysis (Table 1). *Descriptive studies* examine patterns of exposure and disease in defined groups in relation to other demographic, lifestyle, or clinical characteristics. *Cross-sectional studies* are based on a survey of exposures and outcomes in a population in a given period of time. *Case reports* and *case series* describe an unusual relationship between exposure and disease in the clinical setting in an individual or a small group of patients. These studies are inexpensive, may be performed relatively quickly, and often provide useful hypothesis-generating data for further analytic study. However, they are often limited by an inability to determine the strength and temporal relationship between exposure and disease, and they are usually inconclusive regarding the causality of the relationship.

The defining characteristic of a *cohort study* is selection of participants based on their exposures rather than on the occurrence of disease. Cohort studies may be *prospective*, meaning that the patients are selected and followed over time for the development of the outcome, or *retrospective*. In a retrospective cohort study, participants are also selected based on exposure, but both exposure and the outcome of interest occurred in the past, and information is obtained from historical records. The cohort design allows accurate determination of disease incidence and prevalence and is excellent for studying the relationship of candidate risk factors to the development and

Table 1
Study Designs

Study type	Advantages	Disadvantages
Case report/series	Highlights an unusual or interesting relationship between exposure and outcome; typically taken from clinical case material and therefore not costly; generates hypotheses that may be tested in other designs	Evidence is anecdotal; lack of definition of control group or source population prevents measures of frequency or risk ratios
Cross-sectional	Can determine prevalence of diseases and exposures	Cannot determine incidence rates; does not define temporal relationship between variables
Case–control	Sample population selected based on disease (outcome), which is helpful for studying rare diseases; less time consuming and less costly than cohort studies; useful when the outcome is rare	Control selection is vulnerable to bias; exposures are measured after the disease has occurred, so may be influenced by the disease
Cohort	Sample population selected based on exposure; useful when the exposures are rare; temporal relationship between exposure and disease is determined; relationship between multiple exposures and outcome may be studied	May need large cohort or long follow-up period for sufficient outcomes to occur; often costly; if outcome is rare, then statistical power may be insufficient for valid analysis
Clinical trial	Exposure is assigned by the investigator to study groups, and the effect on outcome is observed (analogous to laboratory experimental study); randomization can eliminate bias from both known and unknown confounders	Randomization may fail by chance, especially with smaller sample sizes; may require prolonged follow-up period; often costly; ethical concerns prevent assignment of certain exposures; often difficult to perform in rare diseases

course of disease. This design is particularly efficient for the study of the effects of rare exposures. Disadvantages include the logistical difficulties required in following a large sample over many years, with associated expenses. The cohort design is not ideally suited for studying rare outcomes because the required cohort size and length of follow-up may be prohibitive.

In a *case–control* study, individuals are selected based on their disease status, and their exposure history is determined compared to nondiseased controls. Advantages of this design are its relative efficiency, lack of expense, and ability to study rare diseases that are not feasible for study in a cohort design. However, case–control studies are subject to bias because the investigator determines the participants. To minimize this problem, controls should come from the same source population as cases, and groups should be similar in all respects except for disease status. A further disadvantage is that the temporal relationship between exposure and disease may be unclear because the occurrence of the disease may artificially influence the measurement of the exposure.

Intervention studies or *clinical trials* are used to test interventions designed to modify the course of disease. They may be considered a form of experimental epidemiological study in which the exposure is allocated by the investigator. Most commonly, one group is given the intervention, and a control group is not; both groups are followed for the outcome of interest.

One of the major goals of clinical trial design is the avoidance of bias that could influence the result of the experiment. Differences in important variables between the treatment groups are one major source of bias. Treatment groups should ideally be alike in all aspects and should only differ in the treatment each group receives. Randomly assigning the treatment group (*randomization*) should be done in order to promote an equal distribution of known and unknown potential confounders among the different groups. When demographic or clinical variables exist that could overwhelm the magnitude of the possible treatment effect, *stratification* may be done to avoid an imbalance of the variables among treatment groups. In stratified randomization a separate randomization procedure is done for each defined subset; the subset could be based on age or gender, for example. *Block randomization* is used to ensure balance in numbers between the treatment arms at any point in the trial; for example, trial participants may be grouped in blocks of ten with five receiving study drug and five receiving placebo. To eliminate bias resulting from physicians and patients knowing their treatment assignment, *blinding* (in which the treatment assignment is concealed) and *placebos* (an inactive form of the medicine given to the control group) are frequently used.

Box 2
Relative and Attributable Risk

Disease (e.g., stroke)

Exposure (e.g., obesity)	Disease Present	Disease Absent
Exposure Present	*A*	*B*
Exposure Absent	*C*	*D*

$$\text{Relative risk (risk ratio)} = \frac{\text{Proportion of disease in exposed group}}{\text{Proportion of disease in unexposed group}}$$

$$= \frac{A/(A+B)}{C/(C+D)}$$

Attributable risk = Proportion of disease in exposed group – Proportion of disease in unexposed group

$$= A/(A+B) - C/(C+D)$$

MEASURES OF DISEASE ASSOCIATION

Proportions, Odds, and Ratios

In epidemiological terms, a *proportion* is the ratio of part of a group to the whole group. In contrast, *odds* refers to the ratio of a part of a group (numerator) to the whole group minus the part (denominator). The strength of association between a defined exposure and disease is frequently summarized as a ratio that compares the proportions or odds of disease in exposed and nonexposed groups.

Relative Risk, Attributable Risk, and Odds Ratios

The *risk* of disease is the probability of disease occurrence in a defined population. An exposure (an environmental or inherited factor) that modifies the disease frequency in the exposed group is termed a *risk factor*.

In epidemiological studies of the relationship between exposure and disease, risk is usually quantified in one of several ways. In cohort studies, *relative risk* is frequently used to summarize the strength of an exposure on the development of disease (Box 2). Relative risk may be expressed as a risk ratio or rate ratio. The *risk ratio* is obtained by dividing the cumulative incidence of disease in the exposed group by the cumulative incidence in the nonexposed group. Similarly, the *rate ratio* is calculated by dividing the incidence rate of disease in exposed individuals by the incidence rate in nonexposed

Box 3
Population-attributable Risk

$$\text{Population-attributable risk} = \frac{\text{Prevalence} \times (\text{Relative risk} - 1) \times 100}{\text{Prevalence} \times (\text{Relative risk} - 1) + 1}$$

or

Attributable risk due to exposure × Proportion of population exposed

$$(P_e) = [A/(A + B) - C/(C + D)] \times P_e$$

individuals. This information can be readily expressed by constructing a contingency (2 × 2) table using data from a cohort study (Box 2). It is assumed that the groups compared are identical except for the exposure of interest. A relative risk greater than 1.0 indicates that the exposure is associated with increased frequency of the disease; a relative risk less than 1.0 indicates that the exposure is associated with decreased frequency of the disease.

In addition to the relative risk, the risk associated with an exposure may be expressed in absolute terms by calculating the difference in cumulative incidence of disease between exposed and nonexposed individuals (Box 2). This is termed the *attributable risk* or *risk difference*. The influence of an exposure on the risk of disease throughout an entire population may be estimated if the population prevalence of the exposure is known (Box 3). This measure, the *population-attributable risk*, is useful from a public health perspective as it provides an estimate of the number of cases of disease that may be prevented in a population by eliminating the exposure.

In a case–control study, in which subjects are eligible based on disease status rather than exposure status, it is not possible to calculate the risk ratio directly. The *odds ratio* (OR) is used in this context; it is defined as the odds of exposure in the disease group (cases) divided by the odds of exposure in the nondisease group (controls) (Box 4). For practical purposes, the OR approaches the risk ratio (particularly for rare diseases), assuming that incident cases are enrolled, and subjects are not selected based on their exposure status.

Bias and Confounding

In observational studies, bias refers to a systematic difference in the enrollment of subjects (selection bias) or collection of data (information bias) between individuals with and without the exposure or outcome of interest. Confounding refers to misinterpretation of the relationship between exposure and outcome due to the presence of one or more other factors (con-

Box 4
Odds Ratio

Exposure (e.g., obesity)	Disease (e.g., stroke): Disease Present	Disease (e.g., stroke): Disease Absent
Exposure Present	*A*	*B*
Exposure Absent	*C*	*D*

$$\text{Odds ratio} = \frac{\text{Odds of exposure in cases}}{\text{Odds of exposure in controls}} = \frac{A/C}{B/D} = \frac{A \times D}{B \times C}$$

founders) which are related to the exposure and independently associated with the outcome.

DESCRIPTION OF EPIDEMIOLOGICAL DATA

Types of Data

Data from analytic epidemiological studies must be described and quantified, and statistical methods are employed to test hypotheses that outcomes or exposures are different between groups. Data may be qualitative (discrete) or quantitative (continuous). Discrete data fall into two or more distinct categories without an intervening measure. In the simplest form, discrete data are *dichotomous*, falling into one of only two categories (e.g., male/female). If several categories exist with a natural progression between categories (e.g., the modified Rankin scale), the data are termed *ordinal*. In contrast, continuous data are measured on a scale without a predefined limit and within which intervening measures are possible (e.g., residual carotid lumen diameter on angiography).

Qualitative data are usually presented in terms of proportions (percentages) of each category. In contrast, the distribution of quantitative data is usually summarized as a measure of central tendency and spread around the center. Values often used to describe the central tendency include the mean and median; spread is most commonly measured by the standard deviation (Box 5). The median is less sensitive to influence from extreme data points (outliers) compared to the mean. The data are *normally distributed* if they assume a symmetric, bell-shaped curve. In this case, the mean and median are equal, and the distribution of data is symmetric about the mean. If the

Box 5
Measures of Data Distribution

$$\text{Mean} = \frac{\text{Sum of all values measured}}{\text{Number of measurements}}$$

Median = Value at the 50th percentile
= Value at which 50% of the observations are below it and 50% of the observations are above it

Standard deviation = Square root of the variance, a measure of the spread

$$= \sqrt{\frac{\Sigma\,(\text{Value} - \text{Mean})^2}{\text{Sample size} - 1}}$$

Range = Maximum value – Minimum value

distribution is normal, one and two standard deviations from the mean encompass 67 and 95% of the data points, respectively. Other types of distributions include *skewed* (a "tail" exists at one end of the distribution) and *bimodal* (two separate peaks in frequency of the measures exist).

In many studies, the important end point is the time to a major event, such as the occurrence of stroke. In this situation, the data are described as *time-to-event data* and can be graphed as a Kaplan–Meier plot. In such studies, many patients will not have had the outcome of interest by the time the study results are analyzed; in this case, the patient is said to be *censored* at the last time point for which information is available. Specific statistical methods for analysis are used that account for the amount of time patients are free of the end point before being censored.

Hypothesis Testing

When studies show a difference between two groups, the next step is to determine whether this difference is significant or merely represents a chance random variation. By convention, the null hypothesis that there is no difference between the groups is tested and either rejected or accepted. In general, the null hypothesis is rejected when the *p* value, which is the probability that the observed result could have happened purely by chance, is less than 0.05. The *p* value is equal to the chance of a *type I error*, which is the error of rejecting the null hypothesis when in fact it is true (i.e., obtaining a false-positive result). When multiple comparisons are made, it is appropriate to decrease the *p* value required for significance (the Bonferroni method is often used, in which the usual level of 0.05 is divided by the number of tests made). The opposite error, that of accepting the null hypothesis when in fact it is false (thereby obtaining a false-negative result) is termed a *type II error*. The *power* of the test is 1 minus the type II error; in most studies, it is designed to be between 0.70 and 0.90. The *95% confidence interval* provides useful information about the distribution of the true result by giving the range in which the true result is contained with a probability greater than or equal to 95%.

Selection of the appropriate statistical test is determined by the type of data (qualitative or quantitative, ordinal or continuous, etc.) and is outside the scope of this discussion. The most common statistical tests are the *t*-test for quantitative data, the chi-square test for qualitative data, the Wilcoxon rank sum test for nonparametric distributions, and the log-rank test for time-to-event data.

After significant relationships between exposures and outcome are found in univariate analysis, the next step is to determine whether all the exposures are independently associated with the outcome, or whether one or more exposures are dependent on one another. This can be done using *multivariate analysis*, also referred to as *regression analysis*, by which a statistical model is created to fit the data using multiple variables (also known as *predictors*) entered by the investigator. The analysis is called *logistic regression* when the outcome is qualitative, *linear regression* when the outcome is quantitative, and Cox proportional hazards regression when the outcome is time to event. The model can be used to calculate a *p* value and logistic regression analyses allows calculation of an adjusted odds ratio for each predictor variable. A variable that was significant in univariate analysis may no longer be a significant predictor when other variables are entered into the regression model.

EPIDEMIOLOGY OF STROKE

Incidence

In developed and developing countries, stroke is a common disease with a large impact on the health of the population. In the United States, data from epidemiological studies such as the Greater Cincinnati/Northern Kentucky Stroke Study indicate that the incidence of stroke is approx 700,000 cases per year *(3)*. Of these, approx 500,000 cases are first strokes, and 200,000 cases are recurrent strokes. The age-adjusted annual incidence rates for first stroke are 167 per 100,000 population for white males and 138 per 100,000 population for white females. The age-adjusted rates in black and Japanese American men and women in the United States are approximately twice those in whites.

The most reliable international stroke incidence data are from the World Health Organization (WHO) MONICA Study *(4)*. This project reported standardized data from 18 populations in 10 countries (including eastern and western European countries, Russia, and China) between 1985 and 1987. Age-standardized stroke incidence rates varied widely, from 101 to 285 in men and from 47 to 198 in women (all rates per 100,000 population), with the highest rates in Russia and Finland and the lowest in Italy. In general, rates were higher in eastern than western Europe and in men than in women (male:female range 1.2–2.4). Recurrent stroke accounted for 18–22% of total reported stroke.

Prevalence

The American Heart Association estimated that there are approx 4.7 million stroke survivors in the United States *(5)*. Many of these individuals are elderly and require long-term institutionalized care. Data indicate that the number of noninstitutionalized stroke survivors in the United States is approx 2.4 million *(6)*. These figures underscore the potential impact of measures for primary and secondary prevention of stroke.

Subtype-Specific Frequency Data

The widespread availability of computed tomography and magnetic resonance imaging of the brain has allowed categorization of stroke into distinct subcategories. This has facilitated the emergence of a more detailed understanding of the epidemiology and natural history of stroke based on pathophysiology. This in turn may greatly influence strategies for stroke prevention as some risk factors (e.g., hyperlipidemia) may influence the risk of some, but not all, stroke subtypes.

Stroke may be subdivided into ischemic or hemorrhagic stroke. Hemorrhagic stroke may be further subdivided into intracerebral hemorrhage (ICH) and subarachnoid hemorrhage (SAH). Ischemic stroke accounts for about 80–85% of all stroke in European and North American populations. Although some stroke registries have reported rates as high as 23–27%, hemorrhagic stroke accounts for 10–15% in most studies; of this percentage, 3–6% are caused by SAH, and 8–10% are caused by ICH.

Several classification schemes have been developed to subdivide ischemic stroke further. The scheme developed for the Trial of Org 10172 in Acute Stroke Treatment (TOAST) is one widely accepted method *(7)*. This uses the results of the clinical evaluation and supplemental laboratory testing (including imaging, cardiac imaging, electrocardiography, etc.) to divide stroke into five categories based on etiology: large-artery atherosclerosis, cardioembolism, small-artery occlusion (lacunar stroke), stroke of other determined etiology (e.g., hypercoagulable state), and stroke of undetermined etiology.

Other authors have used similar schemes. In the multiethnic Northern Manhattan Stroke Study, 32% of strokes were cryptogenic (no determined etiology), 20% were cardioembolic, 17% were caused by large-artery atherosclerosis (of which half involved intracranial arteries and half involved extracranial arteries), and 27% were lacunar *(8)*. The incidence of lacunar stroke has been lower in predominantly white population studies, such as the Framingham study.

OUTCOME FOLLOWING STROKE

Mortality

Different studies have shown widely variable case fatality rates for ischemic stroke. Potential reasons for this heterogeneity include regional or international variability in acute medical care and variability in the distribution of stroke types within populations. In the United States, 30-day case fatality rates as low as 5% and as high as 22% have been reported. Data from the multiethnic Northern Manhattan Stroke Study indicated a 30-day mortality of 5%, a 1-year mortality of 18%, and a 5-year mortality of 42% after first-ever ischemic stroke *(9)*. Large hemispheric infarction and major basilar territory infarction have been associated with an increased risk of death *(10)*. Lacunar stroke is associated with a lower risk of death, with a 30-day case fatality rate as low as 1% *(11)*.

The case fatality rate is higher for hemorrhagic stroke, with mortality rates of 40–50% for ICH and SAH. Factors associated with increased early mortality caused by ICH include hemorrhage volume, Glasgow Coma Scale score, and the presence of intraventricular hemorrhage *(12)*.

Outside the United States, the MONICA study reported 28-day case fatality rates of 15–49% for men and 18–57% for women *(4)*. However, comparisons with US data must be performed with caution as the data include both ischemic and hemorrhagic stroke subtypes.

Disability

The Global Burden of Disease project has summarized disease-specific disability in terms of disability adjusted life years (DALYs) lost *(13)*. This measure combines premature mortality with disease-related impairment and allows internally valid disease-specific comparisons to be made between regions. In 1990, it was estimated that stroke was the sixth most common cause of DALY lost worldwide. It is projected to be the fourth most common cause by 2020 *(13)*.

In the developed world, important regional and international variation exists in provision of postacute stroke services. In the United States, 19–32% of ischemic stroke survivors are discharged from the acute hospital to a nursing home or rehabilitation facility. Severity of stroke, age, living alone before stroke, and cognitive impairment are associated with inability to return home following stroke. Approximately 50–70% of survivors return to functional independence, 15–30% remain with permanent disability, and 20% require residential care 3 months after stroke onset. Lacunar and cerebellar ischemic stroke have better prognoses, with higher rates of recovery and decreased rates of discharge to rehabilitation or nursing homes.

Cost

In the United States, the direct health care-related cost of stroke was estimated as $17 billion in 1990 *(14)*. The indirect costs, such as loss of productivity, are even greater and, when added to the direct costs, produced a total of $40 billion in 1990. SAH and ICH are more costly per person than ischemic stroke. The most costly is SAH, in large part because of a younger mean age of onset, which leads to greater loss of lifetime productivity.

RECURRENT STROKE

The rate of early (within 30 days) ischemic stroke recurrence varied from 3 to 10% in reported studies *(15)*. The subtype of ischemic stroke appears to be a major determinant of early recurrence. Sacco and colleagues *(15)* and others reported that patients with stroke resulting from large artery atherosclerosis had the highest recurrence rate (8–18%), lacunar stroke had the lowest recurrence rate (1.4–2%), and cardioembolic stroke and cryptogenic stroke had intermediate rates (3–5%). Reported late recurrence rates varied from 12 to 14% at 1 year and 25 to 40% by 5 years *(10)*. Atrial fibrillation, hypertension, alcohol abuse, and hyperglycemia have all been found as independent predictors of stroke recurrence. Recurrent strokes have a higher rate of mortality and disability than first-ever strokes.

Transient ischemic attack (TIA) identifies a group of patients at high risk for early development of ischemic stroke. In one study, patients diagnosed with TIA in the emergency room had a 10.5% risk of stroke in the next 90 days, of which half occurred in the first 2 days following the index event *(16)*. Older age (>60 years), diabetes, focal weakness or dysarthria, or duration longer than 10 minutes were additive independent predictors of stroke following TIA.

A recent meta-analysis of ICH found a recurrence rate of 2.3% per year *(17)*. Patients with hemorrhages in lobar brain regions, who are at risk for cerebral amyloid angiopathy, had a higher recurrence rate of 4.4% per year. Recurrent lobar hemorrhage has been associated with the presence of the apolipoprotein E ε2 or ε4 allele.

TEMPORAL TRENDS

Stroke incidence declined from the 1950s to the end of the 1970s, but this trend appeared to end in the 1980s. Data from a longitudinal study in Rochester, Minnesota, indicated that rates actually rose between 1985 and 1989 *(18)*. This trend was seen for both ischemic stroke and ICH. The factors that led to the decline in the 1950s to 1970s are not fully known. Improvements in prevention, particularly treatment of hypertension, may have been partly responsible. The recent increasing incidence of stroke may be partly because of improved case finding or the increasing prevalence of survivors of chronic medical problems, such as ischemic heart disease, who are at risk for stroke. It is likely that the recent apparent increase in incidence of ICH is the result of more reliable diagnosis with the use of CT scanning.

Case fatality rates from stroke have been in decline from 1950 to the present. This has been attributed to both improved medical care and increased incidence of less-severe strokes, partly because of improved diagnosis. The improvement in stroke mortality has been balanced by an increase in the number of stroke survivors. Data indicated that the number of noninstitutionalized stroke survivors increased from 1.5 million in the early 1970s to 2.4 million in the early 1990s.

RISK FACTORS

Nonmodifiable Risk Factors: Age, Sex, Race or Ethnicity, and Family History

Advancing age is a strong risk factor for stroke, both ischemic and hemorrhagic. Data from the Framingham study indicated that stroke incidence doubles for each decade after 55 years *(19)*.

In general, stroke is more common in men than in women. After adjusting for age, the male:female incident stroke ratio varies from 1.39 (Framingham study) *(19)* to 2.4 (MONICA) *(4)*. Exceptions include age groups from 35 to 44 and older than 85 years, for which the age-adjusted stroke incidence is slightly higher in women.

Race or ethnicity is also associated with the risk of ischemic and hemorrhagic stroke. African Americans and Hispanic Americans are at increased risk for ischemic stroke, ICH, and SAH. For example, among the residents of northern Manhattan, African Americans had a 2.4-fold and Hispanic Americans had a 2.1-fold increase in the incidence of combined ischemic stroke and hemorrhagic stroke compared to whites *(20)*. Hispanic Americans and African Americans are reported to have a higher proportion of strokes caused by intracranial atherosclerosis and lacunes and a lower proportion of strokes caused by cardioembolism *(8)*. ICH is approximately three times more common in Hispanic Americans and African Americans and almost six times more common in Japanese Americans compared to whites. These racial and ethnic variations in stroke are only partly explained by differences in socioeconomic status and higher prevalence of known stroke risk factors such as diabetes, obesity, and hypertension, suggesting that genetic factors may also play a role.

A role for genetic factors in stroke was further suggested by several studies that found a higher stroke concordance rate for monozygotic compared to dizygotic twins *(21)*. Paternal and maternal history of stroke have also been linked with increased stroke risk *(22)*. In some of these family studies, a history of stroke in a first-degree relative was an independent risk factor for stroke occurrence. Most of these studies did not differentiate between ischemic strokes and hemorrhagic strokes. However, a population-based study of ICH found that a history of ICH in a first-degree relative was a significant risk factor for both lobar and nonlobar hemorrhages *(23)*.

Modifiable Risk Factors

The American Heart Association has published consensus recommendations based on best available evidence for the management of modifiable risk factors for ischemic stroke *(5)*. A summary of potentially modifiable risk factors for ischemic stroke is presented in Table 2; these are grouped according to the level of evidence establishing their connection with stroke (observational studies only vs observational and intervention studies). For many of the stroke risk factors that are less well documented, well-conducted randomized controlled trials addressing the effect of specific interventions on stroke risk are not available.

The concept of population-attributable risk is helpful for understanding the relative impact of different stroke risk factors (discussed in the section on measures of disease association). The population-attributable risk estimates the proportion of total incident stroke cases in the population than can be attributed to a given risk factor (Box 3). It is proportional to the prevalence of the risk factor and the degree of relative risk it confers. Among the well-documented ischemic stroke risk factors, hypertension accounts for the highest proportion of stroke among younger patients *(5)*. For example, it accounts for 40% of stroke in individuals aged 50–60 years. The attributable risk caused by hypertension decreases with increasing age because the increase in the prevalence of hypertension is more than offset by an accompanying decrease in the relative risk. In 80-year-olds, the attributable risk has dropped to 20%. As age increases, atrial fibrillation assumes a more prominent role, accounting for 23.5% of ischemic strokes in 80-year-olds. Hyperlipidemia and diabetes also account for a substantial proportion of ischemic stroke. Among the risk factors that are less well documented, obesity, physical inactivity, and hyperhomocysteinemia may account for a high number of strokes because of their high prevalence.

Table 2
Ischemic Stroke Risk Factors[a]

Nonmodifiable risk factors
Age
Sex
Race or ethnicity
Family history
Well-documented modifiable risk factors (intervention of proven benefit)[b]
Hypertension
Atrial fibrillation
Smoking
Diabetes
Hyperlipidemia
Carotid stenosis
Sickle cell disease
Less well-documented modifiable risk factors (observational studies, benefit of intervention unproven)
Cardiac
Myocardial infarction
Left ventricular dysfunction
Valvular heart diseases
Left ventricular hypertrophy
Patent foramen ovale
Atrial septal aneurysm
Mitral annular calcification
Mitral valve strands
Aortic arch atheroma
Physical inactivity
Poor diet
Lipoprotein (a)
Excessive alcohol consumption
Antiphospholipid antibodies
Hyperhomocysteinemia
Hypercoagulable states
Hormone replacement therapy
Oral contraceptive pill
Hyperfibrinogenemia
Drug abuse
Migraine
Fibromuscular dysplasia
Chronic inflammation/infection

[a]From ref. *1*.
[b]From ref. *5*.

Table 3
Intracerebral Hemorrhage Risk Factors

- Nonmodifiable
  - Age
  - Race or ethnicity
  - Apolipoprotein E ε2 or ε4 allele
  - Cerebral amyloid angiopathy
- Modifiable
  - Hypertension
  - Alcohol use
  - Ischemic stroke
  - Coagulopathy
  - Warfarin use
  - Aspirin use
  - Other anticoagulants and fibrinolytics
  - Cigarette smoking
  - Vascular malformation
  - Sympathomimetic drugs (including cocaine)
  - Vasculitis
  - Intracerebral tumors

Table 4
Subarachnoid Hemorrhage Risk Factors

- Saccular aneurysms
  - Nonmodifiable
    - Family history
    - Aneurysm size
    - Aneurysm location
    - Prior history of aneurysmal bleeding
    - Female gender
    - Autosomal dominant polycystic kidney disease
    - Ehler–Danlos syndrome
    - Associated with arteriovenous malformations
    - Moyamoya disease
    - Aortic coarctation
    - Fibromuscular dysplasia
  - Modifiable
    - Cigarette smoking
    - Hypertension
    - Cocaine use
- Other causes
  - Trauma
  - Mycotic aneurysms
  - Arteriosclerotic aneurysms
  - Arterial dissection (vertebral arteries)

Table 3 lists the known modifiable and nonmodifiable risk factors for ICH. A population-based case–control study found that lobar and nonlobar hemorrhages have different risk factors *(23)*. Hypertension was a significant risk factor for nonlobar ICH, accounting for 54% of the population-attributable risk. Lobar brain hemorrhage was instead associated with the presence of the apolipoprotein E ε2 or ε4 allele (29% population-attributable risk for the presence of either allele). Prior history of ischemic stroke, anticoagulant use, first-degree relative with ICH, and frequent alcohol use were associated with either type of hemorrhage.

Excluding head trauma, SAH is most commonly caused by rupture of a saccular aneurysm. The largest study of the natural history of saccular aneurysms found that aneurysm size, location, and prior history of SAH were associated with an increased risk of rupture *(24)*. Other modifiable and nonmodifiable risk factors for SAH are presented in Table 4.

REFERENCES

1. Batchelor T, Cudkowicz ME. Principles of Neuroepidemiology. Boston, MA: Butterworth-Heinemann, 2001.
2. Hennekens CH, Buring JE, Mayrent SL. Epidemiology in Medicine. Boston, MA: Little, Brown, 1987.
3. Impact of Stroke. Dallas, TX: American Heart Association, 2003. Available at: http://www.strokeassociation.org/. Accessed July 16, 2003.
4. Thorvaldsen P, Asplund K, Kuulasmaa K, Rajakangas AM, Schroll M. Stroke incidence, case fatality, and mortality in the WHO MONICA project. World Health Organization Monitoring Trends and Determinants in Cardiovascular Disease. Stroke 1995;26:361–367.
5. Goldstein LB, Adams R, Becker K, et al. Primary prevention of ischemic stroke: a statement for healthcare professionals from the Stroke Council of the American Heart Association. Stroke 2001;32:280–299.
6. Muntner P, Garrett E, Klag MJ, Coresh J. Trends in stroke prevalence between 1973 and 1991 in the US population 25 to 74 years of age. Stroke 2002;33: 1209–1213.
7. Adams HP, Bendixen BH, Kappelle LJ, et al. Classification of subtype of acute ischemic stroke. Definitions for use in a multicenter clinical trial. TOAST. Trial of Org 10172 in Acute Stroke Treatment. Stroke 1993;24:35–41.
8. Sacco RL. Risk factors, outcomes, and stroke subtypes for ischemic stroke. Neurology 1997;49:S39–S44.
9. Hartmann A, Rundek T, Mast H, et al. Mortality and causes of death after first ischemic stroke: the Northern Manhattan Stroke Study. Neurology 2001;57: 2000–2005.
10. Sacco RL, Shi T, Zamanillo MC, Kargman DE. Predictors of mortality and recurrence after hospitalized cerebral infarction in an urban community: the Northern Manhattan Stroke Study. Neurology 1994;44:626–634.
11. Bamford J, Sandercock P, Jones L, Warlow C. The natural history of lacunar infarction: the Oxfordshire Community Stroke Project. Stroke 1987;18:545–551.

12. Portenoy RK, Lipton RB, Berger AR, Lesser ML, Lantos G. Intracerebral haemorrhage: a model for the prediction of outcome. J Neurol Neurosurg Psychiatry 1987;50:976–979.
13. Murray CJ, Lopez AD. Alternative projections of mortality and disability by cause 1990–2020: Global Burden of Disease Study. Lancet 1997;349:1498–1504.
14. Taylor TN, Davis PH, Torner JC, Holmes J, Meyer JW, Jacobson MF. Lifetime cost of stroke in the United States. Stroke 1996;27:1459–1466.
15. Sacco RL, Foulkes MA, Mohr JP, Wolf PA, Hier DB, Price TR. Determinants of early recurrence of cerebral infarction. The Stroke Data Bank. Stroke 1989;20: 983–989.
16. Johnston SC, Gress DR, Browner WS, Sidney S. Short-term prognosis after emergency department diagnosis of TIA. JAMA 2000;284:2901–2906.
17. Bailey RD, Hart RG, Benavente O, Pearce LA. Recurrent brain hemorrhage is more frequent than ischemic stroke after intracranial hemorrhage. Neurology 2001;56: 773–777.
18. Brown RD, Whisnant JP, Sicks JD, O'Fallon WM, Wiebers DO. Stroke incidence, prevalence, and survival: secular trends in Rochester, Minnesota, through 1989. Stroke 1996;27:373–380.
19. Wolf PA, D'Agostino RB. Epidemiology of stroke. In: Barnett HJM, Mohr JP, Stein B, Yatsu FM, eds. Stroke: Pathophysiology, Diagnosis, and Management. London: Churchill Livingstone, 1998.
20. Sacco RL, Boden-Albala B, Gan R, et al. Stroke incidence among white, black, and Hispanic residents of an urban community: the Northern Manhattan Stroke Study. Am J Epidemiol 1998;147:259–268.
21. Brass LM, Isaacsohn JL, Merikangas KR, Robinette CD. A study of twins and stroke. Stroke 1992;23:221–223.
22. Kiely DK, Wolf PA, Cupples LA, Beiser AS, Myers RH. Familial aggregation of stroke. The Framingham Study. Stroke 1993;24:1366–1371.
23. Woo D, Sauerbeck LR, Kissela BM, et al. Genetic and environmental risk factors for intracerebral hemorrhage: preliminary results of a population-based study. Stroke 2002;33:1190–1195.
24. Unruptured intracranial aneurysms—risk of rupture and risks of surgical intervention. International Study of Unruptured Intracranial Aneurysms Investigators. N Engl J Med 1998;339:1725–1733.

2
Subtypes of Ischemic Stroke

John Sims and Walter J. Koroshetz

INTRODUCTION

Ischemic stroke occurs as a result of an extremely heterogeneous group of vascular pathological events (Table 1). Because treatment is often aimed at attenuating a specific vascular disorder, identifying the underlying cause is critical for optimal stroke prevention. As an example, secondary stroke prevention for a young patient with endocarditis will differ substantially from that for an elderly patient with atrial fibrillation, although both conditions cause cardioembolic stroke.

Therefore, in clinical practice and research studies, ischemic stroke is frequently classified into subtypes. Although different schemes exist, the rationale for their introduction was based on an attempt to resolve the anatomic and pathophysiological heterogeneity of ischemic stroke by grouping individual patients into one of several categories. In this way, the understanding of stroke natural history and pathophysiology could be refined, and hypotheses about the response to interventions targeted at specific stroke mechanisms could be tested. Accurate categorization into subtypes also increases the uniformity of subjects entered into clinical trials, thus facilitating the interpretation and application of results in clinical practice. In practice, the underlying heterogeneity of stroke pathophysiology creates difficulties in determining the pathological basis of the stroke in many individuals. Therefore, most commonly used classification systems separate patients with stroke into broad categories.

COMMON CLASSIFICATION SCHEMES

TOAST and Stroke Data Bank Classifications

One commonly used subtyping scheme is the Trial of Org 10172 in Acute Stroke Treatment (TOAST) classification (Table 2) *(1)*. Following completion of brain imaging and diagnostic testing, this scheme subdivides ischemic

From: *Current Clinical Neurology: Handbook of Stroke Prevention in Clinical Practice*
Edited by: K. L. Furie and P. J. Kelly © Humana Press Inc., Totowa, NJ

Table 1
Pathophysiological Basis of Ischemic Stroke

Pathology	Cause	Ischemic pathophysiology and stroke subtype
I. Intracranial vessels may be normal		
(a) Cardiac thrombus, with embolism	Atrial fibrillation, patent foramen ovale with septal aneurysm, fibroelastoma, atrial myxoma, post-myocardial infarction, ventricular aneurysm, cardiomyopathy, marantic endocarditis, infectious endocarditis, valvular heart disease	Cardioembolic; CE by TOAST
(b) Extracranial arterial disease with distal embolization	Carotid, aortic, vertebral artery atherosclerosis, dissection, or arteritis	Artery-to-artery embolus; LAS or other by TOAST; aortic arch suspected as cause of many "undetermined"
(c) Extracranial arterial stenosis that impedes blood flow to brain	Carotid, vertebral, atherosclerotic plaque; carotid or vertebral dissection; fibromuscular dysplasia; Ehlers Danlos; arteritis (infectious and noninfectious); sickle cell; radiation-induced arteriopathy	Low-flow state; LAS or other by TOAST
(d) Other causes of embolic or thrombotic vessel occlusion; *see* Section IV	*See* Section IV	Embolic or thrombotic
II. Large intracranial vessel disease		
Atherosclerosis, arteritis (infectious and non-infectious), moya-moya, sickle cell, vasoconstriction; *see* Section IV	Intracranial arterial occlusion or stenosis of circle of Willis vessels or more distal arteries	Low-flow, distal embolus; LAS or Other by TOAST; sometimes causes occlusion of small, deep penetrator vessels that arise from the diseased parent vessel; such cases cases can be clinically classified as SVO if intracranial vessels not investigated

III. Small, deep penetrator vessel disease[b]		
Hypertensive occlusion caused by progressive lipohyalinosis, occlusion caused by microatherosclerotic plaque, cerebral autosomal dominant arteriopathy with subcortical infarcts and leukoencephalopathy (CADASIL), amyloid angiopathy; *see also* Section IV	Occlusion of small arteries that originate at right angle from larger parent vessel; vessels supply basal ganglia, thalamus, brain stem, and white matter	Lacunar; SVO by TOAST unless another cause identified
IV. Occlusive disease that may affect the spectrum of intracerebral vessels		
Antiphospholipid antibody syndrome, Thrombotic thrombocytopenic purpura, disseminated intravascular coagulation, leukemia, vasculitis, heparin-induced thrombocytopenia, thrombocytosis, hyperviscosity, migraine, other hypercoagulable disorders, emboli	Thrombosis of intracranial vessels; some may also cause embolic occlusion	Variety of presentations and vessel syndromes; may present diagnostic challenges; other by TOAST when cause identified
V. Venous infarction	Thrombosis of dural venous sinus, cortical vein, or deep venous system	Other by TOAST classification

[a]It is sometimes difficult to distinguish atherosclerotic from nonatherosclerotic cause of intracranial vessel stenosis.

[b]Emboli can also enter and cause strokes in small, deep penetrator vessels, and such strokes are often misclassified as "lacunar" or "small vessel."

CE, cardioembolic; TOAST, Trial of Org 10172 in Acute Stroke Treatment; LAS, large-artery atherosclerosis; SVO, small vessel occlusion.

Table 2
TOAST Classification of Acute Stroke Subtypes

Large-artery atherosclerosis (embolus/thrombosis)[a]: Clinical evidence of cortical, subcortical, brain stem, or cerebellar dysfunction with more than 50% lesion or occlusion in an extracranial or intracranial vessel in the distribution of an infarct larger than 1.5 cm by CT or MRI. This diagnosis cannot be made if arterial studies show no evidence of pathology or if there is reasonable suggestion by history or studies that another mechanism is possible.

Cardioembolism (high risk/medium risk)[a]: Clinical evidence of cortical, subcortical, brain stem, or cerebellar dysfunction with a lesion size larger than 1.5 cm on CT or MRI and the presence of at least one high-risk (e.g., atrial fibrillation or mechanical heart valve) or medium-risk cardiac pathology (e.g., lone atrial fibrillation or patent foramen ovale) on diagnostic studies (electrocardiogram, rhythm strip, 24-hour cardiac monitoring, transthoracic or transesophageal echocardiography). Evidence of transient ischemic attacks or strokes in more than one vascular territory or of systemic emboli support the diagnosis. Finally, other categories (large artery, small artery) must be excluded.

Small-vessel occlusion (lacunar)[a]: A lacunar syndrome (pure motor, sensorimotor, pure sensory, ataxia hemiparesis, dysarthria-clumsy hand) with normal CT or MRI or a lesion smaller than 1.5 cm on CT or MRI in the territories supplied by small-vessel penetrators. Large-artery and cardiac sources must be excluded.

Stroke of other determined etiology[a]: Stroke caused by nonatherosclerotic vasculopathies, hypercoaguable states, or hematologic disorders and other rare causes of stroke after diagnostic testing. Other categories must be excluded.

Stroke of undetermined etiology (cryptogenic): This diagnosis is made if two or more etiologies of stroke are possible, a complete evaluation reveals no possible source, or the patient had an incomplete evaluation.

[a]Category broken into "possible" or "probable" subcategories depending on the weight of ancillary studies.

stroke based on a pathophysiological mechanism. In this regard, it is similar to an earlier classification scheme developed for the National Institute of Neurological Disorders and Stroke (NINDS) Stroke Data Bank, one of the earliest large, multicenter prospective registries of stroke etiology *(2)*.

Oxfordshire Community Stroke Project Classification

Unlike the mechanistic approach employed in the Stroke Data Bank and TOAST classifications, the Oxfordshire Community Stroke Project (OCSP) scheme classifies patients according to their clinical syndrome at the time of stroke onset *(3)*. Cases are categorized by suspected anatomic location as

Table 3
Oxfordshire Community Stroke Project Classification

TACS (total anterior circulation syndrome): This diagnosis is made if the patient presents with the triad of hemiparesis (or hemisensory loss), dysphasia (or other higher cortical dysfunction), and homonymous hemianopia.
PACS (partial anterior circulation syndrome): This diagnosis is made if the patient presents with only two of the three features above or with isolated cortical dysfunction or a restricted motor (or sensory) deficit (e.g., face or hand alone).
LACS (lacunar syndrome): This diagnosis is made if the patient presents with pure motor or sensory loss, sensorimotor stroke, or ataxic hemiparesis.
POCS (posterior circulation syndrome): This diagnosis is made if the patient presents with brain stem or cerebellar signs or isolated homonymous hemianopia.

total anterior circulation syndrome (TACS), partial anterior circulation syndrome (PACS), lacunar syndrome (LACS), or posterior circulation syndrome (POCS) (Table 3). Following brain imaging, patients are then subclassified according to infarction (TACI, PACI, LACI, POCI, respectively, as subclasses of TACS, PACS, LACS, POCS) or hemorrhage. Although the scheme provides limited information regarding the pathophysiological mechanism, it has the advantages of simplicity and speed and does not require extensive diagnostic testing (Table 4). It also identifies the common devastating TACS stroke syndrome. Thus, it is well suited for use in observational epidemiological studies or clinical trials that include patients who do not present to the hospital (approx 5% of strokes in community studies) or in areas where access to diagnostic testing is limited. It may also be useful for initial stratification of patients for clinical trials of potentially risky therapies in the first 3 to 6 hours after stroke, when extensive diagnostic testing for stroke mechanism is usually unavailable (see discussion of the Prolyse in Acute Cerebral Thromboembolism II trial in the section on subtypes in intervention studies).

Validity, Accuracy, and Reliability

TOAST Scheme

As no generally accepted "gold standard" exists for comparison (criterion validity), the degree of certainty of assignment of pathophysiological mechanism in the TOAST scheme cannot be definitively determined for an individual patient. This was recognized when the classification was devised and is reflected in the designation of individual cases as "probable" or "possible" for each category. However, the scheme displays both face and content valid-

Table 4
Comparison of TOAST and OCSP Classification Schemes

TOAST	OCSP
Advantages	
1. Based on pathophysiological mechanism	1. Simple to use
2. Valid (displays content validity)	2. Valid (displays content validity)
3. Provides prognostic information on mortality and disability	3. Provides prognostic information on mortality and disability
4. Provides prognostic information on recurrence	4. Provides some prognostic information on recurrence
5. Allows stratification for targeted interventions in clinical trials (mainly secondary prevention)	5. May assist in stratification of severely affected patients in trials of potentially risky acute therapies (e.g., thrombolysis)
Disadvantages	
1. Diagnostic testing may be expensive and time consuming	1. Limited information on etiology or pathophysiology
2. Variable interrater reliability (overall $\kappa = 0.42$ [95% CI 0.32 to 0.53]	2. Variable interrater reliability (overall $\kappa = 0.54$ [95% CI 0.39 to 0.68])
3. Limited applicability for community-based epidemiological studies	3. Limited (42–72%) sensitivity for detection of imaging-confirmed infarction
4. Limited applicability in acute (<6 hours) stroke trials and practice	4. Limited applicability in mechanism-based secondary prevention stroke trials

ity because it distills knowledge of stroke pathogenesis derived from a large body of prior clinical and clinicopathological studies and incorporates categories for all common and rare stroke etiologies. It also displays construct validity because stroke frequencies and outcomes assigned by TOAST subtype are largely consistent with those assigned by other mechanism-based classification schemes (Table 5).

There is some degree of variability in interobserver reliability of TOAST subtype assignment. Interobserver reliability displays a moderate-to-substantial level of agreement ($\kappa = 0.5–0.7$) even with the standardized TOAST system ($\kappa > 0.8$ is considered excellent agreement) *(9,10)*. Overall, there is poor interobserver agreement on stroke subtype when only the history and physical examination information are known. Other researchers have found poor inter-

Table 5
Distribution of Stroke Subtypes in Stroke Data Banks Using NINDS or TOAST Criteria[a]

Stroke subtype	NINDS	Lausanne	TOAST	SSDB[b]	UCSD	Mayo
	N = 1805	*N* = 1000	*N* = 752	*N* = 1000	*N* = 500	*N* = 454
Ischemic	**71%**	**80%**	**78%**	**71%**	**90%**	**97%**
Large-artery stenosis or occlusion	6%	23%	13%	27%	18%	16%
Tandem arterial embolism	4%	16%				
Lacune	19%	13%	23%	18%	27%	16%
Cardioembolic	14%	16%	27%	14%	22%	29%
Undetermined	28%	12%	35%	11%	23%	36%
Hemorrhagic	**26%**	**11%**	**17%**	**24%**	Not included	Not included
Intracerebral	13%	11%	13%	23%		
Subarachnoid	13%	Not included	3%	2%		
Other	**3%**	**9%**	**6%**	**5%**	**10%**	**3%**

NINDS, National Institute of Neurological Disorders and Stroke Data Bank *(2)*; SSDB, Saudi Stroke Data Bank *(4)*; Lausanne, Lausanne Stroke Registry *(5)*; TOAST, Trial of Org 10172 in Acute Stroke Treatment *(6)*; UCSD, University of California, San Diego, Stroke Data Bank *(7)*; Mayo, Rochester Epidemiology Project Stroke Data Bank *(8)*.

[a]Only bold numbers represent percentage of subtypes of the total *N* for each study. Other percentages give a relative distribution of subtypes within ischemic stroke category except hemorrhage.

[b]Retrospective data collection for 62% of cases.

observer agreement (overall $\kappa = 0.42$) when routine chart abstraction and data interpretation techniques were used *(11)*. This improved substantially with the use of a standardized data abstraction form and operations manual. Again, this demonstrates the difficulty of diagnosing stroke subtype on purely clinical grounds. Diagnostic agreement appears greater for some subtypes than for others. For example, there appears to be greater agreement among observers when the etiology of the stroke is cardioembolic than when the etiology is undetermined *(10)*.

Because the TOAST classification uses both clinical information and additional diagnostic testing to determine the subtype, the final subtype classification often differs from the clinical assessment at the time of hospital admission. Initial clinical impression of subtype agreed with final determination in only 62% of the cases in the TOAST study *(12)*. Other studies have shown that the initial impression is consistent with the final assigned subtype only 50–70% of the time *(5,10,13)*.

These data demonstrate the difficulty of diagnosing the etiology of stroke by clinical findings alone. For example, without appropriate evaluation of the craniocervical vessels and heart, a physician may incorrectly diagnose a pure motor stroke or other lacunar syndrome in 25–33% of cases *(5)*. Because location and size of stroke are inherently linked to the classification scheme, neuroimaging of the acute stroke plays an important role in assignment of stroke subtype.

The contribution of diffusion-weighted magnetic resonance imaging (DWI) to the accuracy of mechanism-based subtyping has been investigated. The sensitivity and specificity of DWI for detection of new ischemic stroke are superior to routine computed tomography (CT) and conventional (T2 and proton density) magnetic resonance imaging (MRI) in both the hyperacute and the subacute phases *(14–16)*. In patients with previous stroke or diffuse nonspecific white matter abnormality, DWI may even identify which lesion is the acute stroke *(14,17)*. In one study, DWI with apparent diffusion coefficient (ADC) maps added clinically significant information in 48% of cases. This included detection of multiple lesions in different vascular territories suggestive of cardiac embolism, even in patients with clinical lacunar syndromes *(18)*.

The classification of stroke as caused by larger artery atherosclerosis also requires identification of a responsible vascular stenosis. Noninvasive means of angiography (CT and magnetic resonance angiography [MRA]) and neurovascular ultrasound are commonly used *(19)*. Lee and colleagues found improved diagnostic accuracy of TOAST subtype assignment using DWI and craniocervical MRA *(20)*. Despite its proven utility in stroke subtype assignment and acute stroke research, current problems with availability of MRI limit its widespread application to acute stroke evaluation. Angiography is a newer, but potentially more available, technology that may improve stroke subtyping in the acute setting *(21)*.

OCSP Scheme

Although the OCSP scheme displays content and construct validity, its precision for accurate prediction of CT-proven stroke location varies by subcategory *(13)*. The OCSP investigators found that the overall accuracy of the scheme was 71–75%, with 71–83% of PACIs, LACIs, and POCIs classified correctly. Using a stringent definition of CT-proven TACIs, only 54% of cases were correctly classified. These data indicate that, although the scheme has advantages for stratification in epidemiological studies and acute stroke trials, it is not a reliable indicator of infarct anatomy or etiology.

The interobserver reliability of the OCSP scheme is similar to that of the TOAST scheme. The OCSP investigators found that the overall interobserver agreement was moderate to good ($\kappa = 0.54$, 95% confidence intervals [CIs] 0.39 to 0.68) *(22)*. Agreement varied for different clinical findings; it was good for hemiparesis and aphasia, moderate for hemianopia, and poor for sensory loss.

FREQUENCY AND OUTCOMES

Frequency of Subtypes

The distribution of subtypes in the OCSP study was 17% TACI, 34% PACI, 25% LACI, and 24% POCI. Other investigators have found differing proportions in their populations. For example, the Perth Community Stroke Study reported 27% TACI and 15% POCI in their sample.

Some of the largest studies on the prevalence of stroke subtypes based primarily on TOAST or NINDS Data Bank criteria are listed in Table 5. Overall, the data suggest that approx 80–85% of strokes are ischemic, and 15–20% are hemorrhagic. Some of the differences in distribution of stroke subtypes are a result of patient selection. That is, NINDS and Lausanne are both hospital-based stroke registries; the University of California, San Diego, and Mayo data are population based, including both hospitalized and nonhospitalized patients. Also, differences may stem from variability in the racial distributions and prevalence of risk factors throughout the studied population. Risk factors such as hypertension and diabetes mellitus appear to be more prevalent in blacks and Caribbean Hispanics, whereas atrial fibrillation and coronary artery disease are more prevalent in Caucasians *(23,24)*.

Subtype-Specific Stroke Outcomes

In the OCSP study, the subtypes displayed some distinct patterns of mortality, disability, and recurrence. As might be expected, TACIs are associated with high early and late mortality and disability (Table 6). These are most commonly caused by embolic occlusion of the middle cerebral or intracranial carotid artery, the latter occluding flow to the anterior and middle cerebral artery territories (so-called T occlusions). The origin of the embolic material varies among cases, but cardioembolic and carotid atherosclerotic origins are common. Most deaths in this group were related to direct neurological complications (e.g., massive cerebral edema) of the stroke. Case fatality and disability rates in the other groups were approximately similar. In contrast, PACIs and POCIs were distinguished by a high recurrence rate. Most recurrences in the PACI category occurred in the first 3 months. These outcome patterns were largely consistent with those reported by the Perth Community Stroke Study, although the high rate of POCI recurrences was not confirmed by the Perth investigators *(25)*.

Table 6
Outcomes by OCSP Subtype

	TACI	PACI	LACI	POCI
Mortality				
30 days	39%	4%	2%	7%
1 year	60%	16%	11%	19%
Dependence				
30 days	56%	39%	36%	31%
1 year	36%	29%	28%	19%
Recurrence				
1 year	6%	17%	9%	20%

Mechanism-based subtypes are associated with different mortality, disability, and recurrence rates following stroke (Table 7). Overall, hemorrhagic stroke carries greater mortality than ischemic stroke *(2,5)*. In the ischemic category, mortality from cardioembolic causes is greater than that for large-vessel causes, which in turn is greater than that for lacunar infarcts at 30 days, 1–2 years, and 5 years *(2,26–28)*. In the population-based Mayo Clinic data set, cardiogenic embolism was an independent predictor of long-term (but not early) mortality. The distribution of disability among stroke subtypes is similar to that of mortality. Disability because of cardiogenic embolism exceeds that caused by large-vessel stroke, which in turn exceeds that caused by lacunar stroke *(27)*. In contrast, several studies have found that the risk of early (<30 days) recurrent stroke is greater for large-vessel disease than for cardioembolic disease, which in turn is greater than for lacunar disease *(26,27,29)*. Large-artery subtype is also a strong independent predictor of stroke recurrence at 30 days *(27)*. Although this hierarchy (large-artery subtype > cardiogenic embolism > small-artery subtype) was maintained for late recurrence in several studies, some groups have found that subtype was not an independent predictor of recurrence at 2 years and 5 years *(27,28)*.

SUBTYPES IN INTERVENTION STUDIES

Important stroke prevention data have been learned from intervention studies targeting progression of atherosclerosis and thrombosis (e.g., trials of lipid-lowering, antihypertensive, and antiplatelet drugs) that considered stroke as a single entity. However, interventions focused on subtype-specific pathophysiologies have also shown benefit in clinical trials.

Table 7
Mechanism-Based Subtype Outcomes (Mortality, Disability, and Recurrence)

	Cardiogenic embolism	Large vessel	Small vessel (lacunar)
Mortality			
30 day[a]	11–30%	8–14%	0–1%
2 year[b]	45–61%	19–42%	13–15%
5 year[c]	68–80%	32–61%	15–35%
Disability			
Rankin IV or V or dead at 1 year[d]	63%	36%	10%
Recurrence			
30 day recurrence[e]	4–6%	8–19%	1–4%
1 year[d]	13.7%	24.4%	7.1%
5 year[d]	31.7%	40.2%	24.8%

[a]From refs. *2*, *26*, and *27*.
[b]From refs. *27* and *28*.
[c]From refs. *26* and *27*.
[d]From ref. *27*.
[e]From refs. *26*, *27*, and *29*.

Partly because of difficulty in accurately assigning subtype by mechanism in the early hours after stroke, relatively few randomized trials have studied subtype-specific acute interventions. Examples include the TOAST study, in which a secondary subgroup analysis demonstrated benefit of the heparinoid danaparoid in patients with large-artery, but not other, ischemic stroke subtypes. The Heparin in Acute Embolic Stroke Trial showed no benefit of subcutaneous dalteparin over aspirin in prevention of recurrent stroke at 14 days in patients with atrial fibrillation *(30)*. The NINDS trial of intravenous tissue plasminogen activator for acute ischemic stroke collected subtype data, but found no interaction of treatment benefit by subtype.

A good example of a successful trial for acute stroke treatment based on pathophysiological subtype is the Prolyse in Acute Cerebral Thromboembolism II study *(31)*. This trial demonstrated benefit of the intervention with a relatively small number of subjects ($N = 180$) for several important reasons. First, it enrolled patients early in the ischemic time window (<6 hours). Second, all patients had defined embolic disease (demonstrated by angiography). Third, the embolic disease was confined to a single arterial distribution (middle cerebral artery). These measures ensured that patients suffered from similar stroke pathophysiology, that the clinical deficit was relatively uniform, and that the intervention was applied to the appropriate pathophysiology. In this case, stratification by a combined subtyping approach based on clinical syndrome (analogous to OCSP TACIs) and pathophysiological mechanism (analogous to TOAST/Stroke Data Bank) was critical in selecting appropriate patients for inclusion. It is likely that a similar approach will be employed in future trials of acute therapies.

Primary and secondary prevention trials have also demonstrated benefit when a mechanism-based approach was used to target the intervention. Examples include anticoagulation to prevent cardiogenic brain embolism in nonvalvular atrial fibrillation, endarterectomy for symptomatic carotid stenosis, and unfractionated heparin for treatment or progression of cerebral venous thrombosis. Ongoing trials targeted to subtype-specific mechanisms include trials of warfarin compared with antiplatelet agents for intracranial large-artery atherosclerosis and cardiogenic embolism associated with left ventricular failure and intracranial–extracranial bypass for occlusion of the internal carotid artery associated with cerebral hypoperfusion as demonstrated by positron emission tomography. An untested, but important, goal is the targeted prevention of small, deep penetrator vessel strokes that occur in the basal ganglia, brain stem, thalamus, and white matter of hypertensive individuals (lacunar strokes). Small-vessel strokes make up 20–30% of all ischemic strokes (Table 5), and most affected individuals suffer multiple such infarcts. Such individuals are likely to benefit more from measures to lower blood pressure (and perhaps cholesterol reduction) than patients with stroke caused by other mechanisms (e.g., cardiac embolism).

SUBCATEGORIZATION OF EXISTING MECHANISM-BASED SUBTYPES

Although requiring greater effort for recruitment in clinical trials, subcategorization of existing subtypes is likely to yield further pathophysiologically specific therapies in the future. For example, anoxic brain injury secondary to cardiac arrest is not readily inserted into the current stroke subtypes, yet specific therapeutic interventions such as hypothermia have proven benefit *(32,33)*. Definition of subcategories within the cardioembolic group may yield successful prevention strategies for dilated cardiomyopathy and patent foramen ovale or atrial septal aneurysm. Further categories in the large-artery group might differentiate carotid occlusion from stenosis and intracranial from extracranial large-artery disease.

Supporting this contention, a TOAST subgroup analysis identified acute carotid occlusion as a group demonstrating benefit from early anticoagulation *(6)*. Natural history studies have demonstrated that patients with carotid occlusion who demonstrate a high oxygen extraction fraction on positron emission tomography are at very high risk of recurrent strokes and may be potential candidates for extracranial–intracranial bypass *(34–36)*. Natural history and uncontrolled trials suggested that patients with large-artery intracranial stenosis may show a differential benefit from acute treatment with hypertensive therapy, anticoagulation, angioplasty, or stenting *(37–39)*. Clearly, the "other" category in TOAST criteria represents a collection of unique pathophysiological mechanisms for study, ranging from central sinus thrombosis, to sickle cell anemia, to arterial dissection, to vasculitis. These unusual causes of stroke are discussed in greater detail in Chapter 14.

REFERENCES

1. Adams HP Jr, Bendixen BH, Kappelle LJ,et al. Classification of subtype of acute ischemic stroke. Definitions for use in a multicenter clinical trial. TOAST. Trial of Org 10172 in Acute Stroke Treatment. Stroke 1993;24:35–41.
2. Foulkes MA, Wolf PA, Price TR, Mohr JP, Hier DB. The Stroke Data Bank: design, methods, and baseline characteristics. Stroke 1988;19:547–554.
3. Bamford J, Sandercock P, Dennis M, et al. Classification and natural history of clinically identifiable subtypes of cerebral infarction. Lancet 1991;337:1521–1528.
4. Awada A, al Rajeh S. The Saudi Stroke Data Bank. Analysis of the first 1000 cases. Acta Neurol Scand 1999;100:265–269.
5. Bogousslavsky J, Van Melle G, Regli F. The Lausanne Stroke Registry: analysis of 1000 consecutive patients with first stroke. Stroke 1988;19:1083–1092.
6. Low molecular weight heparinoid, ORG 10172 (danaparoid), and outcome after acute ischemic stroke: a randomized controlled trial. The Publications Committee for the Trial of ORG 10172 in Acute Stroke Treatment (TOAST) Investigators. JAMA 1998;279:1265–1272.
7. Rothrock JF, Lyden PD, Brody ML, et al. An analysis of ischemic stroke in an urban southern California population. The University of California, San Diego, Stroke Data Bank. Arch Intern Med 1993;153:619–624.
8. Petty GW, Brown RD Jr, Whisnant JP, et al. Ischemic stroke subtypes: a population-based study of incidence and risk factors. Stroke 1999;30:2513–2516.
9. Gross CR, Shinar D, Mohr JP, et al. Interobserver agreement in the diagnosis of stroke type. Arch Neurol 1986;43:893–898.
10. Gordon DL, Bendixen BH, Adams HP Jr, et al. Interphysician agreement in the diagnosis of subtypes of acute ischemic stroke: implications for clinical trials. The TOAST Investigators. Neurology 1993;43:1021–1027.
11. Goldstein LB, Jones MR, Matchar DB, et al. Improving the reliability of stroke subgroup classification using the trial of ORG 10172 in acute stroke treatment (TOAST) criteria. Stroke 2001;32:1091–1097.
12. Madden KP, Karanjia PN, Adams HP Jr, Clarke WR. Accuracy of initial stroke subtype diagnosis in the TOAST study. Trial of ORG 10172 in Acute Stroke Treatment. Neurology 1995;45:1975–1979.
13. Mead GE, Lewis SC, Wardlaw JM, Dennis MS, Warlow CP. How well does the Oxfordshire Community Stroke Project classification predict the site and size of the infarct on brain imaging? J Neurol Neurosurg Psychiatry 2000;68:558–562.

14. Albers GW, Lansberg MG, Norbash AM, et al. Yield of diffusion-weighted MRI for detection of potentially relevant findings in stroke patients. Neurology 2000;54: 1562–1567.
15. Lansberg MG, Albers GW, Beaulieu C, Marks MP. Comparison of diffusion-weighted MRI and CT in acute stroke. Neurology 2000;54:1557–1561.
16. Gonzalez RG, Schaefer PW, Buonanno FS, et. al. Diffusion-weighted MR imaging: diagnostic accuracy in patients imaged within 6 hours of stroke symptom onset. Radiology 1999;210:155–162.
17. Oliveira-Filho J, Ay H, Schaefer PW, et al. Diffusion-weighted magnetic resonance imaging identifies the "clinically relevant" penetrator infarcts. Arch Neurol 2000;57:1009–1014.
18. Ay H, Oliveira-Filho J, Buonanno FS, et al. Diffusion-weighted imaging clarifies a subset of lacunar infarctions associated with embolic source. Stroke 1999;30: 2644–2650.
19. Lev MH, Farkas J, Rodriguez VR, et al. CT angiography in the rapid triage of patients with hyperacute stroke: accuracy in the detection of large vessel thrombus. J Comput Axial Tomogr 2001;25:520–528.
20. Lee LJ, Kidwell CS, Alger J, Starkman S, Saver JL. Impact on stroke subtype diagnosis of early diffusion-weighted magnetic resonance imaging and magnetic resonance angiography. Stroke 2000;31:1081–1089.
21. Ezzeddine MA, Lev MH, McDonald CT, et al. CT angiography with whole brain perfused blood volume imaging: added clinical value in the assessment of acute stroke. Stroke 2002;33:959–966.
22. Lindley RI, Warlow CP, Wardlaw JM, et al. Interobserver reliability of a clinical classification of acute cerebral infarction. Stroke 1993;24:1801–1804.
23. Zweifler RM, Lyden PD, Taft B, et al. Impact of race and ethnicity on ischemic stroke. The University of California at San Diego Stroke Data Bank. Stroke 1995; 26:245–248.
24. Sacco RL, Boden-Albala B, Abel G, et al. Race–ethnic disparities in the impact of stroke risk factors: the Northern Manhattan Stroke Study. Stroke 2001;32:1725–1731.
25. Anderson CS, Taylor BV, Hankey GJ, et al. Validation of a clinical classification for subtypes of acute cerebral infarction. J Neurol Neurosurg Psychiatry 1994;57: 1173–1179.
26. Sacco RL, Shi T, Zamanillo MC, Kargman DE. Predictors of mortality and recurrence after hospitalized cerebral infarction in an urban community: the Northern Manhattan Stroke Study. Neurology 1994;44:626–634.
27. Petty GW, Brown RD Jr, Whisnant JP, et al. Ischemic stroke subtypes: a population-based study of functional outcome, survival, and recurrence. Stroke 2000;31: 1062–1068.
28. Kolominsky-Rabas PL, Weber M, Gefeller O, Neundoerfer B, Heuschmann PU. Epidemiology of ischemic stroke subtypes according to TOAST criteria: incidence, recurrence, and long-term survival in ischemic stroke subtypes: a population-based study. Stroke 2001;32:2735–2740.
29. Sacco RL, Foulkes MA, Mohr JP, et al. Determinants of early recurrence of cerebral infarction. The Stroke Data Bank. Stroke 1989;20:983–989.
30. Berge E, Abdelnoor M, Nakstad PH, Sandset PM. Low molecular-weight heparin vs aspirin in patients with acute ischaemic stroke and atrial fibrillation: a double-

blind randomised study. HAEST Study Group. Heparin in Acute Embolic Stroke Trial. Lancet 2000;355:1205–1210.

31. Furlan A, Higashida R, Wechsler L, et al. Intra-arterial prourokinase for acute ischemic stroke. The PROACT II study: a randomized controlled trial. Prolyse in Acute Cerebral Thromboembolism. JAMA 1999;282:2003–2011.
32. Bernard SA, Gray TW, Buist MD, et al. Treatment of comatose survivors of out-of-hospital cardiac arrest with induced hypothermia. N Engl J Med 2002;346: 557–563.
33. Hypothermia After Cardiac Arrest Study Group. Mild therapeutic hypothermia to improve the neurologic outcome after cardiac arrest. N Engl J Med 2002;346:549–556. Erratum in: N Engl J Med 2002;346:1756.
34. Yamauchi H, Fukuyama H, Nagahama Y, et al. Evidence of misery perfusion and risk for recurrent stroke in major cerebral arterial occlusive diseases from PET. J Neurol Neurosurg Psychiatry 1996;61:18–25.
35. Derdeyn CP, Yundt KD, Videen TO, et al. Increased oxygen extraction fraction is associated with prior ischemic events in patients with carotid occlusion. Stroke 1998;29:754–758.
36. Derdeyn CP, Videen TO, Simmons NR, et al. Count-based PET method for predicting ischemic stroke in patients with symptomatic carotid arterial occlusion. Radiology 1999;212:499–506.
37. Chimowitz MI, Kokkinos J, Strong J, et al. The Warfarin-Aspirin Symptomatic Intracranial Disease Study. Neurology 1995;45:1488–1493.
38. Gomez CR, Orr SC. Angioplasty and stenting for primary treatment of intracranial arterial stenoses. Arch Neurol 2001;58:1687–1690.
39. Rordorf G, Koroshetz WJ, Ezzeddine MA, et al. A pilot study of drug-induced hypertension for treatment of acute stroke. Neurology 2001;56:1210–1213.

3

Hypertension As a Risk Factor for Stroke

Epidemiology of Blood Pressure Risks and Evidence for Treatment Benefit

Donald M. Lloyd-Jones and Christopher J. O'Donnell

INTRODUCTION

Hypertension is a highly prevalent, major risk factor for stroke in both men and women in the developed world. Recent data from population-based studies emphasize the substantial risks conferred by elevated levels of systolic blood pressure (SBP) over and above diastolic blood pressure (DBP) and the risks of borderline elevations in SBP. Decades of randomized treatment trials have demonstrated the clear net benefit on stroke and cardiovascular disease (CVD) conferred by antihypertensive therapy. Recent data emphasize the stroke prevention benefits of treatment of isolated systolic hypertension and the benefits of nonpharmacological dietary and other lifestyle interventions for lowering elevated blood pressure. Many classes of antihypertensive agents are available, and the largest trial comparing the risks and benefits of commonly used agents, the Antihypertensive and Lipid-Lowering Treatment to Prevent Heart Attack (ALLHAT) trial, provided evidence for a net benefit from diuretic therapy as the initial agent. Here, we review the epidemiology of hypertension, the relations of hypertension with risk for stroke, and the evidence for benefit from pharmacological and nonpharmacological treatments.

EPIDEMIOLOGY OF HYPERTENSION

Prevalence and Incidence

Hypertension is the most prevalent modifiable risk factor for CVD, affecting 50 million individuals or one in four adults in the United States, including two-thirds of men and three-quarters of women over the age of 75 years.

From: *Current Clinical Neurology: Handbook of Stroke Prevention in Clinical Practice*
Edited by: K. L. Furie and P. J. Kelly © Humana Press Inc., Totowa, NJ

Hypertension is substantially more common among African American men and women than among other ethnic groups, with a prevalence of 37%. The direct and indirect costs of hypertension total more than $50 billion annually *(1)*. Data from the Framingham Heart Study indicate that, among men and women free of hypertension at age 55 years, the remaining lifetime risk for hypertension is more than 90%, with more than half developing hypertension within 10 years. For subjects free of hypertension at age 65 years, the remaining lifetime risk still exceeds 90%, with two-thirds developing hypertension within the next 10 years *(2)*. Thus, it is a rare individual who escapes the risk of developing hypertension during their life-span.

Temporal Trends

The prevalence of hypertension in the population has been declining over the last five decades *(1,3)*, with gradual declines in levels of both SBP and DBP *(3)*. One explanation for these trends is the dramatic increase in rates of treatment for hypertension *(3,4)*. However, with the emerging major epidemic of obesity *(5)* and the aging of the population, such long-standing trends may slow or reverse, and treatment and control rates remain far below optimal. Data from a nationally representative sample in the United States in 1999–2000 (National Health and Nutrition Examination Survey IV) indicated that 70% of hypertensive individuals are aware of their diagnosis, and 59% are receiving treatment, but only 34% have had their blood pressure controlled to goal levels of less than 140 mmHg systolic and less than 90 mmHg diastolic *(4)*. In cross-sectional studies, rates of control are significantly lower for those who are older and obese individuals *(6)*.

Risk Factor Clustering

Independent of other risk factors, hypertension is associated with increased risk for stroke, congestive heart failure (CHF), coronary heart disease, end-stage renal disease, and total and cardiovascular mortality. However, hypertension rarely occurs in isolation, and clustering of CVD risk factors is well described. Indeed, elevated blood pressure (SBP $\geq$ 130 or DBP $\geq$ 85 mmHg) is one of five components of the metabolic syndrome, related to central adiposity, insulin resistance, and lipid abnormalities, that markedly increases risk for stroke and other CVD events *(7)*. In a recent study of Framingham Heart Study participants with high-normal blood pressure or hypertension, 38.2% had evidence of CVD, target organ damage, or diabetes; 59.3% had at least one other CVD risk factor associated with hypertension; and only 2.4% had no other risk factors *(8)*. Thus, hypertension almost always occurs in subjects who are already at increased risk for stroke and other CVD events.

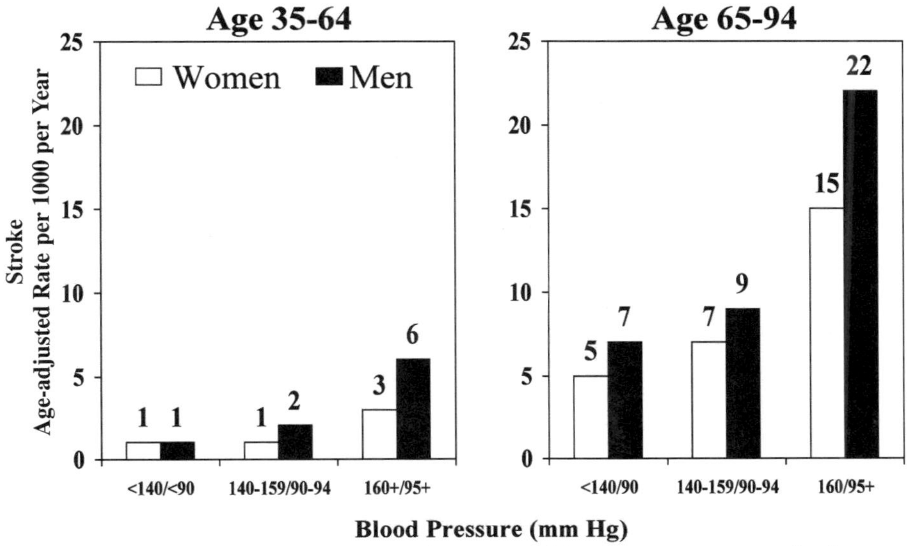

Fig. 1. Age-adjusted rates of stroke by age and blood pressure categories in men and women.

BLOOD PRESSURE AND RISK FOR STROKE

Hypertension is well established as the dominant risk factor for stroke, even when considered in the context of other known risk factors (cigarette smoking, atrial fibrillation, myocardial infarction [MI], diabetes, etc.). The concept of the population-attributable risk percentage is useful in describing what proportion of a disease in a population is caused by an individual risk factor. The attributable risk percentage accounts for the relative risk of disease associated with a risk factor, as well as the risk factor's prevalence. Data from the Framingham Heart Study indicated that hypertension confers a threefold relative risk of stroke compared with levels below 140/90 mmHg, and approx 80% of subjects have hypertension prior to the occurrence of a stroke. Thus, the attributable risk for stroke conferred by hypertension varies between 33 and 53% in different age groups *(9)*.

Hypertension works synergistically with other risk factors to increase risk for stroke and other CVD outcomes. For example, the effect of hypertension on risk for stroke is modified substantially by age. As shown in Fig. 1, data from 30-year follow-up of the Framingham cohort revealed that there is a linear increase in stroke rates with increasing level of blood pressure, but absolute rates of stroke and transient ischemic attack are substantially higher

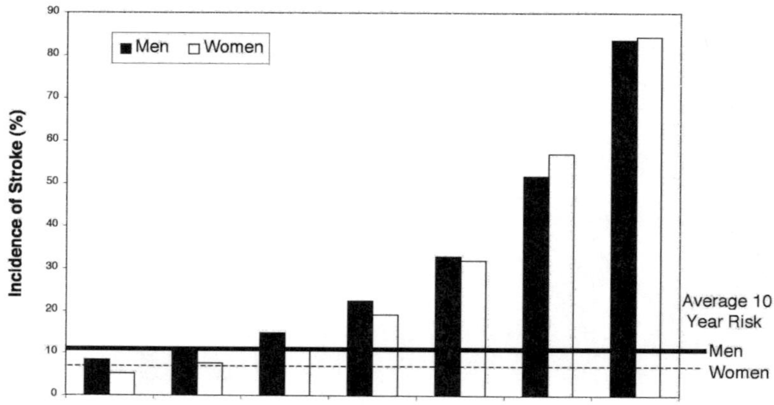

Risk Factor Present							
HTN Rx	-	+	+	+	+	+	+
Diabetes	-	-	+	+	+	+	+
Cigarette Use	-	-	-	+	+	+	+
Cardiovascular Disease	-	-	-	-	+	+	+
Atrial Fibrillation	-	-	-	-	-	+	+
ECG LVH	-	-	-	-	-	-	+

Fig. 2. Ten-year probablility of stroke according to presence of stroke risk factors in men and women aged 65 years with systolic blood pressure 160 mmHg. HTN Rx, hypertension drug therapy; ECG LVH, left ventricular hypertrophy by electrocardiography. (Adapted from ref. *9*.)

for subjects with hypertension in the age range 65 to 94 years compared with 35 to 64 years.

Mutivariable risk formulations provide more precise estimation of the probability of stroke in people with one or more of the major stroke risk factors, allowing quantification of the joint effect of these interrelated factors on the development of stroke. This approach takes into account the multifactorial elements of risk and the continuous gradient of risk. A risk-prediction algorithm was developed by Framingham Heart Study investigators to estimate the absolute 10-year risk of an atherothrombotic brain infarct; the algorithm uses the standard risk factors plus the presence of atrial fibrillation, heart failure, and coronary disease *(9)*. Hypertension represents the predominant risk factor for stroke, but the risk in people with elevated blood pressure varies over as much as a 10-fold range, depending on the degree of exposure to the concomitant predisposing risk factors (Fig. 2).

Risk for stroke is not limited to subjects with frank hypertension, however. There is a linear, graded risk for stroke that extends even to optimal levels of blood pressure. Beginning at 115 mmHg, the risk for stroke mortality doubles for each increase of 20 mmHg in the SBP; likewise, stroke mortality risk doubles for each increase of 10 mmHg in the DBP, beginning at 75 mmHg *(10)*.

Elevated SBP and DBP Relationship to Stroke

The substantial burden of hypertension is largely a function of vascular changes that occur as a result of aging and exposure to environmental and genetic factors that alter vascular function. Specifically, arteriosclerosis, loss of elasticity, and increasing vascular stiffness all contribute to increasing SBP, which rises linearly with age across all segments of the population, beginning at approx 30 years of age. DBP rises gradually until approximately 50 years of age, after which it stabilizes for approx 5–10 years and then declines steadily through the end of the life-span *(11,12)*. The result of increasing SBP and decreasing DBP in middle-aged and older individuals is a steadily increasing *pulse pressure*, which is defined as the SBP minus the DBP.

As discussed in this section, risk for stroke increases linearly with increases in SBP (beginning at 115 mmHg) or DBP (beginning at 75 mmHg) when each blood pressure component is considered individually *(10)*. However, a substantial body of epidemiological evidence has demonstrated that level of SBP is far more important than DBP in determining risk for stroke and other CVD outcomes in the population. Several lines of evidence deserve mention: (1) Isolated systolic hypertension is the most common form of hypertension *(13)*. (2) SBP correctly classifies blood pressure stage far better than DBP, and SBP therefore determines need for treatment among high-normal and hypertensive subjects *(13,14)*; (3) SBP is at least as strong a risk factor as DBP, and often stronger, in prediction of adverse CVD outcomes, including stroke *(15–17)*; and (4) large clinical trials *(18,19)* have demonstrated substantial benefit with treatment of isolated systolic hypertension in patients 60 years and older. The Coordinating Committee of the National High Blood Pressure Education Program and the Seventh Report of the Joint National Committee on Prevention, Detection, Evaluation, and Treatment of High Blood Pressure (JNC 7) therefore recommended that SBP become the major criterion for the diagnosis, staging, and management of hypertension in middle-aged and older patients, who represent the majority of hypertensives *(4,20)*.

Risk for stroke is greater for SBP than DBP whether the two blood pressure components are compared linearly *(17)*, by deciles (Fig. 3) *(16)*, or by JNC stage (Table 1) *(16)*. In addition, SBP predominates when SBP and DBP are considered jointly *(17)*. As shown in Fig. 4, rates of stroke mortality increase dramatically with increasing SBP at any given level of DBP. However, for any given level of SBP, there is only a modest increase in stroke mortality

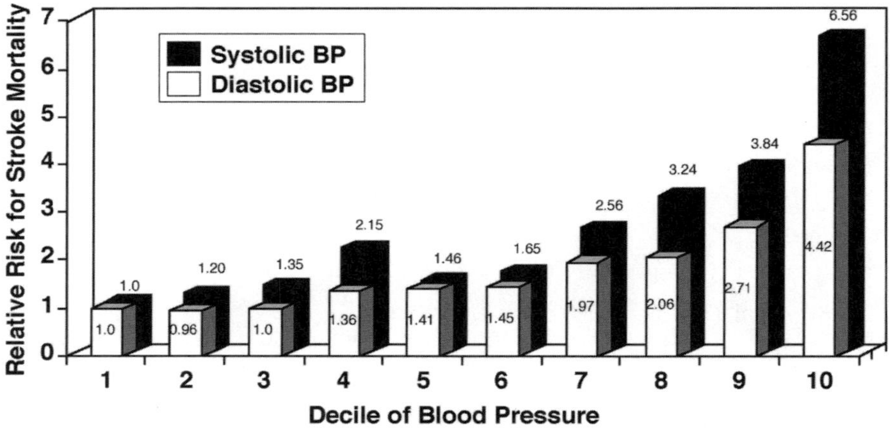

Fig. 3. Relative risk of stroke mortality by decile of systolic or diastolic blood pressure. (Adapted from ref. *16*.)

Table 1
Mutivariable-Adjusted Relative Risk for Stroke Mortality by JNC Stage of Systolic and Diastolic Blood Pressure

JNC stage	SBP (mmHg)	Adjusted RR	DBP (mmHg)	Adjusted RR
Optimal	<120	1.00 (ref)	<80	1.00 (ref)
Normal	120–129	1.68	80–84	1.44
High normal	130–139	2.33	85–89	1.76
Stage 1 HTN	140–159	3.78	90–99	2.54
Stage 2 HTN	160–179	6.57	100–109	4.00
Stage 3 HTN	180–209	10.7	110–119	6.31
Stage 4 HTN	≥210	24.3	≥120	12.6

The risk is higher for systolic blood pressure than for diastolic blood pressure at any given blood pressure stage above optimal.

HTN, hypertension; RR, relative risk.

with increasing DBP, and the trend is nonlinear at higher levels of SBP *(16)*. Furthermore, elevations in SBP are far more prevalent than elevations in DBP *(13,14)*, thus indicating a greater attributable risk for SBP than for DBP.

Risk for stroke is also substantially elevated even at borderline levels of optimum blood pressure, at which current guidelines do not currently support institution of antihypertensive drug treatment. In the Framingham Heart Study, there was a 2.5-fold increased risk for CVD associated with high-

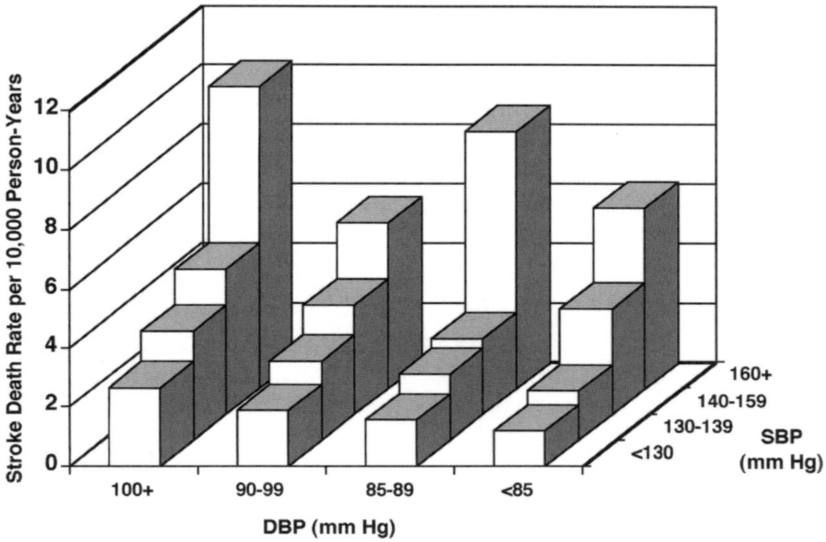

Fig. 4. Stroke death rate by categories of systolic blood pressure and diastolic blood pressure. (Adapted from ref. *16*.)

normal (SBP 130–139 or DBP 80–89 mmHg) levels of blood pressure *(21)*; in the Physicians' Health Study, there was a nearly 2-fold increased risk of stroke associated with borderline elevated SBP *(22)*. Moreover, the risk of new-onset hypertension is elevated for persons with high-normal SBP *(23)*. For these reasons, JNC 7 reclassified the JNC 6 blood pressure categories to place greater emphasis on prevention of hypertension. These previously normal and high-normal levels (i.e., SBP 120–139 or DBP 80–89 mmHg) are now classified as prehypertension *(4)*.

There has been interest in pulse pressure (SBP minus DBP) as a predictor of CVD events. Some studies have found that elevations in pulse pressure predict certain CVD outcomes better than do individual levels of SBP or DBP *(24,25)*, whereas other studies indicated that SBP predicts better *(17)*. For the outcome of stroke, however, it is clear that SBP predominates in risk prediction. Data from a large pooling project of nearly 1 million subjects followed in 61 different cohorts for more than 12.7 million person-years have provided important insights into the relative contributions of SBP, DBP, and pulse pressure to risk for stroke mortality. Of the three single blood pressure measurements, SBP is more informative than DBP in prediction of stroke mortality and markedly more informative than pulse pressure *(10)*.

HYPERTENSION TREATMENT STRATEGIES FOR PREVENTION OF STROKE

Blood Pressure Reduction and Stroke Prevention

As discussed in this chapter, hypertension is the major risk factor for stroke. In addition, data from numerous clinical trials *(18,19,26)* of antihypertensive therapy have documented dramatic reductions in stroke incidence with treatment of hypertension. In a meta-analysis of the three largest trials examining treatment of isolated systolic hypertension in older patients, there was a 37% reduction in stroke incidence with active treatment compared with placebo. The average SBP at entry in these trials was 174 mmHg and average SBP reduction compared with placebo was only 10.4 mmHg *(27)*. Thus, relatively modest reductions in SBP can result in a large decrease in stroke incidence. Nonetheless, treatment to goal blood pressure levels of less than 140 mmHg systolic and less than 90 mmHg diastolic should be the ultimate goal of therapy, with SBP/DBP goal values less than 130/80 mmHg among patients with diabetes or renal disease *(4,28)*.

Lifestyle Modification for Blood Pressure Reduction

The importance of lifestyle modification cannot be overstated in efforts to prevent hypertension and to control blood pressure once hypertension has developed. Drug therapy should not be used as a substitute for, or in the absence of, concomitant lifestyle modification. A number of studies have documented reductions in blood pressure with various changes in dietary habits. For example, sodium restriction alone results in an average reduction in SBP of 2–8 mmHg. Implementing the more comprehensive Dietary Approaches to Stop Hypertension eating plan, including sodium restriction, a focus on fruits and vegetables, and limitation of fats and carbohydrates, has been shown to reduce SBP by 8–14 mmHg. Moderation of ethanol intake from higher amounts to approximately one drink per day can result in SBP reductions of 2–4 mmHg. In concert with dietary changes, increasing physical activity reduces SBP by 4–9 mmHg. Weight reduction can dramatically improve SBP, lowering it by 5–20 mmHg with a 10-kg weight loss *(4)*.

Drug Therapy for Blood Pressure Reduction

The current JNC 7 recommendations for initiation of drug therapy for blood pressure reduction are summarized in Table 2. Several key concepts regarding antihypertensive therapy deserve emphasis. First, several trials in the past decade demonstrated conclusively that treatment of isolated systolic hypertension is associated with substantially lowered risks for stroke and other cardiovascular events *(27)*. However, to date there have been no trials

Table 2
Recommendations for Initiation of Therapy in JNC 7

BP stage	Lifestyle modification	Initial drug therapy[a]: Without compelling indications	With compelling indications
Normal (<120/<80)	Encourage	No drugs indicated	No drugs indicated
Prehypertension (120–139/80–89)	Yes	No drugs indicated	Drug(s) for compelling indications[b]
Stage 1 HTN (140–159/90–99)	Yes	Thiazides for most. May consider ACEI, ARB, BB, CCB, combination	Drug(s) for compelling indications[b]
Stage 2 HTN (≥160/≥100)	Yes	Two-drug combination for most[b]	Other anti-HTN drugs (diuretics, ACEI, ARB, BB, CCB) as needed

[a]Treatment determined by highest BP category.

[b]Treat patients with chronic kidney disease or diabetes to BP goal of <130/80 mmHg.

[c]Initial combined therapy should be used cautiously in those at risk for orthostatic hypotension.

ACEI, angiotensin-converting enzyme inhibitors, ARB, angiotensin$_2$-receptor blocker; BB, β-blocker; CCB, calcium-channel blocker.

specifically examining treatment for borderline isolated SBP or for prehypertension levels of SBP or DBP.

In particular, the PROGRESS trial *(36)* was a dedicated secondary prevention trial in patients with stroke. It included 6105 subjects (mean age 64 years, 70% male) with prior stroke or TIA within the previous 5 years (48% hypertensive, defined as BP ≥160/90), and randomized them to therapy with perindopril (an angiotensin-converting enzyme [ACE] inhibitor) with or without indapamide (a thiazide diuretic) vs placebo. Both groups received other accepted "best medical therapy," consisting of aspirin and other antihypertensive medications. Included stroke categories were: 71% (ischemic), 11% (intracerebral hemorrhage), 4% (unknown), 14% (TIA).

In the treatment arm, 58% of subjects received combination therapy. Perindopril-based therapy was associated with an overall relative risk reduction for recurrent stroke of 28% (confidence interval [CI] 17, 38%), with a striking 50% risk reduction in subjects included because of hemorrhagic stroke. Other subgroups with greater benefit were those with hypertension and subjects treated with combined perindopril–indapamide therapy. Among included subjects, perindopril-based therapy was well-tolerated, although 14% of eligible subjects dropped out during an initial open-label phase owing to adverse effects.

Second, the majority of hypertensive patients will require more than one agent to achieve their goal blood pressure level. In the ALLHAT trial, patients (with average blood pressures of 146/84 mmHg at entry) required an average of two medications to achieve goal blood pressure *(29)*. Diabetic patients with hypertension require, on average, three or more agents to achieve goal blood pressure levels *(30,31)*. It is reasonable to consider monotherapy as initial treatment for patients with only mild or modest elevations of blood pressure *(29)*. In further management, it is often useful to add a second agent rather than pushing a first-line agent to its maximal dose; the additional agent minimizes side effects and takes advantage of synergy between different classes of antihypertensive agents. However, for subjects with stage 2 or higher hypertension (>160 mmHg systolic or >100 mmHg diastolic), initiation of therapy with two agents is recommended *(4)*.

A third key concept in hypertension management is the importance of choosing the appropriate medication class for initial therapy based on a patient's individual characteristics. The recently completed ALLHAT trial *(29)* demonstrated that thiazide diuretics (specifically chlorthalidone) should be the initial agent of choice for almost all patients with hypertension. ALLHAT was the largest antihypertensive trial ever performed, enrolling 42,448 patients aged 55 years and older with hypertension and with at least one other CVD risk factor. Patients with CHF, documented left ventricular ejection fraction less than 0.35, or serum creatinine above 2.0 were excluded. The study was a double-blind trial designed to determine whether newer antihypertensive agents used as first-line therapy could prevent CVD and mortality significantly better than chlorthalidone used as first-line therapy. Patients were randomly assigned to receive chlorthalidone (control), doxazosin (an α-blocker), lisinopril (an ACE inhibitor), or amlodipine (a dihydropyridine calcium channel blocker), and they could receive increased doses of their initial therapy as well as second-line agents (including atenolol) and a third-line agent (hydralazine) as needed. Patients were followed for an average of approx 5 years *(29)*.

Patients randomly assigned to chlorthalidone achieved slightly lower SBP levels on average than patients receiving other agents. Regarding clinical outcomes, none of the newer agents tested in ALLHAT were superior to chlorthal-idone in prevention of any end point (including total mortality; cardiovascular mortality; combined CVD, fatal coronary disease, and nonfatal MI; CHF; and stroke) *(29)*. However, chlorthalidone was superior to each of the other agents in reduction of some end points. The most significant differences were seen regarding the occurrence of CHF. Compared with chlorthalidone, doxazosin therapy was associated with a twofold increased risk of CHF *(32)*, amlodipine with a 38% increased risk, and lisinopril with a 19% increased risk, with similar effects seen across all subgroups *(29)*.

Regarding stroke, doxazosin was associated with a significant 19% increased risk for stroke within 3 years. The combination of this finding and the increased risk for CHF with doxazosin prompted early termination of the doxazosin arm by the study investigators *(32)*. There was no significant difference between amlodipine compared with chlorthalidone in stroke incidence to 7 years (hazards ratio for stroke for amlodipine vs chlorthalidone 0.93, 95% CI 0.81–1.06). There was no difference in the comparison of these two medications regarding stroke across important clinical subgroups stratified by age, sex, ethnicity, and diabetes status. However, there was a significantly higher risk of stroke for patients receiving lisinopril compared with chlorthalidone (hazards ratio 1.15, 95% CI 1.02–1.30); this finding was largely driven by a substantially higher risk for stroke among black patients receiving lisinopril (hazards ratio 1.40, 95% CI 1.17–1.68) that was not observed among nonblacks receiving lisinopril (hazards ratio 1.00, 95% CI 0.85–1.17) *(29)*. Given the low cost of chlorthalidone compared with the newer agents, it is clear that diuretics are the most cost-effective choice for initial therapy of hypertension.

On the strength of the ALLHAT results, the JNC 7 recommendations firmly state that a thiazide diuretic should be first-line therapy for the vast majority of patients with hypertension *(4)*. A subsequent meta-analysis of 42 antihypertensive trials involving 192,478 patients confirmed the finding of ALLHAT (Fig. 5) *(33)*.

Another important concept is that the decision to use other agents as first-line antihypertensive therapy may be driven by compelling clinical indications on a patient-by-patient basis. The JNC 7 recommendations acknowledge a number of compelling indications. For example, in patients with hypertension and CHF, diabetes, or chronic renal disease, initial use of an ACE inhibitor or perhaps an angiotensin$_2$-receptor blocker is supported by a large number of placebo-controlled trials *(4)*. In the Heart Outcomes Prevention Evaluation trial, which included patients with CVD or diabetes plus at least one other risk factor, randomization to ramipril (an ACE inhibitor) was associated with substantially lower risks for stroke *(34)* as well as the overall composite end point of MI, stroke, and cardiovascular death *(35)* despite only a modest effect in lowering blood pressure. Similarly, β-blockers should be strongly considered as a first-line agent in patients with recent MI or with angina pectoris. For secondary prevention of stroke, ACE inhibitors could be considered a first-line agent *(36)*. However, if another agent is chosen as

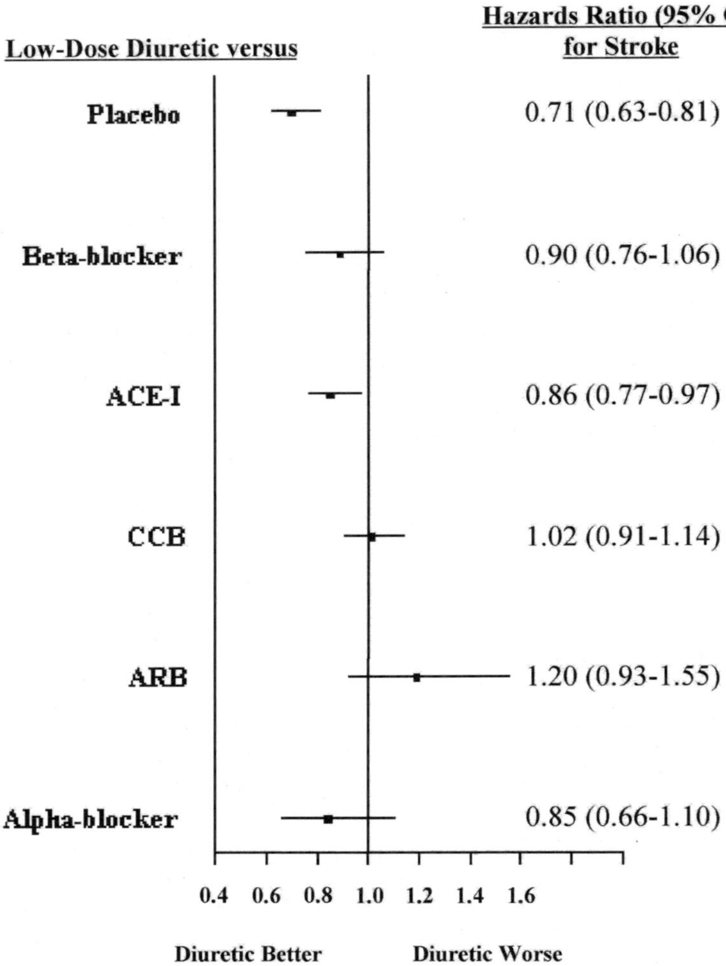

Fig. 5. Relative benefit of thiazide diuretic vs other therapies in antihypertensive trials.

first-line therapy, available data suggest that a thiazide diuretic should be the second agent.

Finally, other key concepts in hypertension management are the importance of lifestyle modification and the emphasis on control of SBP as in this chapter. Patients will require active involvement and support from their entire health care team to achieve blood pressure control. For example, patients with marked elevations in blood pressure cannot expect to achieve goal levels quickly or without side effects related to medications. It is important to explain to the patient that multiple medications will be required. Furthermore, it is important to set realistic goals for controlling blood pressure. For ambulatory patients with marked hypertension, an initial goal of systolic and diastolic levels below 160 and 95, respectively, should be achievable within 1–3 months, and such a reduction can have a dramatic impact in lowering risk for stroke and other CVD. Subsequent efforts should aim to get the patient to their appropriate goal level within 1 year of initiating therapy.

Adjunctive Therapy for Hypertensive Patients

In addition to antihypertensive therapy, strong consideration should be given to initiation of statin therapy in hypertensive patients, regardless of lipid status. The recent Anglo-Scandinavian Cardiac Outcomes Trial-Lipid Lowering Arm (ASCOT-LLA) trial *(37)* randomly assigned 10,305 hypertensive patients with average or lower-than-average cholesterol levels (mean 212 mg/dL) to treatment with atorvastatin 10 mg daily or placebo. Atorvastatin was associated with a significant 36% reduction in the primary end point of fatal CHD or nonfatal MI, but it was also significantly associated with a 27% reduction in stroke and a 21% reduction total CVD events *(37)*. Patients with hypertension should also receive at least 75 mg of aspirin daily. In the Hypertension Optimal Treatment trial, such therapy significantly reduced major CVD events by 15% and MI by 36%, with no major effect on stroke and only a mild increase in nonfatal major and minor bleeding events *(38)*.

CONCLUSION

Hypertension is unequivocally a major stroke risk factor. Mildly elevated SBP confers several-fold elevated risks for stroke and other CVD, and even borderline elevations in SBP confer unacceptably high risks for stroke. The presence of other modifiable stroke risk factors, such as cigarette smoking and diabetes, confer additive risks at any level of blood pressure. The results of multiple, large-scale, randomized controlled trials in tens of thousands of hypertension patients demonstrated beyond a doubt that drug therapy and dietary interventions are well tolerated and reduce risks of stroke and mortality from hypertension. There are modest, but measurable, differences among antihypertensive agents, and the results of available trials, including ALLHAT, support the treatment strategies outlined in the most recent JNC 7 consensus guidelines. The available data justify an aggressive approach by clinicians to identify and treat all patients at elevated risk; to attain or surpass target blood pressure goals, interventions designed to lower blood pressure should be used.

REFERENCES

1. American Heart Association. Heart Disease and Stroke Statistics 2003 Update. Dallas, TX: American Heart Association, 2002.

2. Vasan RS, Beiser A, Seshadri S, et al. Residual lifetime risk for developing hypertension in middle-aged women and men: The Framingham Heart Study. JAMA 2002;287:1003–1010.
3. Mosterd A, D'Agostino RB, Silbershatz H, et al. Trends in the prevalence of hypertension, antihypertensive therapy, and left ventricular hypertrophy from 1950 to 1989. N Engl J Med 1999;340:1221–1227.
4. Chobanian AV, Bakris GL, Black HR, et al. The seventh report of the Joint National Committee on Prevention, Detection, Evaluation, and Treatment of High Blood Pressure: the JNC7 report. JAMA 2003;289:2560–2572.
5. Mokdad AH, Ford ES, Bowman BA, et al. Prevalence of obesity, diabetes, and obesity-related health risk factors, 2001. JAMA 2003;289:76–79.
6. Lloyd-Jones DM, Evans JC, Larson MG, O'Donnell CJ, Roccella EJ, Levy D. Differential control of systolic and diastolic blood pressure: factors associated with lack of blood pressure control in the community. Hypertension 2000;36: 594–599.
7. Third report of the National Cholesterol Education Program (NCEP) Expert Panel on Detection, Evaluation, and Treatment of High Blood Cholesterol in Adults (Adult Treatment Panel III) final report. Circulation 2002;106:3143–3421.
8. Lloyd-Jones DM, Evans JC, Larson MG, O'Donnell CJ, Wilson PW, Levy D. Cross-classification of JNC VI blood pressure stages and risk groups in the Framingham Heart Study. Arch Intern Med 1999;159:2206–2212.
9. Wolf PA, D'Agostino RB, Belanger AJ, Kannel WB. Probability of stroke: a risk profile from the Framingham Study. Stroke 1991;22:312–318.
10. Prospective Studies Collaboration. Age-specific relevance of usual blood pressure to vascular mortality: a meta-analysis of individual data for one million adults in 61 prospective studies. Lancet 2002;360:1903–1913.
11. Burt VL, Whelton P, Roccella EJ, et al. Prevalence of hypertension in the US adult population: results from the Third National Health and Nutrition Examination Survey, 1988–1991. Hypertension 1995;25:305–313.
12. Franklin SS, Gustin W, Wong ND, et al. Hemodynamic patterns of age-related changes in blood pressure. The Framingham Heart Study. Circulation 1997;96: 308–315.
13. Franklin SS, Jacobs MJ, Wong ND, L'Italien GJ, Lapuerta P. Predominance of isolated systolic hypertension among middle-aged and elderly US hypertensives. Hypertension 2001;37:869–874.
14. Lloyd-Jones DM, Evans JC, Larson MG, O'Donnell CJ, Levy D. Differential impact of systolic and diastolic blood pressure level on JNC-VI staging. Hypertension 1999;34:381–385.
15. Neaton JD, Wentworth DN. Serum cholesterol, blood pressure, cigarette smoking, and death from coronary heart disease: overall findings and differences by age for 316,099 white men. Arch Intern Med 1992;152:56–64.
16. Neaton JD, Kuller L, Stamler J, Wentworth DN. Impact of systolic and diastolic blood pressure on cardiovascular mortality. In: Laragh JH, Brenner BM, eds. Hypertension: Pathophysiology, Diagnosis, and Management. New York: Raven Press, 1995:127–144.
17. Psaty BM, Furberg CD, Kuller LH, et al. Association between blood pressure level and the risk of myocardial infarction, stroke, and total mortality. Arch Intern Med 2001;161:1183–1192.

18. SHEP Cooperative Research Group. Prevention of stroke by antihypertensive drug treatment in older persons with isolated systolic hypertension. Final results of the Systolic Hypertension in the Elderly Program (SHEP). JAMA 1991;265:3255–3264.
19. Staessen JA, Fagard R, Thijs L, et al. Randomised double-blind comparison of placebo and active treatment for older patients with isolated systolic hypertension. The Systolic Hypertension in Europe (Syst-Eur) Trial Investigators. Lancet 1997;350: 757–764.
20. Izzo JL, Levy D, Black HR. Importance of systolic blood pressure in older Americans. Hypertension 2000;35:1021–1024.
21. Vasan RS, Larson MG, Leip EP, et al. Impact of high-normal blood pressure on the risk of cardiovascular disease. N Engl J Med 2001;345:1291–1297.
22. O'Donnell CJ, Ridker PM, Glynn RJ, et al. Hypertension and borderline isolated systolic hypertension increase risks of cardiovascular disease and mortality in male physicians. Circulation 1997;95:1132–1137.
23. Vasan RS, Larson MG, Leip EP, Kannel WB, Levy D. Assessment of frequency of progression to hypertension in non-hypertensive participants in the Framingham Heart Study: a cohort study. Lancet 2001;358:1682–1686.
24. Chae CU, Pfeffer MA, Glynn RJ, Mitchell GF, Taylor JO, Hennekens CH. Increased pulse pressure and risk of heart failure in the elderly. JAMA 1999;281:634–639.
25. Franklin SS, Khan SA, Wong ND, Larson MG, Levy D. Is pulse pressure useful in predicting risk for coronary heart Disease? The Framingham heart study. Circulation 1999;100:354–360.
26. Dahlof B, Lindholm LH, Hansson L, Schersten B, Ekbom T, Wester PO. Morbidity and mortality in the Swedish Trial in Old Patients with Hypertension (STOP-Hypertension). Lancet 1991;338:1281–1285.
27. Staessen JA, Gasowski J, Wang JG, et al. Risks of untreated and treated isolated systolic hypertension in the elderly: meta-analysis of outcome trials. Lancet 2000; 355:865–872.
28. Treatment of Hypertension in Adults With Diabetes. Diabetes Care 2003;26:80S.
29. The ALLHAT Officers and Coordinators for the ALLHAT Collaborative Research Group. Major outcomes in high-risk hypertensive patients randomized to angiotensin-converting enzyme inhibitor or calcium channel blocker vs diuretic: the Antihypertensive and Lipid-Lowering Treatment to Prevent Heart Attack Trial (ALLHAT). JAMA 2002;288:2981–2997.
30. Bakris GL. A practical approach to achieving recommended blood pressure goals in diabetic patients. Arch Intern Med 2001;161:2661–2667.
31. UK Prospective Diabetes Study Group. Tight blood pressure control and risk of macrovascular and microvascular complications in type 2 diabetes: UKPDS 38. BMJ 1998;317:703.
32. ALLHAT Collaborative Research Group. Major cardiovascular events in hypertensive patients randomized to doxazosin vs chlorthalidone: the antihypertensive and lipid-lowering treatment to prevent heart attack trial (ALLHAT). JAMA 2000;283: 1967–1975.
33. Psaty BM, Lumley T, Furberg CD, et al. Health outcomes associated with various antihypertensive therapies used as first-line agents: a network meta-analysis. JAMA 2003;289:2534–2544.
34. Bosch J, Yusuf S, Pogue J, et al. Use of ramipril in preventing stroke: double blind randomised trial. BMJ 2002;324:699–703.

35. Yusuf S, Sleight P, Pogue J, Bosch J, Davies R, Dagenais G. Effects of an angiotensin-converting-enzyme inhibitor, ramipril, on cardiovascular events in high-risk patients. The Heart Outcomes Prevention Evaluation Study investigators. N Engl J Med 2000;342:145–153.
36. PROGRESS Collaborative Group. Randomised trial of a perindopril-based blood-pressure lowering regimen among 6105 individuals with previous stroke or transient ischaemic attack. Lancet 2001;358:1033–1041.
37. Sever PS, Dahlof B, Poulter NR, et al. Prevention of coronary and stroke events with atorvastatin in hypertensive patients who have average or lower-than-average cholesterol concentrations, in the Anglo-Scandinavian Cardiac Outcomes Trial—Lipid Lowering Arm (ASCOT-LLA): a multicentre randomised controlled trial. Lancet 2003;361:1149–1158.
38. Hansson L, Zanchetti A, Carruthers SG, et al. Effects of intensive blood-pressure lowering and low-dose aspirin in patients with hypertension: principal results of the Hypertension Optimal Treatment (HOT) randomised trial. Lancet 1998;351: 1755–1762.

4
Evaluation and Management of Hyperlipidemia for Stroke Prevention

Mehmet Akif Topcuoglu,
Ferdinando S. Buonanno, and Peter J. Kelly

EVIDENCE FOR ASSOCIATION BETWEEN HYPERLIPIDEMIA AND RISK OF STROKE

Observational studies and clinical trials have established that lipid disorders (elevated serum total cholesterol [TC], low-density lipoprotein cholesterol [LDLc], or triglycerides [TGs] and reduced serum high-density lipoprotein cholesterol [HDLc]) are independently associated with the risk of coronary heart disease (CHD). Hyperlipidemia was also clearly associated with progression of carotid and peripheral atherosclerosis and intima-media thickness (IMT), a marker of early atherosclerosis.

Despite these data, for years uncertainty existed about whether hyperlipidemia was also associated with risk of stroke, and whether lipid-lowering therapy would be beneficial in preventing first and recurrent stroke *(1,2)*. The association between elevated plasma lipids and ischemic stroke reported in observational studies was not as strong as was reported with CHD. For example, the Framingham study found no overall relationship between lipid status and first stroke. Meta-analyses of large cohorts also did not demonstrate a strong association between hyperlipidemia and stroke. Other data suggested that a J-shaped relationship may exist between lipid status and stroke, with increased ischemic stroke risk occurring at very high lipid levels and increased risk of hemorrhagic stroke associated with very low levels. This pattern was seen in analyses from the Honolulu Heart Study and the Multiple Risk Factor Intervention Trial (MRFIT), raising concerns among some authors that lipid-lowering therapy may prove harmful in patients with cerebrovascular disease by promoting hemorrhagic stroke.

These issues have been clarified with the publication of the results of several randomized trials of lipid-lowering therapies, primarily statins (Table 1).

From: *Current Clinical Neurology: Handbook of Stroke Prevention in Clinical Practice*
Edited by: K. L. Furie and P. J. Kelly © Humana Press Inc., Totowa, NJ

Table 1
Summary of Reported Benefits in Statin and Fibrate Trials for Stroke Prevention

Trial	Intervention	Included	Lipid status at entry	Stroke outcome	Relative risk reduction (95% CI)
Scandinavian Simvastatin Survival Study (4S)	Simvastatin 10–40 mg	Symptomatic CHD (80% men)	High (TC > 270 mg/dL)	Stroke/TIA on post-hoc analysis	30% (4–48%), $p = 0.02$
Cholesterol and Recurrent Events (CARE)	Pravastatin 40 mg	Patients with MI (86% men)	High or average (TC <240 mg/dL, LDLc 115–174 mg/dL)	Stroke/TIA on post-hoc analysis	31% (3–52%), $p = 0.03$
Long-Term Intervention with Pravastatin in Ischemic Disease (LIPID)	Pravastatin 40 mg	Patients with prior MI or unstable angina (83% men)	High or average TC (155–271 mg/dL)	Stroke a specified end point; CT/MRI verified (82%); subtypes defined	19% (0–34%), $p = 0.05$ (ischemic stroke only)
Medical Research Council Heart Protection Study	Simvastatin 40 mg	20,536 adults with high CAD risk[a] (75% men)	Average TC (>135 mg/dL)	Stroke a specified end point; verified by CT/MRI/autopsy	25% (15–34%), $p < 0.0001$ (all strokes); 30% (19–40%), $p < 0.0001$ (ischemic stroke)
ASCOT Lipid-Lowering Arm	Atorvastatin 10 mg	19,342 adults with hypertension plus three other risk factors	Average TC (<250 mg/dL, nonfasting)	Stroke a specified end point	27% (4–46%), $p = 0.02$ (all strokes)
VA-HIT Trial	Gemfibrozil 1200 mg	2,531 adults with CAD (all men)	Low HDLc (<40 mg/dL), average LDLc (≤140 mg/dL)	Stroke a specified end point (adjudication committee)	25% (–6 to 47%), $p = 0.1$ (all strokes)
Bezafibrate Infarction Prevention Study	Bezafibrate 400 mg	3,090 adults with CAD (91% men)	TC 180–250 mg/dL, HDLc <45 mg/dL, LDLc < 180 mg/dL	Stroke a specified end point (adjudication committee)	20% (CIs not provided), $p= 0.36$ (all strokes)

[a]Prior CAD 76%, IS/TIA/CEA 16%, peripheral vascular disease 13%, DM 18%, hypertension + male <65 years 1%.

CAD, coronary artery disease; IS, ischemic stroke; CEA, carotid endarterectomy; CI, confidence interval; MRI, magnetic resonance imaging.

Overall, these trials have demonstrated a reduction in the risk of stroke of approx 30% in high-risk patients (predominantly men) with average or elevated serum cholesterol treated with simvastatin, pravastatin, or atorvastatin. Furthermore, lipid-lowering therapy was safe in patients with cerebrovascular disease in these trials. For example, in the Heart Protection Study, no increase in hemorrhagic stroke occurred among more than 3000 patients with stroke/transient ischemic attack (TIA), despite lowering of LDLc to less than 100 mg/dL in a substantial proportion of these individuals *(3)*. A similar benefit of LDLc-lowering therapy for primary prevention of stroke in high-risk individuals was demonstrated in the lipid-lowering arm of the Anglo-Scandinavian Cardiac Outcomes Trial (Table 1). Other observational studies, such as the Bezafibrate Infarction Prevention Registry, have supported these trial data by reporting a dose-dependent relationship between lipid status (elevated TC and LDLc and reduced HDLc) and first stroke.

DIAGNOSIS OF HYPERLIPIDEMIA FOR PRIMARY AND SECONDARY STROKE PREVENTION

For accurate assessment of lipid status, a complete lipoprotein profile (TC, HDLc, and TG) should be obtained after at least an 8-hour fast. Sampling in the postprandial state is likely to lead to inaccurately depressed LDLc. This is because LDLc is calculated according to Friedewald's formula as TC – (HDLc + TG/5), and TG levels are elevated after meals. If TG levels are over 400 mg/dL, estimation of LDLc by this method is not accurate, and levels must be measured directly by ultracentrifugation. Lipoprotein electrophoresis is very expensive and not necessary for the routine clinical diagnosis of acquired and familial hypercholesterolemia.

The National Cholesterol Education Program (NCEP) Third Report of the Expert Panel on Detection, Evaluation, and Treatment of High Blood Cholesterol in Adults (Adult Treatment Panel III [ATP III]) classification of LDLc, total, and HDLc is summarized in Table 2. Based on experimental data showing that atherosclerosis is related to LDLc and clinical trial data indicating that lowering of LDLc is associated with reduction in the risk of CHD, the panel made recommendations for lipid evaluation primarily in terms of LDLc.

When considering the timing of sampling for lipid measurement for secondary prevention after acute stroke, changes in lipid parameters associated with acute illness must be taken into account. Baseline lipid values change in the setting of pregnancy, weight loss, trauma, and conditions such as stroke, surgery, and infection. During pregnancy, TC levels increase by an average of 75% (mean 315 mg/dL) and return to normal in 6 months. Smoking decreases HDLc levels; alcohol increases HDLc and TG levels. Regular physical activity

Table 2
NCEP Classification of Lipid Status

LDL cholesterol units (mg/dL)	
<100	Optimal
100–129	Above optimal
130–159	Borderline high
160–189	High
≥190	Very high
Total cholesterol	
<200	Desirable
200–239	Borderline high
≥240	High
HDL cholesterol	
<40	Low
≥60	High

Source: From ref. *4*.
Conversion: 1 mmol/L = 38.6 mg/dL.

has been reported to increase HDLc and decrease TG levels. After myocardial infarction (MI) and acute stroke, LDLc and TC levels begin to decline in the first few hours and become significantly decreased by 24–48 hours, returning to baseline by about 6 weeks. For valid interpretation, patients with acute stroke should have phlebotomy for lipid measurement within 24 hours of onset and preferably at the time of admission.

Before initiation of lipid-lowering therapy, any individual with elevated LDLc or other lipid abnormality should be carefully evaluated for causes of secondary dyslipidemia, such as diabetes mellitus (DM), hypothyroidism, obesity, obstructive liver disease, nephrotic syndrome, chronic renal failure, and excess alcohol consumption. Specific inquiry should be made about drugs that increase LDLc or decrease HDLc, such as progestins, anabolic steroids, corticosteroids, β-blockers, thiazides, oral contraceptives, anti-HIV (human immunodeficiency virus) protease inhibitors, or alcohol.

GENERAL CONCEPTS OF PRIMARY AND SECONDARY STROKE PREVENTION

The ATP III details the NCEP's updated guidelines for cholesterol testing and clinical management *(4)*. Most of the recommendations for lipid screening and therapeutic goals in this chapter closely follow these guidelines. More detailed information on risk stratification, dietary modification, and management of specific dyslipidemic disorders may be found in the published summary of the NCEP ATP III report *(4)*.

The general goals of lipid-lowering therapy are to reduce morbidity and mortality caused by first and recurrent stroke (primary and secondary prevention). Lipid-lowering therapy may have long-term and short-term benefits for stroke prevention. The primary long-term benefit is reduction in first stroke by slowing the development and progression of atherosclerosis. This strategy requires early detection of lipid abnormalities in individuals at risk. The NCEP recommends that all adults older than 20 years undergo periodic (every 5 years) testing for serum lipid abnormalities *(4)*. Short-term benefits include reduction in the risk of stroke and other acute manifestations of atherosclerotic disease (e.g., MI) over the 10 years following the first event by contributing to plaque stability, thereby reducing fissuring, rupture, thrombosis, and intramural hemorrhage.

STRATIFICATION OF RISK OF STROKE AND OTHER VASCULAR EVENTS

The NCEP ATP III identified LDLc as the primary target of risk-reduction therapy. NCEP classifications of LDLc, TC, and HDLc levels are summarized in Table 2. Because the intensity of risk-reduction therapy is based on individualized absolute risk assessment, the first step in selecting LDLc management options is the determination of the individual's risk status (Fig. 1). The presence of CHD or other clinical atherosclerotic disease (CHD risk equivalents) (Table 3) is first identified (note that, in the ATP III scheme, craniocervical atherosclerosis and diabetes are regarded as CHD risk equivalents). Next, the presence of major risk factors other than elevated LDLc is determined (Table 4). For individuals without CHD risk equivalents with two or more major risk factors, 10-year (short-term) risk is assessed using the Framingham Point Scores method (Table 5).

Using the information delineated here, the individual is assigned one of the following three risk categories: (1) CHD, CHD equivalent, multiple risk factors conveying 10-year risk above 20%; (2) multiple risk factors conveying 10-year risk less than 20%; or (3) 0–1 risk factor. The LDLc goal and therapeutic strategy are then determined (Table 6).

Other factors not included in the ATP III risk stratification scheme (e.g., obesity, emerging risk markers) may also have utility in selected individuals to guide the intensity of lipid-lowering therapy. Emerging risk factors include lipoprotein(a) [Lp(a)]; homocysteine; lipoprotein remnants such as beta very low-density lipoprotein (β-VLDL) and apolipoprotein C-III; thrombotic (e.g., fibrinogen, plasminogen activator inhibitor-1 [PAI-1]) and inflam-

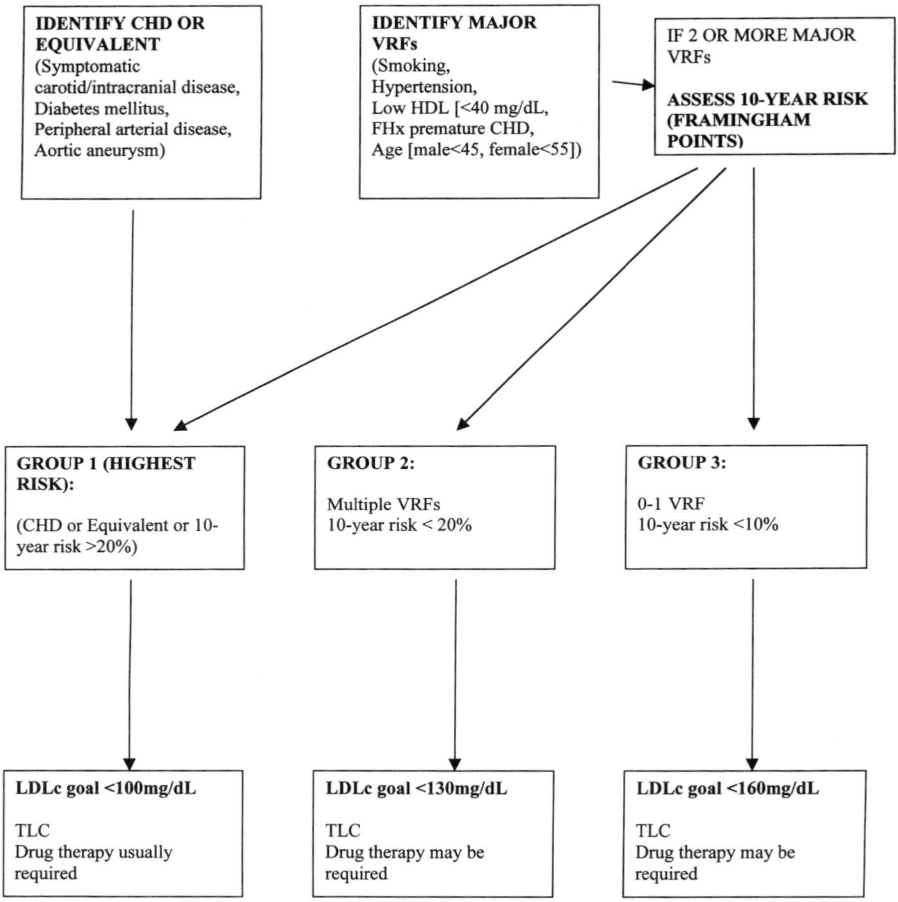

Fig. 1. NCEP risk assessment for intensity of lipid-lowering therapy.

Table 3
NCEP CHD Risk Equivalents

1. Clinical CHD
2. Symptomatic carotid disease[a]
3. Peripheral arterial disease
4. Abdominal aortic aneurysm
5. Diabetes

Source: From ref. *4*.

[a]Symptomatic intracranial parent vessel disease is regarded as CHD risk equivalent.

Table 4
Major Vascular Risk Factors

1. Cigarette smoking (any in the past month)
2. Hypertension (BP≥140/90 mmHg or antihypertensive medication)
3. Low HDLc (<40 mg/dL)
4. Family history of premature CHD[a] (CHD in male first-degree relative younger than 55 years, CHD in female first-degree relative younger than 65 years)
5. Age (men 45 years or older, women 55 years or older)

Source: From ref. *4*.

HDL cholesterol ≥60 mg/dL counts as a negative risk factor; its presence removes one risk factor from the total count.

[a]Myocardial infarction or CHD death.

matory markers (e.g., high-sensitivity C-reactive protein [CRP]); impaired fasting glucose; evidence of subclinical atherosclerotic disease (lowered ankle–brachial blood pressure [BP] index, positive exercise electrocardiogram test or myocardial perfusion imaging); or stress echocardiography and positive tests for atherosclerotic burden (e.g., increased carotid IMT on B-mode ultrasonography, positive coronary calcium on spiral computed tomography [CT]). Among these, detection of subclinical atherosclerosis may be particularly useful for risk assessment in the elderly because the predictive value of standard risk factors declines in this age group *(4)*.

NCEP TREATMENT SELECTION RECOMMENDATIONS APPLIED TO PRIMARY AND SECONDARY STROKE PREVENTION

For individuals with craniocervical atherosclerosis (including carotid and intracranial disease), LDLc levels below 100 mg per day have been recommended as the goal for secondary prevention. The two major modalities of LDL-lowering therapy are therapeutic life-style changes (TLC) and drug therapy. The cut points of lipid levels for initiation TLC and drugs according to the three risk categories are shown in Table 6.

Patients With CHD, CHD Risk Equivalents, or Multiple (Two or More) Risk Factors

If baseline LDLc exceeds 130 mg/dL, intensive TLC and maximal control of other risk factors should be started. For most, an LDL-lowering drug will usually be needed to attain the LDL goal of less than 100 mg/dL. Thus, it is advised to initiate medication simultaneous with TLC.

If LDLc is between 100 and 129 mg/dL either at baseline or after initiation of LDL-lowering therapy, the options are to intensify TLC or to begin drug therapies to lower LDL.

Table 5
Estimated 10-Year CHD Risk

Men		Women	
Age	Points	Age	Points
20–34	–9	20–34	–7
35–39	–4	35–39	–3
40–44	0	40–44	0
45–49	3	45–49	3
50–54	6	50–54	6
55–59	8	55–59	8
60–64	10	60–64	10
65–69	11	65–69	12
70–74	12	70–74	14
75–79	13	75–79	16

	Points						Points				
	Age	Age	Age	Age	Age		Age	Age	Age	Age	Age
Total cholesterol	30–39	40–49	50–59	60–69	70–79	Total cholesterol	30–39	40–49	50–59	60–69	70–79
<160	0	0	0	0	0	<160	0	0	0	0	0
160–199	4	3	2	1	0	160–199	4	3	2	1	0
200–239	7	5	3	1	0	200–239	11	6	5	3	2
240–279	9	6	4	2	1	240–279	11	8	5	3	2
≥280	11	8	5	3	1	≥280	13	10	7	4	2

	Points						Points				
	Age	Age	Age	Age	Age		Age	Age	Age	Age	Age
Smoking	30–39	40–49	50–59	60–69	70–79	Smoking	30–39	40–49	50–59	60–69	70–79
Nonsmoker	0	0	0	0	0	Nonsmoker	0	0	0	0	0
Smoker	8	5	3	1	1	Smoker	9	7	4	2	1

HDL (mg/dL)	Points		HDL (mg/dL)	Points	
≥60	−1		≥60	−1	
50–59	0		50–59	0	
40–49	1		40–49	1	
<40	2		<40	2	
Systolic BP (mmHg)	**Untreated**	**Treated**	**Systolic BP (mmHg)**	**Untreated**	**Treated**
<120	0	0	<120	0	0
120–129	0	1	120–129	1	3
130–139	1	2	130–139	2	4
140–159	1	2	140–159	3	5
≥160	2	3	≥160	4	6
Total points	**10-Year risk (%)**		**Total points**	**10-Year risk (%)**	
<0	<1		<9	<1	
0–4	1		9–12	1	
5–6	2		13–14	2	
7	3		15	3	
8	4		16	4	
9	5		17	5	
10	6		18	6	
11	8		19	8	
12	10		20	11	
13	12		21	14	
14	16		22	17	
15	20		23	22	
16	25		24	27	
≥17	≥30		≥25	≥30	

Source: From ref. *4*.

Note: Automatic downloadable calculator is available at http://hin.nhlbi.nih.gov/atpiii/calculator.asp.

Table 6
NCEP LDL Cholesterol Goals, Thresholds for TLC and Drug Therapy

Risk category	LDL goal	Initiate TLC	Drug recommended
CHD/CHD risk equivalents/ multiple risk factors (10-year risk>20%)	<100 mg/dL	≥100 mg/dL	≥130 mg/dL (100–129 drug optional)[a]
Multiple (2+) risk factors (10-year risk≤20%)	<130 mg/dL	≥ 130 mg/dL	If 10-year risk is 10–20%, ≥130 mg/dL; if 10-year risk <10%, ≥160 mg/dL
0–1 Risk factor[b]	<160 mg/dL	≥160 mg/dL	≥190 mg/dL (if LDLC 160–189 mg/dL, then drug is optional)[a]

[a]Some recommend the use of LDL-lowering drugs if an LDLc of less than 100 mg/dL cannot be achieved by TLC. Others prefer the use of drugs that primarily modify TG and HDL.
[b]10-year risk assessment is not necessary.

If baseline LDLc is below 100 mg/dL, NCEP guidelines do not recommend further LDLc-lowering therapy (although recent trials suggest a benefit even in these individuals).

Multiple Risk Factors Conveying 10-Year Risk of 20% or Less

For the group with multiple risk factors and a 10-year risk of 20% or less, intensification of management is adjusted according to 10-year risk and LDLc (Table 6). In subjects with multiple risk factors and a 10-year risk of 10–20%, the LDLc goal is less than 130 mg/dL, and reduction of short-term as well as long-term risk for CHD is the goal. If LDLc exceeds 130 mg/dL, TLC are started for 3 months. At this time, if LDLc persists above 130 mg/dL, then a hypolipidemic drug is considered. If LDLc decreases to less than 130 mg/dL, TLC alone can be maintained without medication.

In subjects with multiple risk factors and a 10-year risk of less than 10%, the LDLc goal is the same (<130 mg/dL), but the primary aim is to reduce long-term risk. If baseline LDLc is 130 mg/dL or higher, TLC are implemented. If LDLc is below 160 mg/dL on TLC alone, TLC alone may be continued as short-term vascular risk is not high. If LDLc is above 160 mg/dL, a lipid-lowering drug may be initiated.

Subjects With 0–1 Risk Factor

In individuals with 0–1 risk factor, the 10-year risk is generally less than 10%, and the goal is primarily reduction of long-term risk by reducing LDLc to less than 160 mg/dL. NCEP guidelines recommend initiation of TLC and reassessment of LDLc at 3 months. At this time, TLC is continued if LDLc is below 160 mg/dL. However, if LDLc persists between 160 and 189 mg/dL, an LDLc-lowering drug may be initiated. If a major single risk factor (e.g., heavy smoking, poorly controlled hypertension, a strong family history of premature CHD, very low HDLc), multiple life-habit risk factors are present, or if 10-year risk is close to 10%, a lipid-lowering drug can be recommended. If LDLc is 190 mg/dL or above despite TLC, a drug should be added to achieve the LDLc goal of less than 160 mg/dL.

THERAPEUTIC LIFESTYLE CHANGES IN LDL-LOWERING THERAPY

In conjunction with increased physical activity and weight loss, dietary modification remains the cornerstone of lifestyle modification treatment. Reductions in total fat, saturated fat, partially hydrogenated unsaturated (trans) fatty acids, and dietary cholesterol are recommended. Substitution of saturated and trans fats with polyunsaturated and monounsaturated fats is probably more important than reduction of total dietary fat *(5)*.

A stepwise approach, such as the American Heart Association (AHA) Step I or Step II diet, increases adherence and is more effective than other methods *(6)*. The AHA Step I diet includes a daily cholesterol amount less than 300 mg (one egg contains 300 mg cholesterol). Calories from fat and saturated fat must be less than 30% and 10% of the total, respectively. Instead, poly- or mono-unsaturated fats and complex carbohydrates are increased. Given the high prevalence of undesirable lipid profiles in the general population, this diet is recommended for all individuals for primary prevention of vascular disease. The AHA Step II diet, now known as the TLC diet (Table 7) *(1,5–7)*, includes saturated fat as less than 7% of calories and less than 200 mg of cholesterol per day. Overall composition of the TLC diet is consistent with the recommendations of the Dietary Guidelines for Americans 2000 *(8)*.

The physician has an important role in initiating and maintaining adherence to dietary measures. During the first visit, lifestyle changes are started; the emphasis is on reduction of saturated fat and cholesterol intake. Trans fat is particularly important and must be consumed as less than 2% of total energy. Fatty fish is recommended at least once a week, and 400 g or more of vegetables and fruit per day are recommended. Increase of moderate physical activity (Table 7) and incorporation of more physical activity into the daily routine is emphasized. Smoking cessation and moderation of alcohol intake are advised. Low salt consumption (<6 g/day) is advised. Referral to a dietitian or nutritionist at this stage may increase compliance.

Table 7
Therapeutic Lifestyle Changes

Essential components	Recommendations	Approximate LDLc reduction
1. Decrease LDL-raising nutrients		
Saturated fat	Less than 7% of calories	8–10%
Dietary cholesterol	Less than 200 mg per day	3–5%
2. Therapeutic options for LDL lowering		
Plant stanols/sterols	2 g per day	6–15%
Increased viscous (soluble) fiber	10–25 g per day	3–5%
3. Total calories (energy) and weight reductions	Adjust total caloric intake to maintain desirable body weight (lose 10 lb)	5–8%
4. Physical activity	To expend at least 200 kcal per day, perform moderate exercise such as brisk walking (3–4 mph) for 30–40 minutes, swimming with laps for 20 minutes, bicycling (5 miles in 30 minutes), noncompetitive volleyball for 45 minutes, raking leaves for 30 minutes, home care such as heavy cleaning, basketball for 15–20 minutes, social dancing for 30 minutes	
Macronutrients		
1. Polyunsaturated fat	Up to 10% of total calories	
2. Monounsaturated fat	Up to 20% of total calories	
3. Total fat	25–35% of total calories	
4. Carbohydrate	50–60% of total calories	
5. Dietary fiber	20–330 g per day	
6. Protein	Approx 15% of total calories	

Source: From refs. *1* and *5–7*.

After approx 6 weeks, the LDLc response should be evaluated. If the LDLc goal has been achieved or a decreasing trend has been observed, no further dietary modification is needed. If the LDLc goal is not achieved, dietary instructions should be explained again and reinforced. The assistance of nutrition professionals for more formal instruction and counseling is especially valuable at this time. In addition to reinforcement of advice for saturated fat and cholesterol intake reduction, addition of plant stanolsor sterols to 2 g per day and increased viscous (soluble) fiber to 10–25 g per day may be considered. These are currently incorporated into special margarines available in food markets. Dietary viscous fiber can be increased by emphasizing intake of cereal grains, vegetables, dried beans, peas, and legumes.

After another 6 weeks, the response to dietary therapy should be reevaluated. If the LDLc goal is achieved, the current diet should be maintained indefinitely. If not, drug therapy is initiated; weight management, physical activity, and dietary measures are intensified; and a lipid-lowering agent may be prescribed.

LIPID-LOWERING DRUG THERAPY

For secondary prevention among patients with CHD and CHD risk equivalents, lipid-lowering drugs are started simultaneously with TLC. Hospitalized patients with CHD, or with CHD risk equivalents, or with planned cardiac procedure should be discharged on a hypolipidemic drug if the LDLc is 130 mg/dL or above. If the LDLc level is between 100 and 129 mg/dL, the decision to start drug treatment at discharge should be made on a case-by-case basis because LDLc levels diminish in the first few hours after an acute vascular event and may remain low for many weeks. Every effort should be made to measure plasma lipids at hospital admission to avoid problems with interpretation of results. This is important because initiation of lipid-lowering drugs during the hospital stay results in higher compliance and prevents gaps in treatment between the inpatient and outpatient settings.

For primary prevention, drug initiation is considered in the third visit of dietary therapy if LDLc goals have not been reached. Given the current evidence base from randomized trials, a 3-hydroxy-3-methyl-glutaryl-coenzyme A (HMG-CoA) reductase inhibitor (statin) should be the drug of first choice for secondary and primary stroke prevention. Alternatives such as bile acid sequestrants (BASs) or nicotinic acid may be considered for individual patients and are discussed below. In many cases, a moderate dose of simvastatin or pravastatin will be enough to attain the LDLc goal, and higher doses will not be needed. The effect on plasma LDLc should be evaluated after 6 weeks. If the goal is then achieved, the current dose is maintained. If the goal is not achieved, the dose may be increased, or a BAS or niacin may be added. After 12 weeks of drug treatment, the LDLc response is assessed again. If the goal is not achieved at this stage, consultation with a lipid specialist is recommended if such a service is available. Once the LDLc goal is achieved, patients can be monitored every 4–6 months for response to therapy.

HMG-CoA REDUCTASE INHIBITORS (STATINS)

Mechanism and Effects

Statins are the most effective and practical class of drugs for reducing LDLc (Table 8) and are the only class of lipid-lowering drugs consistently proven to reduce the risk of stroke in clinical trials. These drugs are effec-

Table 8
Summary of Statins

Available drugs in US	Lovastatin, pravastatin, simvastatin, fluvastatin, atorvastatin, cerivastatin[a], rosuvastatin
Lipid or lipoprotein effects	LDLc decreased by 18–55% HDLc increased by 5–15% TGs decreased by 7–30%
Major use	To lower LDL cholesterol
Contraindications	*Absolute*: Hypersensitivity to any component of these products, active or chronic liver disease or unexplained persistent elevated liver function tests, pregnancy, lactation, childhood *Relative*: Concurrent use of cyclosporine, macrolide antibiotics, triazole antifungals, other CYP 3A4 inhibitors; in addition, fibrates and niacin should be used with caution
Efficacy	Reduce risk for CHD and stroke
Major side effects	Myopathy and rhabdomyolysis Increases of liver transaminases
Usual starting dose and expected percentage LDLc decrease	Lovastatin 20 mg 24% Pravastatin 20 mg 24% Simvastatin 20 mg 35% Fluvastatin 20 mg 18% Atorvastatin 10 mg 37% Rosuvastatin 20 mg 43%
Maximum FDA-approved dose and expected percentage LDLc decrease	Lovastatin 80 mg 40% Pravastatin 40 mg 34% Simvastatin 80 mg 46% Fluvastatin 80 mg 31% Atorvastatin 80 mg 57% Rosuvastatin 80 mg 65%
Available preparations	Lovastatin 10, 20, and 40 mg tablets Pravastatin 10, 20, and 40 mg tablets Simvastatin 5, 10, 20, 40, and 80 mg tablets Fluvastatin 20 and 40 mg capsules, 80 mg XL tablets Atorvastatin 10, 20, 40, and 80 mg tablets Rosuvastatin 5, 10, 20, 40 mg tablets

FDA, Food and Drug Administration.
[a]Recalled from US market on August 8, 2001.

tive and well tolerated, have few drug interactions, and are relatively safe. Statins inhibit HMG-CoA reductase, the rate-limiting enzyme in cholesterol biosynthesis. A decrease in hepatic cholesterol content results in an increase of hepatic LDL receptor expression, which increases uptake of serum LDLc and triglyceride-rich lipoproteins (TGRLPs; intermediate-density lipoprotein plus VLDL).

Maximum reduction of cholesterol generally occurs when statins are administered with the evening meal or at bedtime. The observed reduction of LDLc (18–55%) is dose dependent and log linear, so each doubling of the dose results in 6% decrease in the LDLc. HDLc rises by 5–10%, but greater increases occur in subjects with low LDLc and elevated TGs. The range of serum TG reduction is 7–30%. In patients with combined hyperlipoproteinemia or atherogenic dyslipidemia, statins reduce both LDL and TGRLP.

Adverse Effects

Statin therapy is generally well tolerated. Hepatic transaminase (TA) elevation occurs in 0.5–2% of individuals in a dose-dependent manner *(9)*. However, clinically apparent hepatotoxicity is exceedingly rare. Reversal of TA elevation is usually observed after reduction of dose. Routine monitoring of TA levels is recommended during statin therapy (baseline, weeks 6 and 12, and twice yearly thereafter). Drugs should be discontinued if a TA increase more than three times the upper limit of normal (ULN) is observed. In these subjects, either readministration of the same drug or selection of another statin does not usually cause a recurrence of TA elevation *(4)*.

The most important side effect of statin therapy is myopathy. The reported incidence of clinical myopathy is 0.08% with lovastatin and simvastatin, and it is 0.09% with pravastatin. Unfortunately, these drugs are frequently stopped unnecessarily because of suspected myopathy, which is not present *(10)*. Nonspecific muscle and joint pains may be inadvertently attributed to statin therapy even if there is no significant increase in serum creatinine kinase (CK). Clinically overt myopathy, characterized by muscle aches, tenderness, weakness, and CK elevation, is very rare. However, life-threatening rhabdomyolysis (CK greater than 10 times the ULN), myoglobinuria, and acute renal failure may develop if this complication is overlooked, and the drug is continued. Myopathy is more common among elderly subjects with complex medical problems who are taking multiple drugs. When combined with statins, some drugs (e.g., cyclosporine, macrolide antibiotics, azole antifungals and other cytochrome P [CYP] inhibitors, fibrates, and niacin) may predispose to myotoxicity.

NCEP and other expert guidelines recommend baseline CK measurements before starting statin therapy. While on therapy, routine monitoring of CK is not recommended, but regular clinical monitoring for symptoms or signs of myopathy is advised. Patients should be instructed to report immediately muscle pain, weakness, or dark urination during statin use, and CK level determination should be performed when clinical suspicion arises. If myopathy is present, the specific statin should be discontinued. In patients with symptoms of muscle pains (myalgia) or asymptomatic elevation of CK, other causes (e.g., strenuous exercise, trauma) should be excluded. For patients with symptomatic moderate CK elevations (between 3 and 10 times the ULN), mon-itoring of symptoms and CK levels is advised until resolution occurs *(10)*.

Clinically Relevant Differences Between Statins and Choice of Agent

Although data suggest that the therapeutic effects of statins may be common to several agents within this class, only simvastatin, atorvastatin, and pravastatin have proven benefit in randomized trials for stroke prevention. Therefore, these should be initially considered in patients at high stroke risk. In patients on warfarin, pravastatin seems the safest drug of choice because it is not metabolized by the P450 system. Atorvastatin and fluvastatin may have cost advantages in some countries *(11)*.

For CHD prevention, the choice of statin in clinical practice mainly relates to pharmacokinetic and pharmacoeconomic considerations. Available statins differ somewhat in the degree of LDLc lowering that can be achieved per milligram dose. In addition, their metabolism is different: Simvastatin and lovastatin undergo metabolic inactivation by the hepatic CYP3A4 isozyme of cytochrome P450; atorvastatin is also a substrate for CYP3A4, but some metabolites remain active; and fluvastatin is metabolized by hepatic CYP2C9. These differences may assume importance when considering drug interactions, particularly for individuals for whom a statin has been discontinued because of myotoxicity.

Statins also differ in the dose needed to produce a given degree of LDLc lowering (Table 8). Although direct comparison data are unavailable, the lower effective doses can be more tolerable because the incidence of side effects increases with the higher dosage for every statin. However, the response of an individual may vary considerably and cannot be predicted definitely because individual factors (diet, compliance, genetic predisposition, gender, hormonal status, apolipoprotein E phenotype) and differences in drug absorption and metabolism may influence statin effects *(12)*.

BILE ACID SEQUESTRANTS (RESINS)

Mechanism and Effects

Resins (Table 9) bind bile acids in the intestinal lumen and form insoluble complexes, thus reducing the enterohepatic recirculation of bile acids. This releases feedback inhibition on the hepatic conversion of cholesterol to bile

Table 9
Summary of Resins

Available drugs in US	Cholestyramine, colestipol, colesevelam	
Lipid or lipoprotein effects	LDLc decreases 15–30% HDLc increases 3–5% Triglycerides: no effect or increase	
Major use	Lower LDL cholesterol	
Contraindications	*Absolute*: Familial dysbetalipoproteinemia, TG > 400 mg/dL, phenylketonuria (cholestyramine) *Relative*: TG > 200 mg/dL, severe constipation	
Efficacy	Clinical trial evidence of CHD risk reduction	
Safety	Lack of systemic toxicity in trials	
Major side effects	Upper and lower gastrointestinal complaints, especially constipation, are common; absorption of other drugs can decrease	
Usual daily dose	Cholestryramine	4–16 g
	Colestipol	5–20 g
	Colesevelam	2.6–3.8 g
Maximum daily dose	Cholestryramine	24 g
	Colestipol	30 g
	Colesevelam	4.4 g
Available preparations	Cholestryramine	9-g packets (4 g of drug), 378 g bulk, 5-g packets (4 g of drug), 210 g bulk (light)
	Colestipol	5-g packets (5 g of drug), 450 g bulk, 1-g tablets
	Colesevelam	625-mg tablets

acids, which decreases hepatocyte cholesterol content. This in turn promotes enhanced LDL receptor expression and reduction of plasma LDLc.

Cholestyramine and colestipol are in the form of powders that must be mixed with water or noncarbonated beverages (i.e., milk, fruit juice). Colestipol and colesevelam are available in tablet form. Cholestyramine 8 to 16 g per day (equivalent with 10–20 g/day colestipol) reduces LDLc by 10–20%.

BAS should be considered as LDLc-lowering therapy for patients with moderate elevations in LDLc, young patients with elevated LDLc, and women with elevated LDLc who are planning pregnancy *(4)*. Resins can also be used in combination with statins in individuals with very high LDLc. This combination is more advantageous than increase of the statin dose; doubling the dose of statin produces a mean 6% further reduction in LDLc, and adding a moderate dose of resin to statin can lower LDLc by 12–16%.

Adverse Effects

Sequestrants may increase serum TG levels. However, unless the TG level is higher than 400 mg/dL, they are not contraindicated in type 2 DM.

The major disadvantages of BASs are the lack of convenience because of their high bulk and gastrointestinal (GI) side effects. GI adverse effects include constipation, heartburn, nausea, flatulence, vomiting, and bloating. Resins can decrease the absorption of a variety of drugs administered concurrently. Therefore, other drugs should be taken 1 hour before or 4 hours after resin administration. (An exception is colesevelam, which may be administered concurrently with other drugs.)

NIACIN

Mechanism and Effects

Niacin is the widest-spectrum hypolipidemic agent and has favorable effects on all dyslipidemic parameters. It modifies atherogenic dyslipidemia by reducing TGRLP, raising HDLc, reducing lipoprotein(a), and transforming small, denser LDL into larger, more buoyant LDL. However, it only results in moderate LDLc reduction (Table 10).

Niacin inhibits lipoprotein synthesis, decreases hepatic VLDL production and secretion, and inhibits peripheral lipolysis and mobilization of free fatty acids. The effects on HDLc and TG levels are log linear, so that smaller doses produce significant effects with fewer adverse effects. However, a dosage of 2 to 3 g per day is usually needed to reduce LDLc by more than 15%.

Adverse Effects

The most frequent side effect of niacin is cutaneous flushing. Although tolerance generally develops if the drug is continued, it frequently leads to discontinuation in the early phase of therapy. It may be alleviated by taking the drug during or after meals, by prior administration of 325 mg aspirin, or by switching to Niaspan®, which causes less flushing than immediate-release forms. Other frequent side effects are GI, including nausea, dyspepsia, flatulence, vomiting, diarrhea, and activation of peptic ulcer disease. Other side effects associated with higher doses (<2 g/day) are hepatotoxicity, hyperuricemia and gout, and hyperglycemia. The risk of hepatotoxicity is higher with sustained-release preparations (excluding Niaspan). Hepatotoxicity should be anticipated if a dramatic reduction in plasma lipids occurs. Higher doses (>3 g/day) of niacin impair insulin sensitivity and worsen glycemic control in type II DM. Other rare side effects are conjunctivitis, nasal stuffiness, acanthosis nigricans, ichthyosis, and toxic amblyopia.

Table 10
Summary of Niacin Group

Available drugs in US	Immediate-release (crystalline) niacin, sustained-release niacin, extended-release niacin (Niaspan), acipimox	
Lipid or lipoprotein effects	LDLc decreases 5–25% HDLc increases 15–35% Triglycerides decrease 20–50%	
Major use	Widest-spectrum hypolipidemic agents useful in almost every type lipid abnormalities	
Contraindications	*Absolute*: Active liver disease, severe gout, documented hypersensitivity *Relative*: Hyperuricemia, higher doses in type 2 DM, active peptic ulcer, arterial bleeding	
Efficacy	Clinical trial evidence of CHD risk reduction	
Safety	Serious long-term side effects are rare for crystalline niacin; hepatotoxicity is higher in sustained-release form	
Major side effects	Flushing, hyperglycemia, hyperuricemia (and gout), gastric distress, hepatotoxicity	
Usual daily dose	Crystalline niacin	1.5–3 g
	Sustained-release niacin	1–2 g
	Extended-release niacin (Niaspan)	2 g
	Acipimox	500–750 mg
Maximum daily dose	Crystalline niacin	4.5 g
	Sustained-release niacin	2 g
	Extended-release niacin (Niaspan)	2 g
	Acipimox	750 mg
Available preparations	Many inexpensive over-the-counter preparations are available for both crystalline and sustained-release niacin as well as acipimox. Niaspan and Advicor® (recently marketed fixed-dose combination of extended-release niacin and lovastatin) are prescription drugs.	

As many niacin preparations are available without a prescription in the United States, patients should be instructed to have regular monitoring by a health professional. In practice, as long-term use of niacin is limited by side effects, it is usually reserved for patients at higher short-term risk, such as those with CHD or CHD risk equivalents. Its use for long-term prevention of CHD in persons with 10-year risk less than 10% is not well established *(4)*.

FIBRATES

Mechanism and Effects

Fibrates are primarily used to lower TG levels because their LDLc-lowering effects are generally less than those of statins. These drugs frequently increase LDLc in patients with severe hypertriglyceridemia. The benefits of fibrates on cardiovascular outcomes reported in some trials have not been consistently observed. Moreover, in large primary prevention trials (clofibrate in a World Health Organization study, gemfibrozil in the Helsinki Heart Study), fibrates were associated with an increase in non-CHD mortality. However, more recent studies (Bezafibrate Infarction Prevention [BIP] trial, Veterans Affairs Lipoprotein Cholesterol Intervention Trial [VA-HIT]) have indicated some benefit to stroke prevention without excess mortality in the treatment arm *(13)*.

The mechanism of fibrates has recently been illuminated: They act as agonists of the nuclear transcription factor peroxisome proliferator activated receptor-α. The activation of this receptor results in downregulation of the C-III gene (an inhibitor of lipoprotein lipase) and upregulation of apolipoprotein A-I, fatty acid transport protein, fatty acid oxidation, and possibly lipoprotein lipase genes. As a result, fibrates enhance the catabolism of TGRLP and decrease production of VLDL triglycerides. Lower serum TGs and increased apolipoprotein A-1 synthesis results in HDLc increase and transformation of small, dense LDL into normal-size LDL.

Fibrates, like niacin, are primarily used to modify atherogenic dyslipidemia (triad of elevated TGs, small LDL particles, and low HDLC). In addition to their TG-lowering effect, they produce moderate HDLc elevation. They are recommended for dysbetalipoproteinemia (increased β-VLDL). Fibrates can also be combined with statins in treatment of combined hyperlipidemia (elevated LDLc plus atherogenic dyslipidemia). In addition, fibrates are recommended for persons with very high TGs to reduce risk of acute pancreatitis. They can also be considered an option for treatment of individuals with established CHD who have atherogenic dyslipidemia and low LDLc levels.

Adverse Effects

Fibrates are usually well tolerated (Table 11). GI complaints such as epigastric pain, dry mouth, constipation, diarrhea, and flatulence are the most common adverse effects. All drugs in this class increase the risk of cholelithiasis.

OTHER DRUGS

Cholesterol Absorption Inhibitors

Ezetimibe specifically inhibits intestinal absorption of dietary and biliary cholesterol. It moderately (<20%) reduces LDLc at a dose of 10 mg per day. As an add-on therapy, it allowed reduction of statin doses in preliminary studies. Further additive effects with Gemfibrozil can also be expected. It has been marketed in the United States as Zetia® *(14)*.

Table 11
Summary of Fibrates

Available drugs in US	Gemfibrozil, fenofibrate, clofibrate	
Lipid or lipoprotein effects	LDLc decreases 5–20% (may be increased in hypertriglyceridemic persons) HDLc increases 10–35% (often in severe hypertriglyceridemia) Triglycerides decrease 20–50%	
Major use	Hypertriglyceridemia, atherogenic dyslipidemia	
Contraindications	*Absolute*: Severe hepatic or renal insufficiency, preexisting gallbladder disease, documented hypersensitivity, biliary cirrhosis, cholelithiasis *Relative*: Concurrent warfarin use	
Efficacy	Clinical trial evidence of moderate CHD risk reduction	
Safety	Serious long-term side effects are rare in long-term use, although early studies indicated an increase in non-CHD mortality	
Major side effects	Dypepsia, various gastrointestinal complaints, cholelithiasis, myopathy	
Usual daily dose	Gemfibrozil	600 mg bid
	Fenofibrate	200 mg
	Clofibrate	1 g bid
Maximum daily dose	Gemfibrozil	1200 mg
	Fenofibrate	200 mg
	Clofibrate	2 g
Available preparations	Gemfibrozil	600-mg tablets
	Fenofibrate	67-, 134-, and 200-mg micronized capsules (160-mg tablets are equal to 200-mg capsules)
	Clofibrate	500-mg capsules

Cholesterol Ester Transfer Protein Inhibitor

JTT-705, a first cholesterol ester transfer protein inhibitor, has been tested in phase 2 studies and found to be well tolerated and very effective in raising HDLc (by about 60%) as well as modestly effective in lowering LDLc (by 10–20%) *(12)*.

Intestinal Bile Acid Transport Inhibitors

The intestinal bile acid transport inhibitor drugs block the ileal sodium-dependent taurocholic acid transport mechanism, preventing enterohepatic recycling, similar to BASs. In phase 2 studies, S-8921 showed modest reduction in LDLc of about 10%. Preliminary experience suggests that these drugs can overcome GI problems, which are very prevalent with BASs *(14)*.

ω-3 Fatty Acids

Omega or n-3 polyunsaturated fatty acids (docosahexaenoic acid, eicosapentaenoic acid, alphalinolenic acid) lower TG by reducing hepatic secretion of TG-rich lipoproteins. They can be used as an alternative to niacin in persons with hypertriglyceridemia, particularly chylomicronemia. They are available as "fish oil" capsules. Dosages of 3 to 13 g per day can be used depending on tolerance and degree of hypertriglyceridemia *(12)*.

Policosanol

Policosanol is a mixture of higher primary aliphatic alcohols. At doses of 10 to 20 mg per day, it lowers TC by 17–21% and LDLc by 21–29% and raises HDLc by 8–15%. A good safety profile and tolerability make this recently introduced drug a viable option as an add-on therapy.

COMBINED DRUG THERAPY

Combination therapy with a statin and BAS can be considered for significant LDLc lowering (by as much as 70%) in some cases of severe polygenic or familial hypercholesterolemia. This combination is more effective than alternatives. Combined therapy should be considered in the early period of treatment of cases with very high LDLc because it is more effective than a maximum dose of statin. The dose of BAS can be maintained at low or moderate levels. The routine instruction is to give the statin at bedtime and the sequestrant with each meal.

The combination of statin and fibrate is highly effective in elevated LDLc plus atherogenic dyslipidemia. This combination can successfully reduce LDLc and VLDL in patients with hypertriglyceridemia. Because the primary aim is to reduce LDLc, statin is usually started before fibrates. The major concern of this combination is increased risk of myopathy. However, with appropriate patient education and clinical monitoring, it can be safely used.

The combined use of statin and niacin offers an attractive potential to correct most dyslipidemias by adding the powerful LDLc-lowering effects of statins to TG-lowering and HDL-raising effects of niacin. The side effect profile of niacin is the only disadvantage. However, there is no known synergism between the agents in producing side effects, particularly myopathy.

FOLLOW-UP AFTER INITIATION OF LIPID-LOWERING THERAPY

Maximum reduction of LDLc and TG and elevation of HDLc are achieved within 6 weeks of initiation of drug therapy. Thus, the first follow-up visit and repeated lipid profile should be done 6–8 weeks after initiation of the

Table 12
ATP III Criteria for Identification of the Metabolic Syndrome

Risk factor	Definition
1. Abdominal obesity	Waist circumference
Men	>102 cm (>40 in)
Women	>88 cm (>35 in)
2. Triglycerides	≥150 mg/dL
3. HDLc	
Men	<40 mg/dL
Women	<50 mg/dL
4. Blood pressure	≥130/≥85 mmHg
5. Fasting glucose	≥110 mg/dL

drug. If the initial dose is increased or another drug is added, a repeat lipid profile and clinical follow-up should be performed 6–8 weeks after the prior dose change. This process should be repeated until the treatment goals are achieved. Then, follow-up intervals may be reduced to every 4–6 months. A lipid profile should be obtained at least once a year, more preferably at each visit, to promote compliance *(4)*. In hypertriglyceridemia, the non-HDLc goal should be addressed after LDLc is sufficiently reduced. Instead of statin dose increase, a TG-lowering drug such as fibrate or niacin is usually required.

DIAGNOSIS AND MANAGEMENT OF METABOLIC SYNDROME

A constellation of abdominal obesity, atherogenic dyslipidemia (lipid triad: elevated TG + small LDL particles + low HDLc), hypertension, insulin resistance (with or without glucose intolerance), and prothrombotic or proinflammatory states constitutes the metabolic syndrome. This is recognized in ATP III as a secondary target of risk-reduction therapy. Clinical diagnosis of the metabolic syndrome is made when three or more criteria summarized in Table 12 are present.

The management of the metabolic syndrome has two objectives: reduction of underlying causes (obesity/overweight and physical inactivity) and treatment of lipid and nonlipid risk factors if they persist after TLC. In this context, intensification of weight management, physical activity increase, hypertension treatment, reduction of prothrombotic state by routine prescription of aspirin at a dose of 325 mg per day in CHD patients, and treatment of elevated TG or reduced HDLc are advised *(1,15)*.

MANAGEMENT OF SPECIFIC DYSLIPIDEMIAS

Very High LDL Cholesterol

A very high LDLc level (≥190 mg/dL after TLC) is usually seen in the monogenic form of familial hypercholesterolemia and rarely in polygenic hypercholesterolemia. Monogenic diseases are known as the "cholesterol quartet": familial hypercholesterolemia (mean LDLc level is 300 mg/dL in heterozygous and 650 mg/dL in homozygous), familial ligand defective apolipoprotein B-100 (mean LDLc level is 270 mg/dL in heterozygous and 320 mg/dL in homozygous), autosomal recessive hypercholesterolemia (mean LDLc level is 470 mg/dL), and sitosterolemia (mean LDLc level is 100–600 mg/dL, depending on diet) *(16)*. Early detection and family screening is vital so that rigorous cholesterol reduction may be begun to prevent premature stroke and CHD. Combination high-dose drug therapy (statin plus BAS) is generally needed. Patients who are unable to reduce LDLc to less than 190 mg/dL despite optimal combination therapy should be referred to a specialist lipid clinic.

Hypertriglyceridemia

Although stroke data are lacking, elevated TGs have been recognized as an independent risk factor for CHD *(17,18)*. The pharmacological management of hypertriglyceridemia is determined by the level of fasting TGs: When the TG level is 150 mg/dL or above, the primary aim is still to reach the LDLc goal. If TG levels are 200 mg/dL or above after the LDLc goal is achieved, a secondary goal for non-HDLc (i.e., TC-HDLc) is set 30 mg/dL higher than the LDLc goal on the premise that a VLDLc level 30 mg/dL or below is normal.

It has become clear that partially degraded VLDL, so-called remnant lipoprotein, is highly atherogenic. VLDLc is the readily available measure of these atherogenic remnants. Thus, VLDLc can be also a target of cholesterol-lowering therapy. If TG levels are 200–499 mg/dL after the LDLc goal is reached, a drug to reduce non-HDLc is considered. Available options include intensification of LDL-lowering therapy or addition of niacin or fibrate to lower VLDLc.

If the TG level is 500 mg/dL or above, the reduction of TGs is more important to prevent pancreatitis. Combination therapy consisting of weight management, increased physical activity, very low fat diet ((15% of calories from fat), and fibrate or nicotinic acid is applied. When TGs have been lowered to below 500 mg/dL, emphasis on LDL-lowering therapy is advised.

Low HDL Cholesterol

Low HDLc is a strong independent risk factor for CHD and has been reported to be independently associated with stroke risk. Low HDLc not only modifies the goal for LDLc lowering, but also is used for a risk factor calculation for 10-year CHD risk. Among many causes of low HDLc, the most common is in conjunction with the metabolic syndrome (Table 13) *(4)*.

Although studies have consistently demonstrated that risk of vascular events decreases with increasing HDL, current data are insufficient to specify a goal *(4)*. Moreover, current lipid-lowering drugs do not raise HDL in a large range (Table 13). Nonetheless, a low HDL should deserve close clinical attention and vigorous management guided by the ATP III recommendations: If HDLc is less than 40 mg/dL, the LDLc goal should be targeted first, using TLC and drug therapy if needed. Low HDLc levels in the presence of low TGs (<200 mg/dL) are considered "isolated low HDLc." Nicotinic acid or fibrates are indicated in subjects with CHD or CHD risk equivalents *(4)* in this situation.

LIPOPROTEIN(a)

Lp(a) is similar in structure to LDL and is characterized by the presence of an additional large, highly glycosylated protein called apolipoprotein(a). The vascular effect of Lp(a) is largely unknown. As a protein with regions homologous to the active sites of plasminogen, apolipoprotein(a) might enhance or inhibit fibrinolysis.

Plasma Lp(a) concentration is weakly associated with blood lipids, fibrinogen, and smoking status. Values have been reported to increase after menopause. Plasma concentrations of Lp(a) are highly skewed and highly variable across studies. Because of very different methodologies to measure Lp(a) levels and the lack of standardization between assays, the interpretation of available data regarding importance of Lp(a) levels as a CHD risk factor is complicated. Despite these factors, the intraindividual correlation between two measurements taken some years apart is good ($r = 0.9$). Lp(a) is an acute phase reactant, and its level rises almost twofold during acute inflammatory and vascular diseases. Therefore, elevated levels detected during acute ischemic stroke should be confirmed 6 weeks later.

Although a recent meta-analysis of 5436 patients in 27 studies *(19)* and a large prospective study (9133 men with 5 years of follow-up) *(20)* have provided more convincing support to the concept that elevated Lp(a) level is an independent risk factor for CHD, measurement of Lp(a) is not currently recommended as a screening tool for cardiovascular risk assessment. Measurement should be considered in patients with premature atherosclerotic vascular disease, patients with a strong family history, or patients with LDLc levels that are borderline for initiation of lipid-lowering drug therapy *(17)*.

Table 13
Low HDL Cholesterol

Causes	Relationship to CHD	HDLc response to therapy	
• Elevated serum triglycerides	• Direct atherogenic effect of low HDL:	• Weight reduction	Increase 5–20%
• Overweight/obesity	— Decreased reverse cholesterol transport	• Physical activity	Increase 5–30%
• Physical inactivity	— Increased LDL oxidation and aggregation	• Smoking cessation	Increase 5%
• Very high carbohydrate intake (>60% of total energy)	— Increased athero-inflammation	• Statin	Increase 5–10%
• Very low fat diet	• Marker for atherogenic dyslipidemia	• Fibrate	Increase 5–15%
• Type 2 DM	• Marker for metabolic syndrome	• Niacin	Increase 15–30%
• End stage renal disease	• Cigarette smoking: Lowers HDLc		
• Chronic inflammatory states like rheumatoid arthritis			
• Drugs: β-blockers, anabolic steroids, progestins, thiazides, probucol			

There are no trial data demonstrating the benefit of Lp(a) lowering on stroke risk reduction. In patients with well-controlled LDLc, elevated Lp(a) may only be a weak risk factor, and further treatment is not warranted. Statins have no effect or might increase Lp(a) concentrations. Niacin is the only hypolipidemic drug that significantly lowers Lp(a) levels, but only at higher doses (3–4 g/day). Some studies have reported that a diet rich in fish, oral estrogen replacement in postmenopausal women, fosinopril, vitamin C, tamoxifen, L-carnitine, neomycine sulfate, and *N*-acetyl cysteine can lower Lp(a) to some extent, but these data are generally poorly substantiated *(21)*.

REFERENCES

1. Amarenco P. Hypercholesterolemia, lipid-lowering agents, and the risk for brain infarction. Neurology 2001;57(Suppl 2):S35–S44.
2. Hachinski V, Graffagnino C, Beaudry M, et al. Lipids and stroke: a paradox resolved. Arch Neurol 1996;53:303–308.
3. Heart Protection Study Collaborative Group. MRC/BHF Heart Protection Study of cholesterol lowering with simvastatin in 20,536 high-risk individuals: a randomized placebo-controlled trial. Lancet 2002;360:7–22.
4. The Third Report of the National Cholesterol Education Program (NCEP) Expert Panel on Detection, Evaluation, and Treatment of High Blood Cholesterol in Adults (Adult Treatment Panel III). Bethesda, MD: National Heart, Lung and Blood Institute, National Institutes of Health, May 2001. NIH Publication 01-3305. (Summary published in JAMA 2001;285(19):2486–2497)
5. Van Horn L, McDonald A, Peters E, Gernhofer N. Dietary management of cardiovascular disease: a year 2002 perspective. Nutr Clin Care 2001;4:314–331.
6. Krauss RM, Eckel RH, Howard B, et al. AHA dietary guidelines. Revision 2000: a statement for health care professionals from the nutrition committee of the American Heart Association. Circulation 2000;102;2284–2299.
7. Kromhout D, Menotti A, Kesteloot H, Sana S. Prevention of coronary heart disease by diet and lifestyle. Evidence from prospective cross-cultural, cohort, and intervention studies. Circulation 2002;105:893–898.
8. US Department of Agriculture and US Department of Health and Human Services. Nutrition and Your Health: Dietary Guidelines for Americans. 5th ed. Washington, DC: US Department of Agriculture, 2000. Home and Garden Bulletin 232.
9. Bernini F, Poli A, Paoletti R. Safety of HMG-CoA reductase inhibitors: focus on atorvastatin. Cardiovasc Drugs Ther 2001;15:211–218.
10. Pasternak RC, Smith SC Jr, Bairy-Merz CN, et al. ACC/AHA/NHLBI advisory on the use and safety of statins. J Am Coll Cardiol 2002;40:568–573.
11. Chong PH, Seeger JD, Franklin C. Clinically relevant differences between the statins: implications for therapeutic selection. Am J Med 2001;111:390–400.
12. Batiste MC, Schaefer EJ. Diagnosis and management of lipoprotein abnormalities. Nutr Clin Care 2002;5:115–123.
13. Lousberg TR, Denham AM, Rasmussen JR. A comparison of clinical outcome studies among cholesterol-lowering agents. Ann Pharmacother 2001;35:1599–1607.
14. Stein EA. Managing dyslipidemia in the high-risk patient. Am J Cardiol 2002; 89(Suppl):50C–57C.

15. Reaven G. Metabolic syndrome. Pathophysiology and implications for management of cardiovascular disease. Circulation 2002;106:286–288.
16. Goldstein JL, Brown MS. The cholesterol quartet. Science 2000;292:1310–1312.
17. Rader DJ, Rosas S. Management of selected lipid abnormalities. Hypertriglyceridemia, low HDL cholesterol, lipoprotein(a), in thyroid and renal disease, and posttransplantation. Med Clin North Am 2000;84:43–61.
18. Jonkers IJAM, Smelt AHM, ven der Laarse A. Hypertriglyceridemia. Associated risks and effect of drug treatment. Am J Cardiovasc Drugs 2001;1:455–466.
19. Danesh J, Collins R, Peto R. Lipoprotein(a) and coronary heart disease. Meta-analysis of prospective studies. Circulation 2000;102:1082–1085.
20. Luc G, Bard JM, Arveiler D, et al. Lipoprotein(a) as a predictor of coronary heart disease: the PRIME Study. Atherosclerosis 2002;163:377–384.
21. Haralampos MJ, Winder AF, Mikhailidis DP. Lipoprotein(a) and stroke. J Clin Pathol 2000;53:487–496.

5
Diabetes

Maria Wormack and Ferdinando S. Buonanno

STROKE RISK AND OUTCOME IN DIABETES

Diabetes mellitus is the sixth leading cause of death in the United States and a major cause of stroke *(1)*. If diabetes were eliminated, 21% of strokes could be prevented *(2)*. Diabetics have both micro- and macrovascular changes caused by thickening of the basement membrane and artherosclerosis *(3)* Coronary heart disease, more prevalent in the diabetic population, results in arrhythmias and ischemic cardiomyopathy, predisposing to cardioembolism. Diabetics also demonstrate hypercoagulability with increased levels of factors V and VII and fibrinogen as well as accentuated platelet aggregation and adhesion *(4)*. Endothelial damage related to hyperglycemia, hyperinsulinemia, increased oxidative stress, and dyslipidemia contribute to vascular remodeling and atherogenesis *(5)*. Consequently, diabetics are at least at twice the risk of the general population to develop arterial hypertension, cardiac disease, and ischemic cerebrovascular disease *(4,6)*.

Both type 1 and type 2 diabetes are associated with an increased risk of stroke. Type 1 diabetes accounts for a relatively smaller proportion of the diabetic population, whereas type 2 diabetes is projected to nearly double over the next 6 years, particularly in cultures that support unhealthy dietary habits and sedentary lifestyle *(7)*. Hyperglycemia without overt diabetes has been associated with a prothrombotic state and is associated with an adverse lipid profile *(8,9)* Hyperglycemia impairs recovery of oligemic brain tissue, measured by MRI as diffusion–perfusion mismatch after stroke and has been associated with poorer stroke outcome *(10,11)*.

The distribution of stroke subtypes among diabetic patients is similar to that in the general population, with the exception of a higher prevalence of lacunar infarcts *(12)*. Transient ischemic attacks are three times more likely in diabetic patients than in nondiabetic patients *(13)*. Diabetes contributes significantly to cerebrovascular disease in the young. Of patients with stroke,

From: *Current Clinical Neurology: Handbook of Stroke Prevention in Clinical Practice*
Edited by: K. L. Furie and P. J. Kelly © Humana Press Inc., Totowa, NJ

76% aged 35–44 years have type 2 diabetes *(14)*. Atherothrombotic brain infarcts are more common and more severe in diabetics *(12)*. Stroke severity may be exacerbated by excess glucose in the ischemic region, producing lactic acid, resulting in further damage to neurons and vascular tissue and triggering of apoptosis *(15)*. Stroke mortality is higher in diabetics. Diabetes is responsible for 7% of deaths among stroke patients, largely in those with ischemic strokes. One in five deaths in both type 1 and type 2 diabetes is stroke related *(16,17)*.

There are subgroups of the population at higher risk of stroke related to diabetes. Minorities, who are more likely to have other vascular risk factors such as hypertension, are particularly vulnerable to diabetes. African Americans and Hispanic Americans are five times more likely to develop diabetes than Caucasians *(18,19)*. Native Americans are thought to be at an even higher risk *(20)*. A major modifier of stroke risk in diabetic patients is hypertension, which has been linked to populations with lower socioeconomic status and effectively less access to consistent quality health care *(18)*.

Risk of stroke can be estimated in an individual diabetic patient based on the clinical profile. A model to estimate the risk of a first stroke was derived from 4549 type 2 diabetic patients in whom there were 188 strokes and who were enrolled in the UK Prospective Diabetes Study *(21)*. The final model to predict the absolute risk of a first stroke included duration of diabetes, age, gender, smoking, systolic blood pressure, ratio of total cholesterol to high-density lipoprotein cholesterol, and atrial fibrillation.

PREVENTION INTERVENTIONS

Management of modifiable risk factors is critically important in diabetic patients and often is suboptimally *(22,23)*. Management strategies are explored in detail in the individual chapters of this book. In diabetics, targets are particularly stringent and reflect the need for more aggressive management in this high-risk population (Tables 1 and 2) *(21–28)*. Intensive risk-factor management (Table 3) can reduce the risk of cardiovascular events in diabetic patients by as much as 20%. Five patients need to be treated to prevent one cardiovascular event. Over a lifetime, these changes can successfully reduce overall stroke risk *(22,27)*.

Overall, a successful diet in diabetics is healthy and well-rounded with a focus on weight loss in type 2 diabetes. Dietary modification should emphasize reduction in fat and cholesterol intake to lower serum cholesterol levels. Carbohydrate content should be noted in an effort to lower serum glucose levels. The target hemoglobin A1c should be less than 6.5% *(28)*. There are no set glucose-lowering guidelines for diabetic patients, but it is suggested

Table 1
Recommended Diet Modifications to Lower Blood Cholesterol Levels

Meats
Fish, poultry without skin, lean cuts of beef, lamb, pork or veal, shellfish
Milk, cheese, dairy
Skim or 1% fat milk (liquid, powdered, evaporated), buttermilk
Nonfat (0% fat) yogurt, low-fat (1–2% fat) cottage cheeses
Sherbet, sorbet
Eggs
Egg whites, cholesterol-free egg substitute
Fruits and vegetables
Fresh, frozen, canned, or dried fruits and vegetables
Breads and cereals
Home-made baked goods using unsaturated oils sparingly
Angel food cake
Low-fat crackers, low-fat cookies
Rice, pasta
Whole grain breads (oatmeal, whole wheat, rye, bran, multigrain) and cereals
Fats and oils
Baking cocoa, unsaturated vegetable oils: corn olive, rapeseed (canola oil), safflower, sesame, soybean, sunflower
Margarine
Low-fat salad dressings
Seeds and nuts (9)

Source: From ref. 22.

that each patient with either type 1 or type 2 diabetes consult a dietician every 6 to 12 months. The total amount of protein consumed should be 10–20% of the total caloric intake (10% in patients with kidney failure). Sodium and fiber can be consumed in normal quantities. Alcohol should be monitored closely in an effort to sustain blood glucose levels; alcohol should not be consumed on an empty stomach *(28)*.

As part of the lifestyle changes and risk-factor intervention, a weight loss program should be included to help reduce the risk associated with obesity and help facilitate better glycemic control *(26)*. Patients should be counseled on a program that incorporates dietary modification, physical activity, and possibly behavioral therapy. Both sibutramine and orlistat have been recommended as drug interventions in weight loss, but these should be reserved for patients who have failed conventional therapy and should be managed by a subspecialty obesity program *(26)*.

Table 2
Modifiable Risk Factors for Stroke: Treatment Specific for Diabetic Patients

Factor	Risk escalation	Population at highest risk	Recommendation
Hypertension: Systolic	Two to four times	40% of African Americans; 20% non-Hispanic whites; 60% of seniors over 60 years are hypertensive	130/80 mmHg for diabetic patients attained via diuretic, ace inhibitor, β-blocker, calcium channel blocker (American Diabetes Association)
Heart disease: Myocardial infarction	3–4% of those who have a myocardial infarction will have an embolic stroke		Reduce blood pressure to 130/80 mmHG, antiplatelet agents, anticoagulation therapy, lipid-lowering agents, lower alcohol consumption, smoking cessation, increased physical activity (American Diabetes Association)
Heart disease: Atrial fibrillation	Overall, 15% of ischemic strokes are attributed to this condition	Seniors aged 65–85 years	Warfarin in patients with atrial fibrillation reduces the overall risk of stroke by 67%; patients who have a lower total stroke risk should use an antiplatelet alternative such as low-dose aspirin *(1)* or clopidogrel; risk of hemorrhagic complications
Hyperlipidemia	Reduction of total and LDL cholesterol reduces stroke risk	Non-Hispanic whites, Mexican Americans, African Americans	Total cholesterol < 200 mg/dL; low-density lipoprotein < 100 mg/dL; high-density lipoprotein > 40 mg/dL for men, high-density lipoprotein > 50 mg/dL for women; <30% calories from fat; <300 mg cholesterol; <10%

			calories from saturated fat; increase physical activity, statins hold important effects on atherosclerotic disease (American Diabetes Association)
Excessive alcohol consumption	1–2 drinks per day lowers risk; >5 drinks per day increases risk for both ischemic and hemorrhagic stroke	General population	Counseling and support groups
Obesity >30.0 body mass index	Doubles the risk of stroke	Prevalence of obesity is over 20% for men and women non-Hispanic whites, African Americans, Mexican Americans, American Indians	Dietary modifications and exercise 30 minutes daily
Cigarette smoking	Risk of stroke is increased 1.5-fold	27.1% men and 22.2% women over the age of 18 years	Smoking cessation
Physical inactivity	Exercise reduces the risk of stroke by improving diabetes, controlling obesity, increasing high-density lipoprotein cholesterol, and lowering blood pressure in some people.	Women more than men, African Americans, Hispanics, seniors, those of lower socioeconomic means	Brisk walking, gardening, swimming, aerobics 30 minutes daily

Table 3
Treatment Goals for Intensive Therapy: Multifactorial Intervention With Type 2 Diabetes

Systolic blood pressure	<130 mmHg
Diastolic blood pressure	<80 mmHg
Glycosylated hemoglobin A1c	<6.5%
Fasting serum cholesterol	<175 mg/dL
Fasting serum triglycerides	<150 mmHg
Treatment with an ACE inhibitor	
Antiplatelet therapy	

Although a daily multivitamin is recommended in addition to a healthy, well-rounded diet, there is no evidence that supplementation of specific vitamins is beneficial. In a 2 × 2 factorial design, the Heart Outcomes Prevention Evaluation (HOPE) trial randomly assigned 3654 diabetics to vitamin E 400 IU per day or placebo with or without ramipril therapy for 4.5 years *(29)*. There was no difference in the primary study outcome of myocardial infarction, stroke, or cardiovascular death (relative risk [RR] = 1.03, 95% confidence interval [CI] 0.88–1.21, $p = 0.70$).

Experimental and clinical evidence suggest that angiotensin-converting enzyme (ACE) inhibition may reduce cardiovascular risk through beneficial effects on blood pressure, endothelial function, and thrombus formation. The Study to Evaluate Carotid Ultrasound Changes in Patients Treated with Ramipril and Vitamin E (SECURE) demonstrated that ramipril, an ACE inhibitor, at a dose of 10 mg per day resulted in a significant reduction in the rate of carotid intimal medial thickening, suggesting a direct effect on atherosclerosis progression *(30)*.

HOPE studied the effect of ramipril in reducing cardiovascular events in 9297 patients older than 55 years who were at high risk of cardiovascular events but did not have left ventricular dysfunction, heart failure, or high blood pressure at the time of study entry. In the overall HOPE population, the risk of the primary composite outcome (cardiovascular death, myocardial infarction [MI], or stroke) was reduced by 22% ($p < 0.001$), and in patients with diabetes plus one other cardiovascular risk, it was reduced by 25% ($p = 0.0004$). In diabetics ($n = 3577$), ramipril lowered the risk of stroke by 33%, MI by 22%, cardiovascular death by 37%, and total mortality by 24%, even after adjusting for the effect of blood pressure reduction *(31,32)*.

In the STOP-NIDDM Trial, patients with impaired glucose tolerance and postprandial hyperglycemia were randomly assigned to acarbose, an α-glucosidase inhibitor, at a dose of 100 mg three times a day, or placebo. There was an overall 49% RR reduction (2.5% absolute RR) in cardiovascular events and a 49% RR reduction (5.3% absolute RR) in hypertension. The stroke benefit–hazard ratio of 0.56 (95% CI 0.1–3.07, $p = 0.51$) was not statistically significant *(33)*.

REFERENCES

1. Thomas RJ, Palumbo PJ, Melton LJ 3rd, et al. Trends in the mortality burden associated with diabetes mellitus: a population-based study in Rochester, Minnesota, 1970–1994. Arch Intern Med 2003;163:445–451.
2. Seshadri S, Wolf P, Beiser A, et al. Elevated midlife blood pressure increases stroke risk in elderly persons: the Framingham Study. Arch Intern Med 2001; 161:2343–2350.
3. Alder A, Stratton I, Neil A, Yudkin J, Matthews D. Association of systolic blood pressure with macrovascular and microvascular complications of type 2 diabetes (UKPDS 36): prospective observational study. BMJ 2000;321:412–419.
4. Biller J, Love B. Diabetes and stroke. Contemp Clin Neurol 1993;77:95–100.
5. Deedwania PC Mechanisms of endothelial dysfunction in the metabolic syndrome. Curr Diab Rep 2003;3:289–292.
6. Sacco RL, Benjamin EJ, Broderick JP, et al. Risk factors panel—American Heart Association Prevention Conference IV. Stroke 1997;28:1507–1517.
7. Watkins PJ, Thomas PK. Diabetes mellitus and the nervous system. J Neurol Neurosurg Psychiatry 1998;65:620–632.
8. Seppo L, Ronnemaa T, Pyorala K, Laakso M. Predictors of stroke in middle-aged patients with non-insulin dependent diabetes. Stroke 1996;27:63–68.
9. Davis T, Millns H, Stratton I, Holman R. Risk factors for stroke in type 2 diabetes mellitus: United Kingdom Prospective Diabetes Study UKPDS 29. Arch Intern Med 1999;159:1097–1103.
10. Parsons M, Barber P, Desmond P, et al. Acute hyperglycemia adversely affects stroke outcome: a magnetic resonance imaging and spectroscopy study. Ann Neurol 2002;52:5–6.
11. Baird TA, Parsons MW, Barber PA, et al. The influence of diabetes mellitus and hyperglycaemia on stroke incidence and outcome. J Clin Neurosci 2002;9:618–626.
12. Megherbi S, Milan C, Minier D, et al. Association between diabetes and stroke subtype on survival and functional outcome 3 months after stroke: data from the European BIOMED Stroke Project. Stroke 2003;34:688–694.
13. Whisnant JP, Brown RD, Petty GW, O'Fallon WM, Sicks JD, Wiebers DO. Comparison of population-based models of risk factors for TIA and ischemic stroke. Neurology 1999;53:532–536.
14. You RX, McNeil JJ, O'Malley HM, Davis SM, Thrift AG, Donnan GA. Risk factors for stroke due to cerebral infarction in young adults. Stroke 1997;28:1913–1918.
15. Muranyi M, Fujioka M, He Q, et al. Diabetes activates cell death pathway after transient focal cerebral ischemia. Diabetes 2003;52:481–486.
16. Tuomilehto J, Rastenyt D, Jousilahti P, et al. Diabetes mellitus as a risk factor for death from stroke: prospective study of the middle-aged Finnish population. Stroke 1996;27:210–215.

17. Laing S, Swerdlow D, Carpenter L, et al. Mortality from cerebrovascular disease in a cohort of 23000 patients with insulin treated diabetes. Stroke 2003;34:418–426.
18. Worrall B, Johnston K, Kongable G, et al. Stroke risk factors in African American women: an interim report from the African American Antiplatelet Stroke Prevention Study. Stroke 2002;33:913–919.
19. Abel GA, Sacco Rl, Lin IF, et al. Race–ethnic variability in etiologic fraction for stroke risk factors: The Northern Manhattan Stroke Study. Stroke 1998;29:277.
20. Galloway JM. The epidemiology of atherosclerosis and its risk factors among Native Americans. Curr Diab Rep 2002;2:274–281.
21. Kothari V, Stevens R, Adler A, Stratton M. UKPDS60 risk of stroke in type 2 diabetes estimated by the UK Prospective Diabetes Study Risk Engine. Stroke 2002; 33:1776–1789.
22. Gaede P, Vedel P, Larsen N, et al. Multifactor intervention and cardiovascular disease in patients with type 2 diabetes. N Engl J Med 2003;348:383–393.
23. Mourdain M, Majumdar S, Senthilselvan A, et al. How well are hypertension, hyperlipidemia, diabetes, and smoking managed after a stroke or transient ischemic attack? Stroke 2002;33:1656–1659.
24. Ozer M, Materson RS, Caplan LR. Prevention of recurrent stroke. In: Management of Persons with Stroke. St. Louis, MO: Mosby, 1994.
25. Tuomilehto J, Lindstrom J, Eriksson J, Timo V. Prevention of type 2 diabetes mellitus by changes in lifestyle among subjects with impaired glucose tolerance. N Engl J Med 2001;344:1343–1392.
26. Wadden T, Pories W, Blair S, et al. The Practical Guide Identification, Evaluation, and Treatment of Overweight and Obesity in Adults. October 2000. National Institutes of Health Publication 00-4084.
27. Laakso, M. Perspectives in diabetes hyperglycemia and cardiovascular disease n type 2 diabetes. Diabetes 1999;48:937–942.
28. Folsom A, Rasmussen M, Chambless L, et al. Prospective associations of fasting insulin, body fat distribution, and diabetes with risk of ischemic stroke. Diabetes Care 1999;22:1077–1083.
29. Lonn E, Yusuf S, Hoogwerf B, et al. Effects of vitamin E on cardiovascular and microvascular outcomes in high-risk patients with diabetes: results of the HOPE study and MICRO-HOPE substudy. Diabetes Care 2002;25:1919–1927.
30. Lonn E, Yusuf S, Dzavik V, et al. Effects of ramipril and vitamin E on atherosclerosis: the Study to Evaluate Carotid Ultrasound Changes in Patients Treated with Ramipril and Vitamin E (SECURE). Circulation 2001;103:919–925.
31. Yusuf S, Sleight P, Pogue J, Bosch J, Davies R, Dagenais G. Effects of an angiotensin-converting-enzyme inhibitor, ramipril, on cardiovascular events in high-risk patients. The Heart Outcomes Prevention Evaluation Study investigators. N Engl J Med 2000;342:145–153.
32. Heart Outcomes Prevention Evaluation Study Investigators. Effects of ramipril on cardiovascular and microvascular outcomes in people with diabetes mellitus: results of the HOPE study and MICRO-HOPE substudy. Lancet 2000;355:253–259.
33. Chiass JL, Josse RG, Gomis R, Hanefeld M, Karasik A, Laakso M. Acarbose treatment and the risk of cardiovascular disease and hypertension in patients with impaired glucose tolerance. JAMA 2003;290:486–494.

6
Tobacco and Alcohol

Mehmet Akif Topcuoglu and Karen L. Furie

TOBACCO

Tobacco use is the single most important cause of preventable illness and premature death. Currently, tobacco use causes an estimated 3 million annual deaths worldwide *(1,2)*. The financial burden of smoking-related diseases is also substantial.

Smoking and Cardiovascular Disease

Tobacco consumption doubles the risk of coronary heart disease (CHD). Compared to nonsmokers, the incidence of acute myocardial infarction (AMI) is increased sixfold in women and threefold in men who smoke at least 20 cigarettes per day. Smoking is estimated to cause one-third of CHD in women and one-half of the CHD in men younger than 65 years of age. Furthermore, smokers have higher mortality from vascular causes and from all causes at all ages *(3)*.

In smokers with AMI, left ventricular dysfunction and arrhythmias are more common. Ventricular fibrillation and sudden death are more likely to complicate AMI in smokers. In contrast to these negative effects of smoking on AMI prognosis, the response to thrombolytic therapy is actually better in smokers. This effect is known as the *smoker's paradox*. The mortality rates after thrombolysis for AMI seems to be inversely related to the numbers of cigarettes consumed per day. Smokers have shorter length of stay, fewer in-hospital vascular complications (including reinfarction), and lower 6-month mortality rates. The smoker's paradox may be explained by the more favorable risk profile and younger age of smokers with AMI. The incidence of other complicating factors, including diabetes, hypertension, previous infarction, and severe CHD are lower in smokers.

From: *Current Clinical Neurology: Handbook of Stroke Prevention in Clinical Practice*
Edited by: K. L. Furie and P. J. Kelly © Humana Press Inc., Totowa, NJ

Smoking and Stroke Risk

Cigarette smoking is an important and prevalent stroke risk factor with a relative risk (RR) of 1.5 (95% confidence interval [CI] 1.4–1.6) for all strokes *(4)*. Up to one-quarter of all strokes can be attributed to smoking *(5)*. Smoking is a more potent risk factor for subarachnoid hemorrhage (RR 2.0–3.0) than for ischemic stroke (RR 2.0). However, its effect on the intracerebral hemorrhage is less clear. Furthermore, the smoking related risk of ischemic stroke is higher in the young. There is a slightly increased risk in women compared to men. The effect of smoking on development of stroke persists after adjustment for other risk determinants (i.e., it is an independent risk factor), and a dose relationship is apparent in virtually every study. Stroke risk increases twofold in heavy smokers (more than 40 cigarettes per day) in comparison to light smokers (fewer than 10 cigarettes per day) *(3,4)*.

Passive and environmental smoking has also been linked to higher risk of stroke. The relative risk of stroke in nonsmoking individuals whose partners smoke was reported to be 2.12 (95% CI 1.17–3.89). There did not appear to be an increased risk associated with parental smoking, however *(6,7)*.

Mechanisms

The mechanism of stroke risk associated with smoking is complex and not completely understood. The main mechanism appears to be through the development and progression of atherosclerosis. Smoking results in elevations of triglycerides and decrease of high-density lipoprotein (HDL) cholesterol. Free radicals in cigarette smoke result in oxidation of low-density lipoprotein cholesterol, increasing atherogenicity. Moreover, smoking reduces the paraoxonase activity of the HDL molecule, a lipid-protective enzyme with significant antioxidant effects. Smoking also increases insulin resistance.

In coronary and extracranial internal carotid arteries, smoking is related to atheroma plaque thickness and burden of atheroma *(8)*. Smoking increases tissue factor expression, inhibits endothelial tissue plasminogen activator (tPA) release by increasing concentrations of plasminogen activator inhibitor 1 and fibrinogen, and increases platelet reactivity. In smokers, increased thrombocyte aggregability is not inhibited by aspirin. Chronic lung diseases related to smoking produce secondary polycythemia, which increases blood viscosity. Smoking decreases prostacyclin production in the endothelium, which increases platelet adhesiveness to the vessel wall. Nicotine also enhances leukocyte transmigration mediated by P-selectin. These changes create a prothrombotic milieu within the vessel lumen and increase the risk of artery-to-artery, and possibly cardiac, embolism.

Cigarette smoking results in enhanced sympathetic activity, increasing heart rate and blood pressure. Vasomotor tone is generally increased in smokers. This results in continuous vasoconstriction in coronary and cerebral arteries as well as platelet activation. Smoking, even in a passive form, impairs endothelium-dependent vasodilation of coronary and cerebral arteries via reduction of nitric oxide generation and increase of endothelin *(5)*.

The smoker's paradox phenomenon has not been reported in patients with acute ischemic stroke who are undergoing thrombolytic therapy. However, prior cigarette smoking is associated with a decreased risk of symptomatic or asymptomatic intracerebral hemorrhage in patients treated with intravenous tPA *(9)*. This effect is related to a nicotine-associated decrease in endogenous tPA activity and increased plasminogen activator inhibitor 1 activity in the cerebral microcirculation, which reflects resistance to thrombolysis. Overall, smoking status before stroke does not affect survival, but persistent smoking after stroke increases risk of all-cause mortality and recurrent hospitalization.

Active smoking history is an independent risk factor for cerebral vasospasm (odds ratio 4.7) and is associated with a worse prognosis after aneurysmal subarachnoid hemorrhage *(10)*. Furthermore, recurrence rate after aneurysm obliteration is higher in patients who continue smoking.

Beneficial Effect of Smoking Cessation on Stroke and Vascular Risk

Although there has been no randomized trial of smoking cessation, epidemiological evidence confirms that there is a benefit to quitting. Primary prevention studies have shown that smoking cessation diminishes coronary event rates by 7 to 46% in persons without CHD. This effect occurs very soon after quitting and continues to fall with increased abstinence. A meta-analysis of secondary prevention studies showed a 20% increase in mortality rates after AMI in persons who continued smoking and demonstrated that 13 patients must stop smoking to save 1 life after AMI *(11)*.

Overall, the excess risk of CHD halves within 1 year of smoking cessation and after 15 years becomes equivalent to that in nonsmokers. Likewise, the excess risk of stroke has been reported to return to that of nonsmokers within 2 to 5 years of smoking cessation *(2,12,13)*. However, one study suggested that an elevated risk persists for at least 20 years after cessation *(14)*. Progression of internal carotid artery atherosclerosis, which is directly related to total pack-years of tobacco exposure, is a cumulative phenomenon and may be irreversible *(8)*.

The early reduction in stroke risk related to smoking cessation may result from improved coagulation parameters or reversal of endothelial dysfunc-

Table 1
Basic Strategies to Help Patients Willing to Stop Smoking: The Five As

- Ask: Ask systematically to identify all tobacco users at every visit
- Advise: Strongly urge all smokers to quit
- Assess: Assess willingness to quit
- Assist: Help the patient with a quitting plan
  Provide intratreatment social support and help the patient obtain extratreatment social support
  Recommend the use of approved pharmacotherapy when appropriate
  Provide supplementary educational materials
- Arrange: Schedule follow-up contact, either in person or via telephone

Source: Adapted from refs. *15, 18–20.*

tion. Late benefits may result from the slowing or reversal of atherosclerotic progression.

Methods of Cessation

Physicians are in an ideal position to identify tobacco users and to facilitate patients' attempts to quit. Questions about smoking should be asked of all patients with transient or fixed cerebral ischemic symptoms or stroke risk factors, and clear, strong, personalized advice on smoking cessation should be provided *(15)*. Brief (less than 3 minutes) advice from a medical practitioner significantly increases the possibility of quitting compared to no advice (odds ratio 1.69, 95% CI 1.45–1.98). In addition, more intensive advice further increases the quitting rate compared to opportunistic advice (odds ratio 1.44, 95% CI 1.23–1.68) *(16)*. Physicians should assess the patient's interest in quitting; assist by counseling and developing a plan for quitting; arrange follow-up and referral to special programs or pharmacotherapy; and urge avoidance of second-hand smoke at work or home (Table 1) *(15,17–20)*.

Nicotine dependence and the development of characteristic withdrawal symptoms make smoking cessation very difficult. Many relapse after trying to stop or need several attempts (the average is six) before successfully quitting (Table 2). In the absence of contraindications, all patients attempting to quit smoking should use one or more medications approved by the Food and Drug Administration, the so-called first-line medications, including nicotine gum, nicotine transdermal patches, nicotine inhaler, or sustained-release bupropion hydrochloride. These approved medicines at least double the likelihood of quitting. Second-line medications, which have not been approved,

Table 2
Enhancement of Motivation to Quit Smoking: The Five Rs

- Relevance: Encourage the patient to indicate why quitting is personally relevant
- Risks: Ask the patient to identify negative results of smoking
- Rewards: Ask the patient to identify potential benefit of smoking cessation
- Roadblocks: Ask the patient to identify barriers or impediments to quitting and identify elements of treatment that could address these
- Repetition: Repeat the motivational intervention at every possible opportunity

Source: Adapted from refs. *15* and *18*.

include clonidine and nortriptyline. The efficacy of medications is clearly increased when coupled with nonpharmacological (behavioral) interventions, such as coping skills training and support groups *(18,20)*.

Medications for Smoking Cessation

Nicotine Replacement Therapy

The rate of successful cessation almost doubles (odds ratio 1.71, 95% CI 1.60–1.82) with nicotine replacement therapy (NRT) *(21)*. NRT reduces nicotine withdrawal symptoms and allows the focus to shift to the behavioral and psychological aspects of smoking *(19)*.

NRT is available in numerous formulations (Table 3). All formulations are thought to be equally effective *(22)*. Choice is guided by factors such as clinician's familiarity with the formulation, contraindications in selected patients, patient preferences, tolerance, and characteristics such as history of depression and concerns about weight gain. Patients who are unable to tolerate one NRT type may benefit from another. Combining NRTs is not recommended by the manufacturers, although an additive effect has been demonstrated in some trials *(21)*. NRT is usually continued for 3 months before withdrawal. Of note, gradual withdrawal, as suggested by the manufacturers, has not been proven superior to abrupt withdrawal. NRT can be used long-term in individuals at high risk of recidivism or in those with persisting withdrawal symptoms.

Nicotine polacrilex gum is a nonprescription gum available in 2- and 4-mg strengths. Its nicotine content is absorbed across the oral mucosa because of the high pH. Patients should use the gum on a fixed regimen, not with an acute urge to smoke. Individuals smoking 24 or fewer cigarettes per day should start with the 2-mg strength gum chewed slowly over 30 minutes. Nicotine

Table 3
First-Line Medication for Smoking Cessation[a]

	NRT				
	Gum	Transdermal patch	Nasal Spray	Oral Inhaler	Bupropion HCl SR
Preparations	Nicorette® and generic 2 or 4 mg	Nicotrol® 15 mg/16 hours; Nicoderm CQ® 7, 14, or 21 mg/24 hours; generic 7, 14, or 21 mg/24 hours; generic 11 or 22 mg/ 24 hours	Nicotrol metered spray (0.5 mg nicotine in 50 μL aqueous nicotine solution)	Nicotrol inhaler (10 mg cartridge delivers 4 mg nicotine vapor)	Zyban® SR tablets
Dosing	Nicorette®: <25 cigarettes, 2 mg; ≥25 cigarettes, 4 mg Generic: w 1-6: piece q1-2h, w 7-9: piece q2-4h, w 10-12: piece q4-8h.	Nicotrol: ≥10 cigarettes, 15mg/day for 6 weeks; <10 cigarettes, not recommended Nicoderm: >10 cigarettes: 21 mg/day for 6 weeks; 14 mg/day for 2 weeks, 7 mg/day for 2 weeks; ≥10 cigarettes: 14 mg/day for 6 weeks, 7 mg/day for 2 weeks Generic 7, 14, or 21 mg: ≥10 cigarettes: 21 mg/day for 4 weeks, 14 mg/day for 2 weeks, 7 mg/day for 2 weeks; <10 cigarettes: 14 mg/day for 6 weeks, 7 mg/day for 2 weeks Generic 11 or 22 mg: >15 cigarettes: 22 mg/day for 6 weeks; ≥15 cigarettes: 11 mg/day for 6 weeks	1–2 doses/hour (8–40 doses/day); 1 dose= 2 puffs (1 in each nostril); each spray delivers 0.5 mg nicotine to the nasal mucosa	6–16 cartridges/day individualized dosing	150 mg po every morning for 3 days, then increase to 150 mg po twice per day

Treatment duration	Up to 12 weeks	Nicotrol, 6 weeks; Nicoderm, 8–10 weeks; Generic 7, 14, or 21 mg, 8 weeks; Generic 11 or 22 mg, 6 weeks	3–6 months	Up to 6 months	7–12 weeks after quit date; maintenance up to 6 months
Side effects	Mouth and jaw soreness, hiccups, dyspepsia, hypersalivation, diarrhea, dry mouth, decreased lower esophageal sphincter pressure Associated with incorrect chewing technique: lightheadedness, nausea, vomiting, throat or mouth irritation.	Local skin reactions: erythema, pruritis, edema, burning Others: headache; insomnia	Nasal irritations, rhinitis, lacrimation, epistaxis, sneezing, coughing, sensations in the ear, headache	Mouth or throat irritation, unpleasant taste, coughing, rhinitis, aphthous ulceration, stomatitis, sinusitis, dyspepsia, dry mouth, hiccups, headache	Insomnia, tremor, headache or migraine, dizziness, nervousness, agitation, anxiety, concentration difficulty, dry mouth; nausea or vomiting, constipation, skin rashes, sweating, fever, hypersensitivity reactions, seizure (0.1%)
Precautions	Pregnancy, AMI (in 2 weeks), arrhythmia, angina pectoris, temporomandibular joint disorders	Pregnancy; AMI (in 2 weeks); arrhythmia; angina pectoris; dermatologic diseases such as psoriasis, eczema, atopic dermatitis	Pregnancy; AMI (in 2 weeks); arrhythmia; angina pectoris; nasal disorders such as rhinitis, polyp, sinusitis; severe reactive airway disease	Pregnancy, AMI (in 2 weeks), arrhythmia, angina pectoris, reactive airway disease	Pregnancy, seizures or tendency to seizure such as drugs or intracranial pathologies, bulimia or anorexia nervosa, monoamine oxidase inhibitor therapy in the last 2 weeks

(continued)

Table 3 (Continued)

	NRT				
	Gum	Transdermal patch	Nasal Spray	Oral Inhaler	Bupropion HCl SR
Advantages	Satisfaction of oral cravings, weight gain delay, individual dose titration to overcome withdrawal symptoms	Ease of use, unobtrusiveness, good compliance, consistent rate of exposure; 24-hour preparations may reduce the morning cravings	User-controlled dose titration, most rapid delivery and highest blood concentrations	Mimics hand-to-mouth ritual of smoking; dosages can be titrated to manage withdrawal symptoms	Easy to use; combination with NRT is safe; beneficial for depression if available
Disadvantages	Social nonacceptance of chewing; difficult to use with dentures; impaired absorption when taken with coffee and acidic beverages; proper chewing technique is needed to minimize side effects	Patient cannot titrate the dose during craving surge; particularly Nicotrol may cause cravings on awakening; allergic reaction to adhesive patch	Bothersome nasal irritation; dependence; tearing and sneezing may complicate driving or skilled jobs; avoidance of contact with skin is needed	Bothersome nasal or throat irritation; frequency of puffing is high, so social visibility of device sometimes is a problem	Seizure risk, wide drug interactions

Source: From refs. *15*, *18*, *19*, and *21*.

[a]Trade names are used for identification purposes only and do not imply any endorsement.

gum is more viscous than ordinary gums, and a specific chewing technique is needed. Individuals who smoke 25 or more cigarettes per day or require more than 15 pieces of 2-mg gum per day should use the 4-mg strength. The maximum dosage is 15 pieces per day. Use of the gum is contraindicated in patients with temporomandibular disorders and dental prostheses. This agent is useful for individuals desiring oral stimulation, identifying boredom as a trigger for smoking, and expressing concern about weight gain after quitting.

Transdermal nicotine patches are available as both prescription and nonprescription preparations. Available agents (Table 3) produce continuous low-level transdermal nicotine delivery. One patch is applied daily to the hip, trunk, or upper arm, usually beginning with the highest strength or a dose determined by the previously consumed number of daily cigarettes. A different site of administration is recommended each day, with several days elapsing before the patch is applied again on the same area. Treatment is usually withdrawn by tapering every 2 to 8 weeks. The 16- and 24-hour patches have similar efficacy. However, the 16-hour patch may be better in patients with sleep disturbances. The 24-hour patches can be used if there are strong morning cravings. These agents are appropriate in subjects with compliance problems.

Nicotine nasal spray is an aqueous nicotine solution delivering 500-μg nicotine with each puff. The absorption takes less than 10 minutes, which is rapid compared to other formulations. The advised initiation dosage is one spray into each nostril up to twice per hour as required, up to a maximum 80 sprays per day for the first 8 weeks, and dosage is gradually reduced thereafter. Tolerance to the initial frequent side effects, such as nose or throat irritation, tearing, sneezing, and coughing, is expected after several weeks. This preparation provides rapid suppression of withdrawal symptoms because of its fast onset of action.

Nicotine inhaler cartridges contain 10 mg of nicotine. The recommended initial dose is 6 to 16 cartridges per day for up to 12 weeks, reduced gradually over a further 6 to 12 weeks. This inhaler is suitable for individuals seeking a motor substitute for cigarettes because use recapitulates the hand-to-mouth ritual of cigarette smoking.

Nicotine sublingual tablets and lozenges have recently become available. Sublingual tablets contain 2 mg nicotine as β-cyclodextrine complex. The recommended dose is 1–2 mg every hour, increased to a maximum of 40 tablets per day if needed, for at least 3 months. Lozenges containing 1 mg nicotine as the tartrate are recommended at a dose of 1 lozenge every 1–2 hours, increased to a maximum of 25 lozenges per day. Treatment is continued for 3 months and thereafter gradually reduced and withdrawn.

The most common side effect of transdermal nicotine patches is skin irritation, characterized by erythema, pruritis, and edema (Table 3). Gastrointestinal side effects, including decreased lower esophageal sphincter pressure, diarrhea, dry mouth, dyspepsia, hiccups, and nausea, are frequent with nicotine gums. Adverse respiratory effects of NRT preparations include bronchitis, coughing, throat irritation, and rhinitis. The spectrum of neurological side effects is wide and includes headaches, paresthesias, nervousness, dizziness, lightheadedness, sleep disturbances, depression, and psychosis. Dependence is low with transdermal application, but may be high with use of the aerosol form. The rare adverse effects are hot flashes, lacrimation, nystagmus, arthralgia, myalgia, and exacerbation of myasthenia gravis. Of note, NRT should be used with caution in patients with serious arrhythmias, unstable angina pectoris, acute or subacute MI because nicotine augments cardiac work by increasing heart rate and blood pressure. Nicotine is also known as a coronary vasoconstrictor. However, the risk of NRT is lower than that for continued smoking *(18)*. Nicotine preparations should not be used during the acute period after cerebrovascular events. They should be used with caution in peripheral arterial disease; in endocrine disorders, including hyperthyroidism and diabetes mellitus; in peptic ulcer; and in hepatic and renal impairment. Their use in pregnancy and lactation is contraindicated.

Sustained-Release Bupropion

Sustained-release bupropion (bupropion SR) is the first nonnicotine drug approved for use in smoking cessation. It is primarily a selective dopamine and noradrenaline reuptake inhibitor and is thought to work by enhancing dopaminergic activity. The drug appears equally effective in smokers with and without depression, suggesting that its efficacy is not only from its antidepressant effect *(20)*. Bupropion SR clearly reduces both nicotine craving and withdrawal symptoms *(23)*. The odds ratio for quitting using bupropion SR compared to placebo is 2.73 (95% CI 1.93–3.94) *(24)*.

Patients should initiate bupropion SR 1–2 weeks before their quit date. The recommended dose schedule begins at 150 mg daily for the first 3 days, then increases to 300 mg daily for 7 to 12 weeks.

Treatment with bupropion is generally well tolerated, and adverse events, including insomnia (30–40%), anxiety, dry mouth (11%), vascular-type headache, tremors (3.4%), and rash (2.4%), are mild. Furthermore, most patients develop tolerance to insomnia and mouth dryness. To diminish sleep disturbance, dosing at bedtime is discouraged. The most serious side effect is seizures (0.1%). Bupropion SR is contraindicated in patients with seizure history or tendency to seizure (Table 3). This side effect is concentration dependent, and separating doses by at least 8 hours and limiting the doses to 300 mg daily are suggested *(25)*. Bupropion is also not suggested in patients taking other antidepressants *(26)*.

The advantages of bupropion SR are ease of use, lack of risk of nicotine toxicity in subjects who continue smoking, and potential additive benefit of depression relief in affected individuals. Furthermore, bupropion SR attenuates the weight gain associated with smoking cessation *(27)*. Its combination with NRT provides safe additive benefit. Bupropion SR is also effective for relapse prevention in patients who successfully quit and for treating relapses *(23)*. Trials of bupropion have included intensive behavioral support; consequently, there is no evidence that it can be used effectively without this additional intervention *(26)*.

Of note, bupropion, like NRT, should be prescribed for a relatively short duration, and prescriptions should only repeated if there are ongoing issues regarding cessation.

Second-Line Agents

Although no Food and Drug Administration approval is available, clonidine and nortriptyline may be useful in some individuals.

Clonidine is a centrally acting α_2-receptor agonist antihypertensive drug that doubles (odds ratio 1.89, 95% CI 1.30–2.74) the rate of smoking cessation *(28)*. The recommended oral dose is initially 0.1 mg po twice a day for 1 week; later, it is 0.15–0.75 mg per day for 3 to 10 weeks. For the patch, the dosage is 0.1 mg per day, followed by 0.1 to 0.2 mg daily for 3–10 weeks.

Nortriptyline is a tricyclic antidepressant agent that significantly (odds ratio 3.83, 95% CI 1.59–5.03) enhances smoking cessation efforts *(24)*. The recommended dose is 25 mg at bedtime initially, gradually increasing to a target dose of 75 to 100 mg daily for 12 weeks.

Other Agents

Mecamylamine is a ganglion blocker antihypertensive agent with nicotinic receptor antagonistic properties. It suppresses nicotine craving alone and in combination with NRT *(29)*. The usual initial dose is 2.5 mg twice daily, with titration to the mean effective dose of 10 mg daily made over the first week of therapy. Divided doses as large as 20 mg can be tried.

Lobeline, a nicotinelike alkaloid, and silver acetate, which produces an aversive taste when combined with cigarette smoke (a smoking deterrent), have been used, but there is insufficient evidence to provide firm recommendations *(20)*.

Glucose has also been identified as a potentially cheap and modestly efficacious smoking cessation aid. There is enough evidence to suggest that chewing glucose tablets can reduce the desire to smoke during the cessation period *(30)*.

Possible Deleterious Effects of Smoking Cessation

Depression can occur as a result of quitting of tobacco. It is usually mild, but may be sufficiently severe to require antidepressant treatment. Weight gain after smoking cessation is common, but the weight increase is usually no more than 5 kg *(31)*.

Some beneficial effects of smoking are less well known *(32)*. An inverse association between smoking and endometriosis, endometrial cancer, Parkinson's disease, severity of Tourette's syndrome, and ulcerative colitis has been reported. In some of these conditions, such as ulcerative colitis, nicotine is now being evaluated as a therapeutic agent. Smoking in these conditions can be considered a minimally effective therapy with a very poor side-effect profile and therefore should not provide a rationale for ongoing cigarette use.

Cost-Effectiveness of Smoking Cessation

Smoking-cessation treatments ranging from brief clinician advice to specialist-delivered intensive programs are not only clinically effective, but also enormously cost-effective compared to other common disease-prevention measures, such as detection and treatment of hypertension or hypercholesterolemia. Treating nicotine dependence is particularly important economically because it can prevent highly costly chronic diseases such as heart disease, stroke, cancer, pulmonary diseases, and delayed wound healing. Smoking-cessation treatments are also cost-effective in hospitalized patients with other diseases. Abstinence not only reduces general medical costs in the short term, but also reduces the number of future hospitalizations *(33)*.

Summary

Cigarette smoking is a highly addictive behavior; even after an AMI or stroke, half of smokers continue the habit. As most smokers who do attempt to quit require multiple attempts before success, tobacco dependence can be considered a chronic relapsing disorder. To improve smoking-cessation rates, effective management is crucial. Current smoking-cessation interventions include behavioral and pharmacological methods. Physicians can play a pivotal role in helping patients choose the level of required support appropriate to their needs. Because smoking duration is a risk factor for smoking-related morbidity, the treatment should be initiated as soon as possible after detection, but pharmacotherapy initiation is not recommended in the peri-stroke period.

Clinicians caring for patients at risk of stroke should determine the patient's level of motivation to quit and the number of cigarettes consumed daily. For motivated light smokers (fewer than 10 cigarettes per day on average), pharmacotherapy is not the first-line approach. These patients ideally should be offered more intensive support by a physician or local smoking-cessation services. For motivated heavy smokers (more than 10 cigarettes daily), NRT should be prescribed in addition to intensive behavioral support. If this fails, bupropion can be considered. For smokers who are not motivated to try smoking cessation, advice from treating doctors can be effective. It is important to raise the topic of smoking repeatedly, wherever and whenever possible. An objective approach and family support are useful in persuading a reluctant smoker to quit.

ALCOHOL

Although alcohol consumption has secondary effects, such as blood pressure elevation and increased plasma osmolarity and plasma homocysteine, cardiomyopathy, and arrhythmias, which are all capable of increasing stroke risk, moderate alcohol consumption may have a beneficial effect. Alcohol inhibits thrombosis by reducing fibrinogen and platelet aggregation; beneficially modifies lipids by decreasing lipoprotein(a) and increasing HDL; enhances insulin sensitivity; and promotes vasodilation, thereby potentially conveying a cardiovascular protective effect.

The relationship between alcohol consumption and ischemic stroke risk remains controversial. Acute heavy alcohol consumption has been associated with a four- to sevenfold increase in cardiac and artery-to-artery embolic stroke risk *(34,35)*. With chronic use, the association most commonly described is "J shaped" (Fig. 1). Moderate alcohol consumption of one to two drinks per day (<24 g; Table 4) has been shown to have a protective effect, reducing risk of stroke by 20–60% *(36–41)*. In contrast, imbibing in three or more drinks per day has been associated with increased risk. The quantity of alcohol in a specific beverage should be taken into account (Table 4). There are conflicting data as to whether wine may convey greater benefit than other types of alcohol, possibly related to antioxidant effects, but it is difficult to eliminate the confounding effects of socioeconomic conditions and lifestyle on alcohol preference *(36,37,42,43)*. Still other studies have not found a consistent association across age groups; therefore, it is not recommended that individuals be encouraged to begin drinking alcoholic beverages if it is not their routine practice *(42,44,45)* (Table 5).

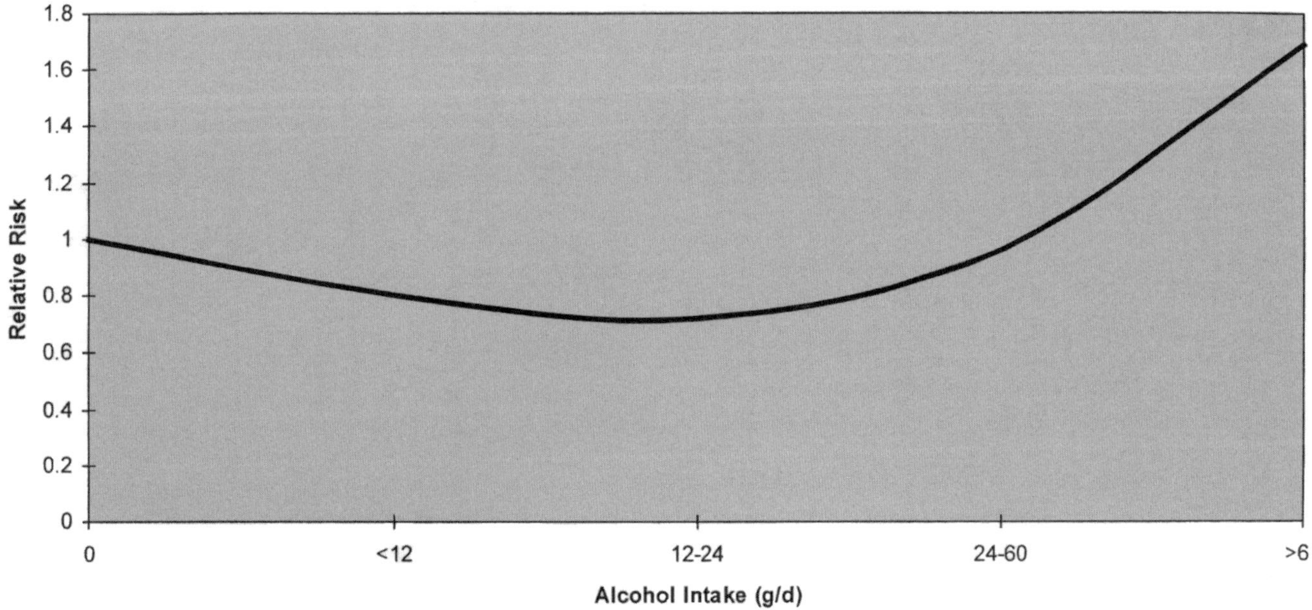

Fig. 1. J-shaped curve for alcohol and stroke. (From ref. *36*.)

Table 4
Alcohol Equivalence

Type of drink	Alcohol content (g)
12 ounces beer	13.7
5 ounces wine	14.2
1.25 ounces vodka	14.2
1.25 ounces whiskey	14.7

Table 5
Recommendations for Alcohol Consumption

1. Do not encourage nondrinkers to begin drinking.
2. If there are no contraindications, patients can be counseled that mild–moderate alcohol consumption may be protective for ischemic stroke.
3. Heavy alcohol use (>3 drinks/day) should be avoided.

REFERENCES

1. Peto R. Smoking and death: the past 40 years and the next 40. Br Med J 1994; 309:937–939.
2. Fagerstrom K. The epidemiology of smoking. Health consequences and benefits of cessation. Drugs 2002;62(Suppl 2):1–9.
3. Mitchell BE, Sobel HL, Alexander MH. The adverse health effects of tobacco and tobacco-related products. Primary Care 1999;26:463–499.
4. Shinton R, Beeves G. Meta-analysis of relation between cigarette smoking and stroke. Br Med J 1989;298:789–794.
5. Hawkins BT, Brown RC, Davis TP. Smoking and ischemic stroke: a role for nicotine? TIPS 2002;23(2):78–82.
6. You RX, Thrift AG, McNeirl JJ, Davis SM, Donnan GA. Ischemic stroke risk and passive exposure to spouses' cigarette smoking. Am J Pub Health 1999;89:572–575.
7. Law MR, Hackshaw AK. Environmental tobacco smoke. Br Med Bull 1996;52: 22–33.
8. Howard G, Wegenknecht LE, Cai J, et al. Cigarette smoking and progression of atherosclerosis; the Atherosclerosis Risk In Communities (ARIC) Study. JAMA 1998; 279:119–124.
9. The NINDS t-PA Stroke Study Group. Intracerebral hemorrhage after intravenous t-PA therapy for ischemic stroke. Stroke 1997;28:2109–2118.
10. Weir BK, Kongable GL, Kassell NF, et al. Cigarette smoking as a cause of aneurysmal subarachnoid hemorrhage and risk for vasospasm. A report of the Cooperative Aneurysm Study. J Neurosurg 1998;89:405–411.
11. Wilson K, Gibson N, Willan A, Cook D. Effect of smoking cessation on mortality after myocardial infarction: metaanalysis of cohort studies. Arch Intern Med 2000; 160:939–944.

12. Kawachi I, Colditz GA, Stampfer MJ, et al. Smoking cessation and the decreased risk of stroke in women. JAMA 1993;269:232–236.
13. Wannamethee SG, Shaper AG, Whincup PH, Walker M. Smoking cessation and the risk of stroke in middle-aged men. JAMA 1995;274:155–160.
14. Shinton R. Lifelong exposures and the potential for stroke prevention: the contribution of cigarette smoking, exercise, and body fat. J Epidemiol Community Health 1997;51;138–143.
15. The Tobacco Use and Dependence Clinical Practice Guideline Panel, Staff, and Consortium Representatives. A clinical guideline for treating tobacco use and dependence. A US Public Health Service Report. JAMA 2000;283:3244–3254.
16. Silagy C, Stead LF. Physician advice for smoking cessation. Cochrane Database Syst Rev 2002;(2):CD000165.
17. Pearson TA, Blair SN, Daniels SR, et al. AHA guidelines for primary prevention of cardiovascular disease and stroke: 2002 update. Consensus panel guide to comprehensive risk reduction for adult patients without coronary and other atherosclerotic vascular diseases. Circulation 2002;106:388–391.
18. West R, McNeill A, Raw M. Smoking cessation guidelines for health professionals. Thorax 2000;55:987–999.
19. Corelli RL. Medications for smoking cessation. West J Med 2002;176:131–135.
20. Sutherland G. Current approaches to the management of smoking cessation. Drugs 2002;62(suppl 2):53–61.
21. Henningfield JE, Fant RV, Gitchell J, et al. Tobacco dependence: global public health potential for new medications development and indications. Ann NY Acad Sci 2000;909:247–256.
22. Silagy C, Lancaster T, Stead L, Mant D, Fowler G. Nicotine replacement therapy for smoking cessation. Cochrane Database Syst Rev 2002;(4):CD000146.
23. Jorenby D. Clinical efficacy of bupropion in the management of smoking cessation. Drugs 2002;62(Suppl 2):25–35.
24. Hughes JR, Stead LF, Lancaster T. Antidepressants for smoking cessation. Cochrane Database Syst Rev 2002;(1):CD000031.
25. Aubin HJ. Tolerability and safety of sustained-release bupropion in the management of smoking cessation. Drugs 2002;62(Suppl 2):45–52.
26. Coleman T. Smoking cessation: Integrating recent advances into clinical practice. Thorax 2001;56:579–582.
27. Gatte KM, Parker CB, Maner LG, et al. Bupropion for weight loss: an investigation of efficacy and tolerability in overweight and obese women. Obesity Res 2001;9: 544–541.
28. Gourlay SG, Stead LF, Benowitz NL. Clonidine for smoking cessation. Cochrane Database Syst Rev 2000;(2):CD00058.
29. Lancaster T, Stead LF. Mecamylamine (a nicotine antagonist) for smoking cessation. Cochrane Database Syst Rev 2000;(2):CD001009.
30. West R. Glucose for smoking cessation: does it have a role? CNS Drugs 2001;15: 261–265.
31. Schoenberger JS. Preventive cardiology: cardiovascular risk of smoking and benefits of smoking cessation. UpToDate Online. Version 10.2, 2002. Available at: http://uptodateonline.com. Accessed July 7, 2002.
32. Baron JA. Beneficial effects of nicotine and cigarette smoking: the real, the possible and the spurious. Br Med Bull 1996;52:58–73.

33. Godfrey C, Fowler G. Pharmacoeconomic considerations in the management of smoking cessation. Drugs 2002;62(Suppl 2):63–70.
34. Hillboom M, Numminen H, Juvela S. Recent heavy drinking of alcohol and embolic stroke. Stroke 1999;30:2307–2312.
35. Hillbom M, Juvela S, Numminen H. Alcohol intake and the risk of stroke. J Cardiovasc Risk 1999;6:223–228.
36. Reynolds K, Lewis B, Nolen JD, Kinney GL, Sathya B, He J. Alcohol consumption and risk of stroke: a meta-analysis. JAMA 2003;289:579–588.
37. Sacco RL, Elkind M, Boden-Albala B, et al. The protective effect of moderate alcohol consumption on ischemic stroke. JAMA 1999;281:53–60.
38. Malarcher AM, Giles WH, Croft JB, et al. Alcohol intake, type of beverage, and the risk of cerebral infarction in young women. Stroke 2001;32:77–83.
39. Caicoya M, Rodriguez T, Corrales C, Cuello R, Lasheras C. Alcohol and stroke: a community case-control study in Asturias, Spain. J Clin Epidemiol 1999;52:677–684.
40. Camargo CA Jr. Moderate alcohol consumption and stroke. The epidemiologic evidence. Stroke 1989;20:1611–1626.
41. Jackson VA, Sesso HD, Buring JE, Gaziano JM. Alcohol consumption and mortality in men with preexisting cerebrovascular disease. Arch Intern Med 2003;163: 1189–1193.
42. Djousse L, Pankow JS, Arnett DK, et al. Alcohol consumption and risk of ischemic stroke: the Framingham Study. Stroke 2002;33:907–912.
43. Truelsen T, Gronbaek M, Schnohr P, Boysen G. Intake of beer, wine, and spirits and risk of stroke: the Copenhagen City Heart Study. Stroke 1998;29:2467–2472.
44. Wannamethee SG, Shaper AG. Patterns of alcohol intake and risk of stroke in middle-aged British men. Stroke 1996;27:1033–1039.
45. Hansagi H, Romelsjo A, Gerhardsson de Verdier M, Andreasson S, Leifman A. Alcohol consumption and stroke mortality. 20-year follow-up of 15,077 men and women. Stroke 1995;26:1768–1773.

7
Diet, Obesity, and Physical Activity

Karen L. Furie

The statistics concerning weight, diet, and exercise in the United States are grim. Seventy-five percent of Americans fail to exercise at least 30 minutes a day. Obesity, low levels of physical activity, and Western diets rich in lipids and carbohydrates and poor in fruits and vegetables contribute to the intermediate medical conditions that increase stroke risk: hypertension, diabetes, and hyperlipidemia. The heartening aspect, however, is that these risk factors are potentially modifiable if clinicians identify and address the issues and patients comply with current recommendations.

PHYSICAL ACTIVITY

Several acute benefits to exercise contribute to reducing stroke risk. Exercise results in reduced blood pressure, glucose levels, and triglyceride levels *(1–4)*. Additionally, physical activity has been shown to be inversely related to levels of hemostatic and inflammatory biomarkers: fibrinogen, factors VIII and IX, blood viscosity, platelet count, von Willebrand factor, fibrin D-dimer, tissue plasminogen activator, C-reactive protein, and white blood cell count *(5)*.

An inherent problem in observational studies on exercise and cardiovascular risk is the potential confounding of other "healthy lifestyle" factors. That is, individuals who exercise regularly are also more likely to eat a healthy diet and may be more compliant with other health recommendations. Conversely, there is also the potential that people with greater cardiovascular risk, either because of their personal or family history, may increase their exercise activity. As a result, the only scientific method of assessing the effect of exercise on stroke risk is through a randomized controlled trial. As yet, there has not been a definitive randomized controlled trial to establish exercise as a modifiable risk factor for stroke.

Many epidemiological studies quantify physical activity in metabolic equivalent (MET) hours; 1 MET is equivalent to oxygen consumption at rest. More

From: *Current Clinical Neurology: Handbook of Stroke Prevention in Clinical Practice*
Edited by: K. L. Furie and P. J. Kelly © Humana Press Inc., Totowa, NJ

vigorous activities are expressed as a factor of this baseline energy expenditure. For example, brisk walking has a MET score of 3.3 because it utilizes 3.3 times the energy expended at rest.

The Oslo Study, Framingham Study, Atherosclerosis Risk in Communities Study (ARIC), and Copenhagen City Heart Study have all demonstrated an inverse association between level of physical activity and risk of stroke, but the strength of the association and the results across age, gender, and socioeconomic strata have not been consistent *(6–9)*.

Physical Activity and Stroke Risk in Men

In the Physicians' Health Study (PHS), 21,823 men aged 40–84 years were randomly assigned to receive aspirin and β-carotene and followed for 11 years. The study found an inverse relationship between vigorous exercise (enough activity to sweat) at least once a week and stroke, especially for hemorrhagic stroke. There was no increased benefit with exercising vigorously more than once a week. The most active men had a 26% lower risk of stroke than the least active men. The effects of vigorous physical activity disappeared after controlling for hypertension, high cholesterol, diabetes, and body mass index (BMI), indicating that these are the intermediates of risk. A 21% (nonsignificant) stroke reduction in thromboembolic stroke was seen in active nonsmoking men in the Honolulu Heart Study, but again there was greater than 69% reduction in hemorrhagic stroke *(10)*.

In the Health Professionals Follow-Up Study, men who ran at least 1 hour a week had a 42% reduction in risk of fatal and nonfatal myocardial infarction. The risk reduction varied by activity. For example, compared to men who did not exercise, weight lifters had a 23% reduction, and brisk walkers and weekly rowers an 18% risk reduction. Exercise intensity, independent of the duration, was associated with reduced risk *(11)*.

The Harvard Alumni Health Study studied 11,130 men aged 43–88 years and found a benefit to moderate intensity (>4.5 MET), but not light (<4.5 MET), physical activity in reducing incidence of stroke by as much as 40%. However, there appeared to be a U-shaped response to exercise that could not be explained by physical activity misclassification or higher risk in the more active group. It may be that the definition of stroke in this study, which included intracerebral hemorrhage and subarachnoid hemorrhage, may have obscured the effects of more intense exercise on ischemic stroke *(12)*.

Physical Activity and Stroke Risk in Women

In the Women's Health Initiative Observational Study, 73,743 healthy women aged 50–79 years were followed for approx 3 years. Walking and vigorous exercise conveyed a similar benefit, but vigorous exercise did effect an additional risk reduction in women who were already walking on a regular basis. Reductions in cardiovascular risks were seen regardless of age, BMI, or race. Women in the highest quintile of physical activity, equivalent to 1 hour of brisk walking each day, had approx 50% lower risk of a first cardiovascular event than those in the lower quintiles *(13)*. Walking or exercising at least 2.5 hours a week reduced cardiovascular events by 30%. In another study focusing on women, the highest quintile of physical activity (>21.7 MET-hours/week) was associated with a 48% reduction in ischemic, but not hemorrhagic, stroke risk. Walking alone was associated with a 34% ischemic stroke risk reduction and brisk walking with an even greater benefit, which was comparable to the reduction seen with vigorous exercise *(14)*.

Race, Physical Activity, and Risk of Stroke

In the Northern Manhattan Stroke Study (NOMASS), a multiracial cohort, there was a protective effect of leisure-time physical activity (odds ratio [OR] 0.37, 95% confidence interval [CI] 0.25–0.55) even after controlling for intermediates such as hypertension, diabetes, and obesity. Additionally, there was greater benefit with increasing exercise intensity (light–moderate vs heavy) and duration (<2 hours/week, 2–4.9 hours/week, ≥5 hours/week). In the NOMASS study, walking, calisthenics, dancing, golf, bowling, horseback riding, and gardening were classified as light–moderate exercise, whereas heavy exercise included hiking, tennis, swimming, bicycle riding, jogging, aerobic dancing, handball, racquetball, or squash *(15)*.

Trials of Physical Activity and Cardiovascular Risk

A meta-analysis of 51 studies examining the effects of cardiovascular rehabilitation found a 31% reduction in cardiovascular mortality over a 2-year follow-up period *(20)*. Counseling alone has not been proven to enhance physical activity, but more targeted interventions, which need not be physician driven, may be useful. In a randomized trial, both a structured exercise program and a lifestyle intervention were effective in increasing levels of physical activity and reducing blood pressure *(21)*. One interesting study randomly assigned overweight subjects to either self-help (two 20-minute counseling sessions with a nutritionist and self-help resources) or free commercial weight loss program (Weight Watchers). Although the absolute magnitude of change was small in both groups, those in the commercial program lost significantly more weight (–2.9 kg vs –0.2 kg) and had greater BMI reduction (–1.1 vs –0.2) in 2 years *(22)*.

OBESITY

There are several ways of measuring obesity. The most commonly used measure is the BMI, calculated as weight in kilograms divided by the square of the height in meters. A table for calculating BMI can also be used (Table 1). Waist-to-hip ratio, waist circumference, and skinfold thickness have also been used in epidemiological studies.

Obesity is an established risk factor for coronary heart disease and, now, for stroke. In the PHS, compared to men with BMIs less than 23, those with BMIs of 30 or above had double the risk of stroke, both ischemic and hemorrhagic. Each unit increase of BMI was associated with a 4–6% increase in the relative risk of stroke independent of other risk factors *(16)*. In NOMASS, subjects with above-median waist-to-hip ratios had three times the risk of ischemic stroke independent of other stroke risk factors and BMI *(17)*. Another study in the elderly found that waist circumference of 99 cm or higher and BMI of 28 or above were associated with a 65% higher risk of stroke in men, but not women *(18)*.

In the Nurses' Health Study (NHS), compared to women with BMI less than 21 kg/m^2, women with BMI of 27 kg/m^2 or higher had a 75–200% higher risk of ischemic stroke. Additionally, weight gain during midlife, as opposed to staying within 5 pounds of body weight at age 18 years, was associated with an increased relative risk for ischemic stroke of 2.52 (95% CI 1.80–3.52) for a gain of 20 kg or more *(19)*.

DIET

Calcium, Potassium, and Magnesium

Dietary calcium is inversely related to blood pressure and is believed to have a beneficial effect on lipid metabolism; therefore, it is reasonable to consider whether increased calcium intake reduces risk of stroke. In the Honolulu Heart Program, the role of calcium was explored by examining the relationship between milk intake and stroke risk in 3150 men of Japanese ancestry aged 45–68 years followed for 22 years *(23)*. These men drank, on average, roughly half the quantity of milk consumed by the average American. The study found that there was almost a 50% reduction in stroke risk associated with drinking 16 oz or more of milk per day, but calcium intake correlated with sodium and potassium intake and higher levels of physical activity and was inversely related to alcohol consumption and BMI. The "milk effect" persisted even after adjustment for these factors as well as for systolic blood pressure. Milk consumption in this population was likely a marker of better nutrition and a healthier lifestyle. There did not appear to

Table 1
BMI Calculation Chart

	Normal						Overweight					Obese										Extreme Obesity										
BMI	19	20	21	22	23	24	25	26	27	28	29	30	31	32	33	34	35	36	37	38	39	40	41	42	43	44	45	46	47	48	49	50
Height (inches)														Wt (pounds)																		
58	91	96	100	105	110	115	119	124	129	134	138	143	148	153	158	162	167	172	177	181	186	191	196	201	205	210	215	220	224	229	234	239
59	94	99	104	109	114	119	124	128	133	138	143	148	153	158	163	168	173	178	183	188	193	198	203	208	212	217	222	227	232	237	242	247
60	97	102	107	112	118	123	128	133	138	143	148	153	158	163	168	174	179	184	189	194	199	204	209	215	220	225	230	235	240	245	250	255
61	100	106	111	116	122	127	132	137	143	148	153	158	164	169	174	180	185	190	195	201	206	211	217	222	227	232	238	243	248	254	259	264
62	10	109	115	120	126	131	136	142	147	153	158	164	169	175	180	186	191	196	202	207	213	218	224	229	235	240	246	251	256	262	267	273
63	107	113	118	124	130	135	141	146	152	158	163	169	175	180	186	191	197	203	208	214	220	225	231	237	242	248	254	259	265	270	278	282
64	110	116	122	128	134	140	145	151	157	163	169	174	180	186	192	197	204	209	215	221	227	232	238	244	250	256	262	267	273	279	285	291
65	114	120	126	132	138	144	150	156	162	168	174	180	186	192	198	204	210	216	222	228	234	240	246	252	258	264	270	276	282	288	294	300
66	118	124	130	136	142	148	155	161	167	173	179	186	192	198	204	210	216	223	229	235	241	247	253	260	266	272	278	284	291	297	303	309
67	121	127	134	140	146	153	159	166	172	178	185	191	198	204	211	217	223	230	236	242	249	255	261	268	274	280	287	293	299	306	312	319
68	125	131	138	144	151	158	164	171	177	184	190	197	203	210	216	223	230	236	243	249	256	262	269	276	282	289	295	302	308	315	322	328
69	128	135	142	149	155	162	169	176	182	189	196	203	209	216	223	230	236	243	250	257	263	270	277	284	291	297	304	311	318	324	331	338
70	132	139	146	153	160	167	174	181	188	195	202	209	216	222	229	236	243	250	257	264	271	278	285	292	299	306	313	320	327	334	341	348
71	136	143	150	157	165	172	179	186	193	200	208	215	222	229	236	243	250	257	265	272	279	286	293	301	308	315	322	329	338	343	351	358
72	140	147	154	162	169	177	184	191	199	206	213	221	228	235	242	250	258	265	272	279	287	294	302	309	316	324	331	338	346	353	361	368
73	144	151	159	166	174	182	189	197	204	212	219	227	235	242	250	257	265	272	280	288	295	302	310	318	325	333	340	348	355	363	371	378
74	148	155	163	171	179	186	194	202	210	218	225	233	241	249	256	264	272	280	287	295	303	311	319	326	334	342	350	358	365	373	381	389
75	152	160	168	176	184	192	200	208	216	224	232	240	248	256	264	272	279	287	295	303	311	319	327	335	343	351	359	367	375	383	391	399
76	156	164	172	180	189	197	205	213	221	230	238	246	254	263	271	279	287	295	304	312	320	328	336	344	353	361	369	377	385	394	402	410

be a benefit of nondairy calcium intake. Calcium was also not associated with stroke risk in the PHS, although in the NHS cohort, there was a nonlinear association between calcium, especially dairy intake, and atherosclerotic stroke risk *(24,25)*.

Potassium and magnesium may help mediate stroke risk by reducing blood pressure, inhibiting free radicals, preventing vascular smooth muscle proliferation, or preventing arrhythmias. Magnesium may also help reduce lipid peroxidation. Both the NHS and the Health Professionals Follow-up Study found an inverse relationship between intake of potassium and magnesium and risk of stroke, stronger in men with hypertension and only significant for noncardioembolic stroke in women *(24,25)*. Adding a serving of fruit or vegetable was associated with a 4% reduction in risk.

Flavonoids and Antioxidants

Flavonoids, most commonly found in tea, have been associated with reduced risk of coronary heart disease and stroke. Their mechanism of action appears related to reduced lipid peroxidation and decreased platelet aggregability. Other food sources of flavonoids include fruits and vegetables. In one study, men who drank 4.7 cups of tea per day had a 69% lower risk of stroke compared to those who drank less than 2.6 cups per day *(26)*.

Lipid peroxidation contributes to the development and progression of atherosclerosis. Antioxidant vitamins, such as vitamins C and E and β-carotene, could potentially modify this risk. Studies showing a benefit to fruit and vegetable consumption support the notion that these vitamins might be beneficial. Studies that examined dietary constituents and supplement use showed that only vitamin E is associated with reduced risk of fatal and nonfatal stroke in women, but the effect of supplements alone remains controversial *(27,28)*.

Results have been less conclusive in men. A Finnish study found that men with the lowest quartile of vitamin C levels have twice the risk of ischemic stroke as men with the highest levels after adjusting for other stroke risk factors *(29)*. Those overweight or hypertensive are at even higher risk with low vitamin C levels *(29)*. In contrast, in the PHS, men aged 40–75 years did not appear to benefit from higher levels of dietary and supplemental vitamins E and C *(30)*.

A Finnish study that randomly assigned patients to supplementation with 50 mg α-tocopherol, 20 mg β-carotene, both, or placebo examined the substudy of male smokers aged 50–69 years who suffered stroke during the 6 years of follow-up. Vitamin E reduced the risk of ischemic stroke in hypertensive men, but it was overshadowed by an increased risk of subarachnoid hemorrhage. There was no effect in those without hypertension. Hypertensive men with diabetes or coronary heart disease had risk reductions of 67 and 24%, respectively, in ischemic stroke without a higher risk of subarachnoid hemorrhage. Similarly, β-carotene, its effect modified by alcohol use, did not have a consistent or robust beneficial effect on stroke risk *(31)*.

The Medical Research Council/British Heart Foundation Heart Protection Study randomly assigned 20,536 high-risk individuals aged 40–80 years with coronary disease, occlusive arterial disease, or diabetes to receive 600 mg vitamin E, 250 mg vitamin C, 20 mg β-carotene, or placebo. There was no difference in stroke rates between the vitamin- and placebo-treated patients after 5 years of follow-up *(32)*.

At present, there is no value to measuring blood levels of antioxidant vitamins. Although it is recommended that individuals take a multivitamin daily for chronic disease prevention, it must be emphasized that vitamin supplements do not replace a healthy diet *(33)*.

Fiber

Epidemiological studies have linked dietary fiber intake with reduced risk of cardiovascular disease. Whole grains contain antioxidants, minerals, fiber, and phytochemicals, including folate, vitamin E, potassium, and magnesium. The NHS explored the association between whole-grain intake and risk of ischemic stroke in 75,521 women aged 38–63 years who were followed for 12 years *(34)*. The study found an inverse relationship between whole-grain intake and ischemic stroke, with a 28–31% reduction in stroke risk with one to three servings per day after adjusting for other cardiovascular risk factors. Women with high whole-grain intake were more active, consumed more fruits and vegetables, had lower fat intake, smoked and drank alcohol less, and more often used hormone replacement therapy. Still, the benefits appeared consistent in women with and without these positive lifestyle attributes.

Fish

Fish consumption is believed to modify ischemic stroke risk through favorable effects of long-chain omega-3 polyunsaturated fatty acids on lipids as well as through platelet and endothelial function. They also reduce the threshold for arrhythmias. The use of omega-3 fatty acid supplements (850 mg/day) has been shown to reduce mortality and sudden death in patients with existing coronary heart disease. In the Health Professionals Follow-up Study, there was a 40% lower risk of ischemic stroke in men who consumed fish once a month *(35)*. There was no dose response effect with higher intake of fish. Again, high fish consumption was higher in physically active nonoverweight nonsmokers, but also with a history of hypertension and hypercholesterolemia. Fish intake was also more common in men taking aspirin and multivitamins, although the benefit persisted after controlling for these variables.

In the NHS cohort, 79,839 women aged 34 to 59 years were compared by category of fish intake and quintile of omega-3 polyunsaturated fatty acid intake and followed for 14 years *(36)*. Women who ate fish at least once a month had a lower risk of stroke. A significantly reduced risk of thrombotic infarction was found among women who ate fish two or more times per week (relative risk 0.49, 95% CI 0.26–0.93). Women in the highest quintile of long-chain omega-3 polyunsaturated fatty acids intake had lower risk of all strokes and thrombotic infarction, with relative risks of 0.72 (95% CI 0.53–0.99) and 0.67 (95% CI 0.42–1.07), respectively.

Neither the Health Professionals Follow-up Study nor the NHS found an association between fish intake and risk of hemorrhagic stroke.

Fruits and Vegetables

Eating more fruits and vegetables will increase dietary fiber, flavonoids, antioxidants, folate, and potassium. In both men and women, fruit intake has a protective effect on ischemic stroke risk. Those with the highest intake of fruits and vegetables had a 60% lower risk of stroke compared with the lowest quintile. There is a 17–25% reduction in risk for eating three servings of fruits or vegetables each day *(37,38)*. Green leafy vegetables, cruciferous vegetables, and citrus fruit or juice, but not legumes or potatoes, were found to be beneficial *(38)*.

RECOMMENDATIONS

The Centers for Disease Control and Prevention and the American College of Sports Medicine recommend at least 30 minutes of moderate exercise on most, and preferably all, days of the week. *Moderate* is defined as exercise resulting in mild shortness of breath. Obviously, the fitness of the individual plays a role in establishing this parameter *(39)*. This target should be considered a minimal level of activity, and patients able and willing to do more should be encouraged to increase their exertion. Recommendations are outlined in Table 2. More recent studies suggest that more intense exercise, such as 1 hour of brisk walking a day, may convey greater benefit. The challenge in instituting this prevention strategy after a first stroke, particularly in patients with other comorbidities limiting mobility, is to define an activity other than walking that is convenient and affordable.

Healthy dietary practices as described in Table 3 should be a long-term commitment throughout the life-span. Although there is evidence that the dietary elements outlined in this chapter may be beneficial for reducing risk of stroke, it should be emphasized that it is more important to maintain a well-rounded diet that includes these food groups rather than to take individual supplements.

Table 2
Physical Activity Recommendations

1. Individuals of all ages should participate in 30 minutes of physical activity of moderate intensity (such as brisk walking, mowing the lawn, dancing, swimming, or bicycling) on most, if not all, days of the week.
2. Previously inactive individuals should start with short amounts of moderate intensity and gradually increase the duration or intensity until the target is achieved.
3. Assess men over age 40 years and women over 50 years as well as individuals with cardiovascular or other chronic disease before advising on exercise. If there are no contraindications, start with short amounts of moderate intensity and gradually increase the duration or intensity until the target is achieved.
4. Aerobic activity should be supplemented with strengthening exercises at least twice per week to improve musculoskeletal health and reduce the risk of falling.

Source: Adapted from ref. *40*.

Table 3
American Heart Association General Dietary Guidelines

1. Consume a variety of fruits and vegetables; choose five or more servings per day.
2. Consume a variety of grain products, including whole grains; choose six or more servings per day.
3. Achieve and maintain a healthy weight (BMI 25).
4. Limit intake of foods with high content of cholesterol-raising fatty acids:
   - saturated fatty acids (dairy products, fatty meats, tropical oils): <7% total calories
   - trans fatty acids (baked goods, fried foods, some margarine): 2–3% total calories
   - cholesterol (egg yolks, shellfish): <300 mg per day, <200 mg per day if low-density lipoprotein is elevated or in the presence of diabetic or cardiovascular disease
5. Substitute grains and unsaturated fatty acids from fish, vegetables, legumes, and nuts.
6. Limit salt intake (6 g/day).
7. Limit alcohol intake (fewer than three drinks/day).

Source: Adapted from ref. *41*.

REFERENCES

1. Thompson PD, Crouse SF, Goodpaster B, et al. The acute versus the chronic response to exercise. Med Sci Sports Exerc 2001;33(6 Suppl):S438–S445; discussion S452–S453.
2. Williams PT. High-density lipoprotein cholesterol and other risk factors for coronary heart disease in female runners. N Engl J Med 1996;334:1298–1303.

3. Mayer-Davis EJ, D'Agostino R Jr, Karter AJ, et al. Intensity and amount of physical activity in relation to insulin sensitivity: the Insulin Resistance Atherosclerosis Study. JAMA 1998;279:669–674.
4. Kraus WE, Houmard JA, Duscha BD, et al. Effects of the amount and intensity of exercise on plasma lipoproteins. N Engl J Med 2002;347:1483–1492.
5. Wannamethee SG, Lowe GD, Whincup PH, et al. Physical activity and hemostatic and inflammatory variables in elderly men. Circulation 2002;105:1785–1790.
6. Haheim LL, Holme I, Hjermann I, Leren P. Risk factors of stroke incidence and mortality. A 12-year follow-up of the Oslo Study. Stroke 1993;24:1484–1489.
7. Kiely DK, Wolf, PA, Cupples LA, Beiser AS, Kannel UB. Physical activity and stroke risk: the Framingham Study. Am J Epidemiol 1994;140:608–620.
8. Lindenstrom E, Boysen G, Nyboe J. Lifestyle factors and risk of cerebrovascular disease in women. The Copenhagen City Heart Study. Stroke 1993;24:1468–1472.
9. Evenson KR, Rosamond WD, Cai J, et al. Physical activity and ischemic stroke risk. The atherosclerosis risk in communities study. Stroke 1999;30:1333–1339.
10. Abbott RD, Rodriguez BL, Burchfiel CM, Curb JD. Physical activity in older middle-aged men and reduced risk of stroke: the Honolulu Heart Program. Am J Epidemiol 1994;139:881–893.
11. Tanasescu M, Leitzmann MF, Rimm EB, et al. Exercise type and intensity in relation to coronary heart disease in men. JAMA 2002;288:1994–2000.
12. Lee IM, Paffenbarger RS Jr. Physical activity and stroke incidence: the Harvard Alumni Health Study. Stroke 1998;29:2049–2054.
13. Manson JE, Greenland P, LaCroix AZ, et al. Walking compared with vigorous exercise for the prevention of cardiovascular events in women. N Engl J Med 2002;347: 716–725.
14. Hu FB, Stampfer MJ, Solomon C, et al. Physical activity and risk of stroke in women. JAMA 2000; 283:2961–2967.
15. Sacco RL, Gan R, Boden-Albala B, et al. Leisure-time physical activity and ischemic stroke risk: the Northern Manhattan Stroke Study. Stroke 1998;29:380–387.
16. Kurth T, Gaziano JM, Berger K, et al. Body mass index and the risk of stroke in men. Arch Intern Med 2002;162:2557–2562.
17. Suk SH, Sacco RL, Boden-Albala B, et al. Abdominal obesity and risk of ischemic stroke: the Northern Manhattan Stroke Study. Stroke 2003;34:1586–1592.
18. Dey DK, Rothenberg E, Sundh V, et al. Waist circumference, body mass index, and risk for stroke in older people: a 15 year longitudinal population study of 70-year-olds. J Am Geriatr Soc 2002;50:1510–1518.
19. Rexrode KM, Hennekens CH, Willett WC, et al. A prospective study of body mass index, weight change, and risk of stroke in women. JAMA 1997;277:1539–1545.
20. Jolliffe JA, Rees K, Taylor RS, et al. Exercise-based rehabilitation for coronary heart disease. Cochrane Database Syst Rev 2001;1:CD001800.
21. Dunn AL, Marcus BH, Kampert JB, et al. Comparison of lifestyle and structured interventions to increase physical activity and cardiorespiratory fitness: a randomized trial. JAMA 1999;281:327–334.
22. Heshka S, Anderson JW, Atkinson RL, et al. Weight loss with self-help compared with a structured commercial program: a randomized trial. JAMA 2003;289: 1792–1798.

23. Abbott RD, Curb JD, Rodriguez BL, et al. Effect of dietary calcium and milk consumption on risk of thromboembolic stroke in older middle-aged men. The Honolulu Heart Program. Stroke 1996;27:813–818.
24. Ascherio A, Rimm EB, Hernan MA, et al. Intake of potassium, magnesium, calcium, and fiber and risk of stroke among US men. Circulation 1998;98:1198–1204.
25. Iso H, Stampfer MJ, Manson JE, et al. Prospective study of calcium, potassium, and magnesium intake and risk of stroke in women. Stroke 1999;30:1772–1779.
26. Keli SO, Hertog MG, Feskens EJ, Kromhout D. Dietary flavonoids, antioxidant vitamins, and incidence of stroke: the Zutphen study. Arch Intern Med 1996;156: 637–642.
27. Manson JE, Gaziano JM, Spelsberg A, et al. A secondary prevention trial of antioxidant vitamins and cardiovascular disease in women. Rationale, design, and methods. The WACS Research Group. Ann Epidemiol 1995;5:261–269.
28. Yochum LA, Folsom AR, Kushi LH. Intake of antioxidant vitamins and risk of death from stroke in postmenopausal women. Am J Clin Nutr 2000;72:476–483.
29. Kurl S, Toumainen TP, Laukkanen JA, et al. Plasma vitamin C modifies the association between hypertension and risk of stroke. Stroke 2002;33:1568–1573.
30. Ascherio A, Rimm EB, Hernan MA, et al. Relation of consumption of vitamin E, vitamin C, and carotenoids to risk for stroke among men in the United States. Ann Intern Med 1999;130:963–970.
31. Leppala JM, Virtamo J, Fogelholm R, et al. Vitamin E and beta carotene supplementation in high risk for stroke: a subgroup analysis of the Alpha-Tocopherol, Beta-Carotene Cancer Prevention Study. Arch Neurol 2000;57:1503–1509.
32. MRC/BHF Heart Protection Study of antioxidant vitamin supplementation in 20,536 high-risk individuals: a randomised placebo-controlled trial. Lancet 2002; 360:23–33.
33. Fairfield KM, Fletcher RH. Vitamins for chronic disease prevention in adults: scientific review. JAMA 2002;287:3116–3126.
34. Liu S, Manson JE, Stampfer MJ, et al. Whole grain consumption and risk of ischemic stroke in women: a prospective study. JAMA 2000;284:1534–1540.
35. He K, Rimm EB, Merchant A, et al. Fish consumption and risk of stroke in men. JAMA 2002;288:3130–3136.
36. Iso H, Rexrode KM, Stampfer MJ, et al. Intake of fish and omega-3 fatty acids and risk of stroke in women. JAMA 2001;285:304–312.
37. Gillman MW, Cupples LA, Gagnon D, et al. Protective effect of fruits and vegetables on development of stroke in men. JAMA 1995;273:1113–1117.
38. Joshipura KJ, Ascherio A, Manson JE, et al. Fruit and vegetable intake in relation to risk of ischemic stroke. JAMA 1999;282:1233–1239.
39. Pate RR, Pratt M, Blair SN, et al. Physical activity and public health. A recommendation from the Centers for Disease Control and Prevention and the American College of Sports Medicine. JAMA 1995;273:402–407.
40. Estabrooks PA, Glasgow RE, Dzewaltowski DA. Physical activity promotion through primary care. JAMA 2003;289:2913–2916.
41. Krauss RM, Eckel RH, Howard B, et al. Revision 2000: a statement for healthcare professionals from the Nutrition Committee of the American Heart Association. J Nutr 2001;131:132–146.

8

Stroke Prevention With Antiplatelet Therapy

Dominick J. H. McCabe, Peter J. Kelly, and J. Philip Kistler

INTRODUCTION

Community-based stroke studies have shown that approx 80% of all strokes are ischemic *(1,2)*. The majority of patients survive their first ischemic stroke, with 95% alive at 7 days poststroke and 90% alive at 1 month *(3)*. These patients subsequently have an increased risk of stroke recurrence of approx 5% per annum and an increased risk of serious coronary events of about 3% per annum over the following 5 years *(4,5)*.

Because there is some evidence that platelets are excessively activated in patients with ischemic stroke and transient ischemic attack (TIA) *(6–8)* and because platelets have a pivotal role in thromboembolism, antiplatelet agents have the potential to play an important role in secondary stroke prevention.

ASPIRIN

Mechanism of Action

Prostaglandin (PG) H synthase is the key enzyme involved in PG biosynthesis *(9)*. The enzyme possesses both cyclooxygenase (COX) and hydroperoxidase activities. Two isoforms exist: PGH synthase-1 and PGH synthase-2 (also known as COX-1 and COX-2, respectively) *(9–11)*. Aspirin selectively and irreversibly inhibits the COX-1-mediated breakdown of arachidonic acid *(12)*, thus inhibiting the subsequent formation of thromboxane A_2 (a potent platelet aggregator and vasoconstrictor) (Fig. 1). Because platelets are anucleate cells, the inhibitory effects of aspirin on platelet function should last for the life-span of the platelet (10 days) *(12)*.

From: *Current Clinical Neurology: Handbook of Stroke Prevention in Clinical Practice*
Edited by: K. L. Furie and P. J. Kelly © Humana Press Inc., Totowa, NJ

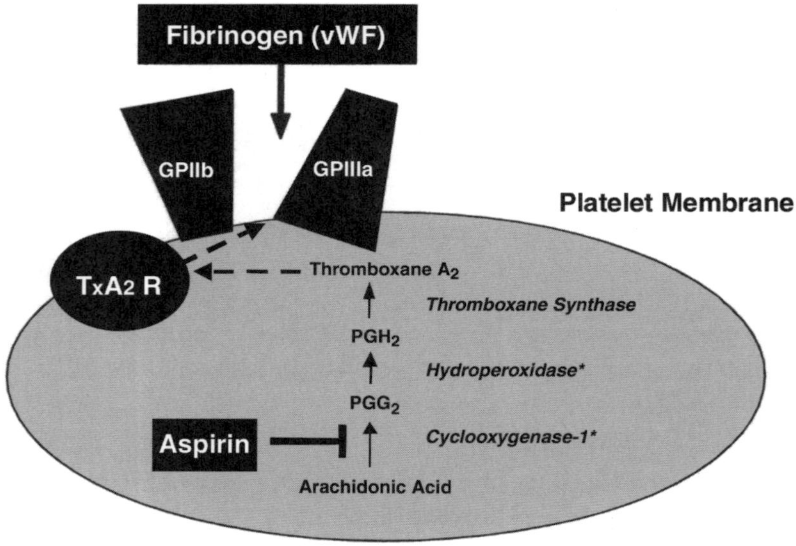

Fig. 1. Mechanism of action of aspirin in platelets. After release from phospholipid membranes, the conversion of arachidonic acid into prostaglandin (PG) G_2 and PGH_2 is catalyzed by PGH synthase*. PGH_2 can be converted into thromboxane A_2, and the subsequent binding of thromboxane A_2 to the thromboxane A_2 receptor (TxA_2 R) can trigger intracellular signaling events that activate the glycoprotein (Gp) IIb/IIIa receptor. This undergoes a conformational change to facilitate binding of fibrinogen or vWF, thus mediating platelet-to-platelet aggregation. Aspirin irreversibly inhibits the cyclooxygenase-1 mediated breakdown of arachidonic acid to PGG_2, but does not affect the peroxidase function of PGG/H synthase.

Early Prevention of Recurrence With Aspirin in Ischemic Stroke and TIA

Until recently, antiplatelet therapy was not routinely given in the acute phase of ischemic stroke, and the benefits of early secondary prevention were unknown. However, large trials of aspirin therapy given within 48 hours of acute ischemic stroke have confirmed that aspirin does have a small, but important, benefit for early secondary prevention *(13,14)*. It is important to recognize that these studies considered ischemic stroke in the aggregate and did not rigorously identify the location of the arterial lesion, the stroke pathophysiology, or the collateral circulation. This is a pervasive issue across the clinical trials that limits generalization to specific stroke subtypes.

Table 1
Outcome Events (%) at the End of 4 Weeks or Earlier Discharge or Death in CAST

	Aspirin (n = 10,335)	Placebo (n = 10,320)
Deaths		
Caused by initial stroke	1.4	1.7
Caused by recurrent stroke (any type)	1.0	1.2
Caused by other or unknown causes	1.0	1.1
Total	3.3	3.9[a]
Recurrent stroke (fatal or nonfatal)		
Ischemic	1.6	2.1[b]
Hemorrhagic[c]	1.1	0.9
Unknown	0.5	0.4
All	3.2	3.4
Death or recurrent nonfatal stroke	5.3	5.9[a]

[a] $p < 0.05$.
[b] $p \leq 0.01$; all other differences between the aspirin and placebo groups were nonsignificant.
[c] Includes cerebral hemorrhage or hemorrhagic transformation of the original infarct.

In the Multicenter Acute Stroke Trial–Italy (MAST-I) study *(15)*, patients with acute (<6 hours) ischemic stroke were randomized to receive 1.5 mU of intravenous streptokinase, 300 mg aspirin daily, streptokinase plus aspirin, or no treatment in a 2 × 2 factorial design. This study was prematurely discontinued after 622 subjects (approx 150 patients in each subgroup) had been randomly assigned because of an excess 10-day case fatality in the streptokinase–aspirin group. The number of early recurrent cerebral infarcts in the aspirin alone (1 patient) and control groups (0 patients) was too limited to make any meaningful conclusions about the efficacy of aspirin for early secondary prevention.

In the Chinese Acute Stroke Trial (CAST), daily aspirin (160 mg, started within 48 hours of onset, for up to 4 weeks) was compared with placebo *(14)*. Outcome data were available for 10,335 patients randomly assigned to receive aspirin and 10,320 randomly assigned to receive placebo; patients were followed up for 4 weeks unless they died or were discharged earlier. Although 13% of patients did not have brain computed tomography (CT) before randomization, the diagnosis of ischemic stroke was eventually confirmed in 98% of patients overall *(14)*.

In CAST, there was a significant reduction in the rate of death (0.54% absolute risk reduction [RR], $p = 0.04$) (Table 1) and in the combined end point of death or nonfatal stroke (0.68% absolute RR, $p = 0.03$) in the aspirin group compared with those allocated the placebo. Although aspirin significantly reduced the absolute rate of recurrent ischemic stroke by 0.47% compared with placebo ($p = 0.01$), its beneficial effect on recurrent stroke overall was reduced by a nonsignificant increase in hemorrhagic stroke (0.21%, $p > 0.1$). Aspirin did not significantly reduce the percentage of patients who died or were dependent at discharge ($p = 0.08$) and was associated with an excess of transfused or fatal extracranial bleeding compared with placebo (0.27%, $p = 0.02$). Concomitant therapy with thrombolysis (22%) and anticoagulants (17%) was not contraindicated in CAST; both could have increased the risk of hemorrhage and reduced the benefit of early aspirin therapy.

The International Stroke Trial (IST) *(13)* randomly assigned 19,345 patients to receive one of six different treatment regimens: 300 mg aspirin daily; 5000 IU (low-dose) subcutaneous heparin twice daily; 12,500 IU (medium-dose) subcutaneous heparin twice daily; aspirin plus low-dose heparin; aspirin plus medium-dose heparin; or no aspirin and no heparin (control group). Treatment was administered within 48 hours of acute stroke onset and was continued for 14 days or until death or discharge.

The major outcome events in patients allocated aspirin vs those allocated to avoid aspirin are outlined in Table 2. When the outcome in patients on aspirin is compared with that in patients randomly assigned to avoid aspirin (regardless of whether they received subcutaneous heparin), early secondary prevention with aspirin was beneficial. Aspirin therapy was associated with an absolute reduction of 1.1% in the rate of recurrent ischemic stroke ($p < 0.001$), and this benefit was not offset by an increased risk of hemorrhagic stroke. However, aspirin did significantly increase the risk of transfused or fatal extracranial bleeding by 0.5% ($p = 0.0004$). In contrast to CAST, aspirin did not reduce the rate of death during the study period in IST. The effect on the unadjusted percentage of patients dead or dependent at 6 months just failed to reach statistical significance ($p = 0.06$). In IST, 33% of patients did not have brain CT before randomization, and concomitant use of other nonsteroidal anti-inflammatory drugs (which theoretically could increase the risk of hemorrhagic complications associated with aspirin) was not prohibited. Additionally, patients randomly assigned to receive heparin did not have obligatory monitoring of their Activated Partial Thromboplastin Time (APTT). The authors justified this decision on the basis of the "low" bleeding rates on medium-dose heparin in two previous trials, despite a significant excess of bleeding on this dose of heparin in both of these studies *(16,17)*.

The trend in CAST and IST toward a beneficial effect of aspirin on the rate of death or dependency became significant in a meta-analysis that included

Table 2
Outcome Events (%) During the First 14 Days in IST

	Aspirin ($n = 9719$)	Avoid aspirin ($n = 9714$)
Deaths and likely causes		
Initial stroke	6.1	6.2
Recurrent ischemic stroke	0.9	0.9
Hemorrhagic stroke	0.2	0.2
Other	1.8	2.1
Total (any cause)	9.0	9.4
Fatal and non-fatal events		
Recurrent ischemic stroke	2.8	3.9[a]
Hemorrhagic stroke	0.9	0.8
Recurrent ischemic stroke or hemorrhagic stroke[b]	3.7	4.6[c]
Death or nonfatal stroke	11.3	12.4[d]
Transfused or fatal extracranial hemorrhage	1.1	0.6[a]

[a] $p < 0.001$.

[b] Hemorrhagic stroke includes symptomatic intracranial hemorrhage or symptomatic hemorrhagic transformation of infarct confirmed by CT scan, magnetic resonance imaging, or necropsy.

[c] $p < 0.01$.

[d] $p < 0.05$.

From ref. *13*.

the Multicenter Acute Stroke Trial–Italy data and was published with the CAST results *(14)*. Early aspirin (160–300 mg daily) significantly reduced the rate of recurrent ischemic stroke by 7 per 1000 ($p < 0.001$), the rate of death or nonfatal stroke by 9 per 1000 ($p = 0.001$), and the rate of death or dependency by 13 per 1000 ($p = 0.007$) compared with the control group. Thus, roughly 1 in 100 acute stroke patients benefits substantially from early aspirin treatment. Because aspirin is cheap and stroke is common, this small relative benefit translates into substantial clinical and cost benefit when applied in routine practice.

Long-Term Secondary Prevention With Aspirin in Ischemic Stroke and TIA

Four large randomized trials studied the benefit of aspirin in late secondary stroke prevention. The United Kingdom Transient Ischemic Attack (UK-TIA) trial compared the outcome of treatment with aspirin (300 or 1200 mg daily) or placebo in patients with a recent history of TIA or minor stroke; the mean duration of follow-up was 4 years *(18)*. There was no significant difference in efficacy between the two different doses of aspirin. After combining the two aspirin groups, there was a nonsignificant reduction of 15% in the odds of major stroke, myocardial infarction (MI), or vascular death with aspirin compared with placebo. More upper gastrointestinal (GI) symptoms occurred with 1200 mg compared with 300 mg aspirin daily (41 vs 31%, odds ratio 1.54).

The Swedish Aspirin Low-Dose Trial (SALT) compared the outcome of treatment with 75 mg of aspirin daily with placebo in patients with a recent TIA, minor ischemic stroke, or retinal artery occlusion *(19)*. Patients were followed up for a median duration of 32 months. Aspirin reduced the relative risk of stroke, MI, and vascular death by 17% compared with placebo ($p = 0.03$), the benefit of which outweighed the excess risk of severe bleeding ($p = 0.04$) and fatal hemorrhagic stroke ($p = 0.03$). However, for the end point of stroke, there was no significant reduction in risk associated with aspirin therapy ($p = 0.11$).

The Dutch TIA Trial compared the efficacy and tolerability of 30 vs 283 mg aspirin daily in patients with a TIA or minor ischemic stroke in the preceding 3 months; the mean follow-up period was 2.6 years *(20)*. The two doses of aspirin were equally effective at preventing nonfatal stroke, nonfatal MI, or vascular death, but minor bleeding, GI discomfort, and other minor adverse effects were significantly less common in the 30-mg group (17% risk reduction).

In the Second European Stroke Prevention Study (ESPS-2), 6602 patients with recent stroke or TIA were randomly assigned to one of four treatment arms: placebo, aspirin (25 mg twice daily), modified-release dipyridamole (200 mg twice daily), or aspirin plus dipyridamole *(21)*. This was the first study to show that very-low-dose aspirin (50 mg daily) was more effective than placebo in secondary stroke prevention. The relative risk of recurrent stroke (fatal or nonfatal) was reduced by 18.1% ($p = 0.013$), and the combined risk of stroke or death was reduced by 13.2% ($p = 0.016$). Bleeding from any site was approximately twice as common in the two aspirin groups (8.2% in the aspirin-alone group; 8.7% in the aspirin plus dipyridamole group) compared with placebo (4.5%). However, this was responsible for treatment withdrawal in only 1.2% of patients on aspirin alone, and 1.3% of patients on aspirin plus dipyridamole.

In a meta-analysis of 10 randomized trials of aspirin compared with placebo for TIA or nondisabling stroke *(22)*, the relative risk reduction for subsequent vascular events was 13% with low-dose (<100 mg daily), 9% with medium-dose (300 mg daily), and 14% with high-dose aspirin treatment (>900 mg daily). The authors concluded that doses of aspirin between 30 and 1500 mg daily were equally effective for secondary prevention after cerebral ischemia, but cautioned that true differences in efficacy between the treatment regimens could not be excluded because of wide confidence intervals. These findings are also consistent with those of a meta-regression analysis *(23)*.

Furthermore, these benefits were quantified in the latest meta-analysis by The Antithrombotic Trialists Collaboration *(24)*. This group analyzed data from 197 trials of short- or long-term antiplatelet therapy for any vascular indication available by September 1997. Aspirin (≤75 mg to 1500 mg daily) was the most widely tested drug included in the analysis *(25)*. The reported odds reductions in outcome events associated with treatment translate into slightly lower relative risk reductions cited in other studies *(22,26)*. Antiplatelet therapy was associated with a proportional odds reduction in important vascular events (nonfatal stroke, nonfatal MI, vascular death, or death of indeterminate etiology) of 22% in patients with a history of TIA or stroke ($p < 0.0001$) *(24)*. Low-dose (75–150 mg daily) or medium-dose (160–325 mg daily) aspirin were similarly effective at preventing recurrent vascular events during follow-up as higher doses (500–1500 mg daily) among patients at high risk of vascular events (but not specifically those with prior TIA or stroke) *(18,24)*. The benefit of secondary prevention with daily aspirin doses of less than 75 mg was less clear ($p = 0.05$) *(24)*.

Summary of Aspirin Trials

One hundred-sixty to 300 mg of aspirin daily, administered within 48 hours of an acute ischemic stroke, reduces the relative risk of recurrent ischemic stroke in the first 14 to 28 days by 24–28% *(13,14)*. However, long-term secondary prevention with 30 to 1500 mg of aspirin daily reduces the relative risk of subsequent vascular events (including ischemic stroke) by only 13 to 18% *(21,22)*. Given the uncertainty about the efficacy of very-low-dose aspirin (<75 mg daily) in patients at high risk of vascular events, low- or medium-dose aspirin should be used in patients with ischemic stroke or TIA.

Secondary Prevention With Aspirin Therapy in Subtypes of Ischemic Stroke and Asymptomatic Carotid Stenosis

Symptomatic Severe Carotid Stenosis

Both the European Carotid Surgery Trial (ECST) and the North American Symptomatic Carotid Endarterectomy Trial (NASCET) compared the outcome of treatment with carotid endarterectomy to best medical care in patients who had a recent ischemic stroke, TIA, or amaurosis fugax in association with more than 70% angiographic internal carotid artery stenosis.

Of medically treated patients, 79 and 94% were taking aspirin therapy during follow-up in ECST and NASCET, respectively *(27,28)*. Despite aspirin therapy in the majority of these patients, the risk of major ipsilateral stroke was 20.6% over 3 years in ECST and 26% over 2 years in NASCET. This may be partly related to the fact that an ulcerated atherosclerotic plaque causing vessel stenosis exposes platelets to increased shear stress *(29)*, and aspirin has been reported to be relatively ineffective at preventing shear-induced platelet aggregation *(30)*.

Recently, the Aspirin and Carotid Endarterectomy (ACE) Trial Collaborators reported that patients undergoing carotid endarterectomy benefit more from lower than higher doses of aspirin in the perioperative period *(31)*. The combined rate of stroke, MI, or death at 3 months was significantly lower at 6.2% in patients receiving lower dose aspirin (81 or 325 mg) compared with 8.4% with higher doses of 650 or 1300 mg daily ($p = 0.03$).

Cardioembolic Ischemic Stroke in Association With Nonvalvular Atrial Fibrillation

Primary stroke prevention in patients with atrial fibrillation is discussed in Chapter 12. Warfarin is significantly more effective than aspirin at preventing further stroke in patients who have had a recent TIA or minor ischemic stroke associated with nonvalvular atrial fibrillation *(32)*. In the European Atrial Fibrillation Trial, 1007 patients were randomly assigned to receive anticoagulation (target international normalized ratio 3.0, $n = 225$), aspirin (300 mg daily, $n = 404$), or placebo ($n = 378$) within 3 months (43% within 2 weeks) of experiencing a TIA or minor ischemic stroke *(32)*. The annual risk of recurrent stroke was reduced from 12% with placebo to 4% with warfarin ($p < 0001$) *(32)*, but aspirin did not significantly reduce the risk of recurrent stroke compared with placebo (10 vs 12% per annum, $p = 0.31$).

In a meta-analysis of the IST and CAST data, early aspirin therapy significantly reduced the risk of recurrent ischemic stroke in patients without atrial fibrillation, but the risk reduction in stroke patients with atrial fibrillation did not reach statistical significance *(33)*.

Lacunar Ischemic Stroke and Stroke of Indeterminate Etiology

A meta-analysis of the data from CAST and IST suggests that early aspirin therapy is similarly effective in patients with lacunar or nonlacunar ischemic stroke syndromes *(33)*. There are no reliable data on the efficacy of long-term aspirin therapy in patients with lacunar stroke or stroke of indeterminate etiology. Furthermore, the diagnosis of lacunar stroke may be inaccurate as a small, but significant, percentage of small vessel strokes are caused by emboli.

Aspirin Therapy in Patients With Asymptomatic Carotid Stenosis

The Asymptomatic Cervical Bruit Study investigated the outcome of treatment with aspirin compared with placebo in patients with asymptomatic carotid stenosis *(34)*. Three hundred seventy-two patients with more than 50% carotid stenosis on duplex ultrasonography were randomly allocated to receive 325 mg aspirin daily (n = 188) or placebo (n = 184). The mean duration of follow-up was 2.4 years. The primary end point was the composite outcome of TIA, stroke, MI, unstable angina, or death; the rates of stroke and TIA were included among the secondary end points in the study. Approximately one-third of patients in each group had 80 to 99% carotid stenosis. There was no significant difference in the rate of occurrence of the primary (composite) outcome, or the rates of stroke or TIA considered separately, between groups. The low rate of outcome events, the small sample size, and the small proportion of patients with more than 80% carotid stenosis limit the applicability of these results to patients with asymptomatic severe (>70%) carotid stenosis. Therefore, it is reasonable to treat asymptomatic severe carotid stenosis patients with long-term aspirin therapy unless data become available to suggest an alternative therapeutic strategy.

DIPYRIDAMOLE

Mechanism of Action

Dipyridamole exerts its antiplatelet effects by inhibiting phosphodiesterase E5 in platelets, thus increasing intraplatelet levels of cyclic guanosine monophosphate and cyclic adenosine monophosphate (cAMP) *(21)*, and by inhibiting the uptake and metabolism of adenosine by erythrocytes and endothelial cells *(34)* (Fig. 2). This increases the availability of adenosine (a platelet-inhibiting vasodilator) in the vascular microenvironment. Dipyridamole has also been reported to inhibit cAMP phosphodiesterases in platelets, thus increasing intraplatelet cAMP levels even further *(35)*. Additionally, there is in vitro evidence to suggest that dipyridamole mediates some of its antithrombotic effect by its action on the endothelium itself, perhaps by enhancing the effects of nitric oxide *(36)*. Dipyridamole also inhibits lipid peroxidation and may protect the endothelium from damage by peroxiradicals *(36)*.

Dipyridamole Monotherapy and Combination Therapy With Aspirin and Dipyridamole

Early trials investigating the relative effects of the combination of dipyridamole and aspirin vs aspirin alone were inconclusive, mainly because of their small sample size *(37,38)*. However, the European Stroke Prevention Study (ESPS) found that the combination of 225 mg dipyridamole and 990 mg aspi-

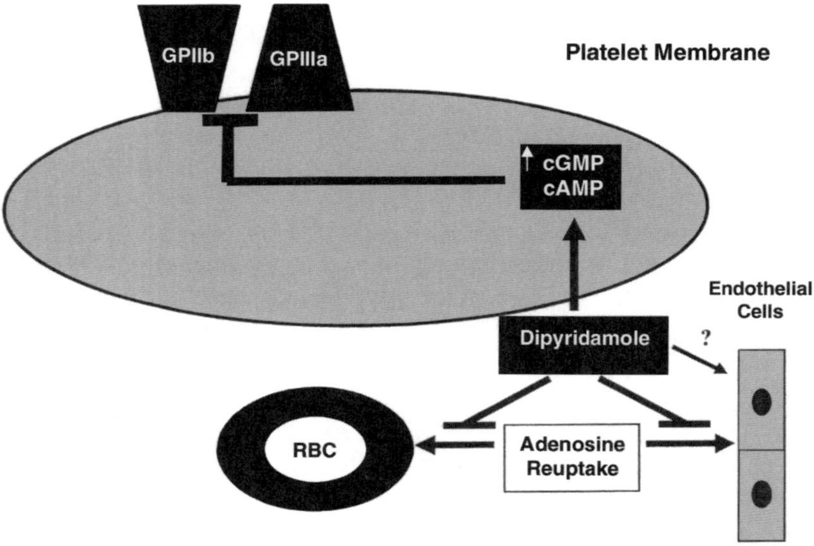

Fig. 2. Mechanisms of action of dipyridamole (RBC, red blood cell).

rin daily reduced the relative risk of death or recurrent stroke by 33.5% compared with placebo in patients with a recent TIA or ischemic stroke ($p < 0.001$) *(38)*. However, this study had a number of methodological flaws and did not include a dipyridamole-only or an aspirin-only arm.

ESPS-2 showed that modified-release dipyridamole (200 mg twice daily), aspirin (25 mg twice daily), or a combination of dipyridamole and aspirin were superior to placebo in secondary stroke prevention *(21)*. The trial design and the results from the aspirin-alone arm of the trial were discussed in the section on long-term secondary prevention with aspirin in ischemic stroke and TIA. Modified-release dipyridamole is available as monotherapy in Europe, but only as a combination tablet with 25 mg of aspirin in the United States (Aggrenox®). In comparison with placebo, the overall reduction in stroke risk was 16% with dipyridamole alone, which was very similar to the 18% reduction associated with aspirin alone. The combination of dipyridamole and aspirin led to a 37% reduction in stroke risk compared with placebo; this represented greater benefit than treatment with either agent alone (Fig. 3). The relative risk reductions for the combined end point of stroke or death were 15% with dipyridamole and 24% with combination therapy. However, there was no significant reduction in the rate of subsequent MI with any of the treatment regimens.

Treatment withdrawal occurred in 22% of patients in the placebo or aspirin-only groups and in 29% of patients on dipyridamole (alone or in combi-

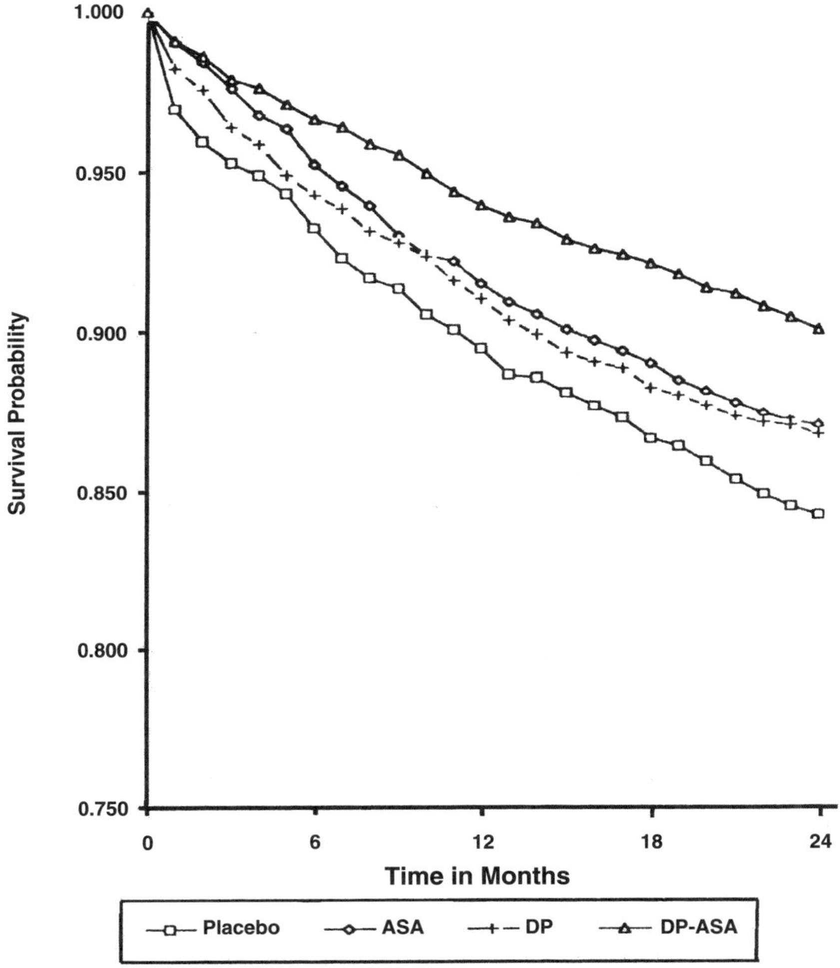

Fig. 3. Survival curves showing the probability of survival free of stroke over a 2-year treatment period on treatment with placebo, aspirin (ASA), dipyridamole (DP), or combination therapy (DP-ASA) in ESPS-2. (Redrawn from ref. *21*.)

nation with aspirin). The most common adverse events leading to treatment withdrawal were headache (8%) and gastrointestinal disturbance (6–7%) in the dipyridamole groups. There was no excess bleeding in patients treated with dipyridamole alone compared with placebo (4.7 vs 4.5%).

A meta-analysis of 15 trials supported the view that the combination of dipyridamole and aspirin is superior to aspirin alone in preventing nonfatal stroke in patients with a history of vascular disease *(39)*. Combination therapy significantly reduced the odds of nonfatal recurrent stroke by 23% compared with aspirin alone, but did not significantly reduce the odds of having a subsequent MI or other vascular events. Because ESPS-2 was the first study to show an unequivocal benefit of combination therapy with dipyridamole and aspirin over aspirin alone and because of the unexplained and disparate effects of dipyridamole on the cerebrovascular and coronary circulation, further studies are warranted to confirm these findings. An ongoing study (European and Australian Stroke Prevention in Reversible Ischemia Trial [ESPRIT]) is addressing these issues *(40)*.

THIENOPYRIDINE DERIVATIVES: TICLOPIDINE AND CLOPIDOGREL

Mechanism of Action

Adenosine diphosphate (ADP) is a platelet agonist with actions that are mediated by three distinct platelet receptors *(41–43)*. Ticlopidine and clopidogrel are thienopyridine derivatives that selectively and irreversibly inhibit the $P2Y_{12}$ ADP receptor on platelets, thus interfering with ADP-induced activation of the GPIIb/IIIa receptor complex (Fig. 4). These agents may have the potential to be particularly useful in stroke patients with platelet activation induced by shear stress, in whom elevated circulating levels of ADP are expected *(44)* (e.g., in patients with symptomatic severe carotid stenosis or in patients undergoing carotid endovascular treatment).

Ticlopidine

Ticlopidine is inactive in vitro and must undergo hepatic metabolism by the cytochrome P450-1A enzyme system to exhibit its antiplatelet effects *(45,46)*. It is rapidly and extensively metabolized after oral administration, with 13 metabolites identified in humans *(12)*. Its maximal antiplatelet effects occur after 5 to 6 days of repeated oral therapy *(44)*. It has been shown to be more effective than placebo in reducing vascular events *(47)* and more effective than aspirin in secondary stroke prevention in patients with recent TIA or minor stroke *(48)*.

In the Canadian American Ticlopidine Study, patients with recent noncardioembolic ischemic stroke were randomly assigned to receive either 250 mg ticlopidine twice daily (n = 525) or placebo (n = 528) (average follow-up 24 months) *(47)*. Ticlopidine reduced the combined risk of stroke, myocardial infarction, or vascular death by 23% compared with placebo ($p = 0.02$).

In the Ticlopidine Aspirin Stroke Study, the outcome of treatment with ticlopidine (250 mg twice daily) was compared with that of aspirin (650 mg twice daily) in patients with a history of TIA or minor stroke (excluding

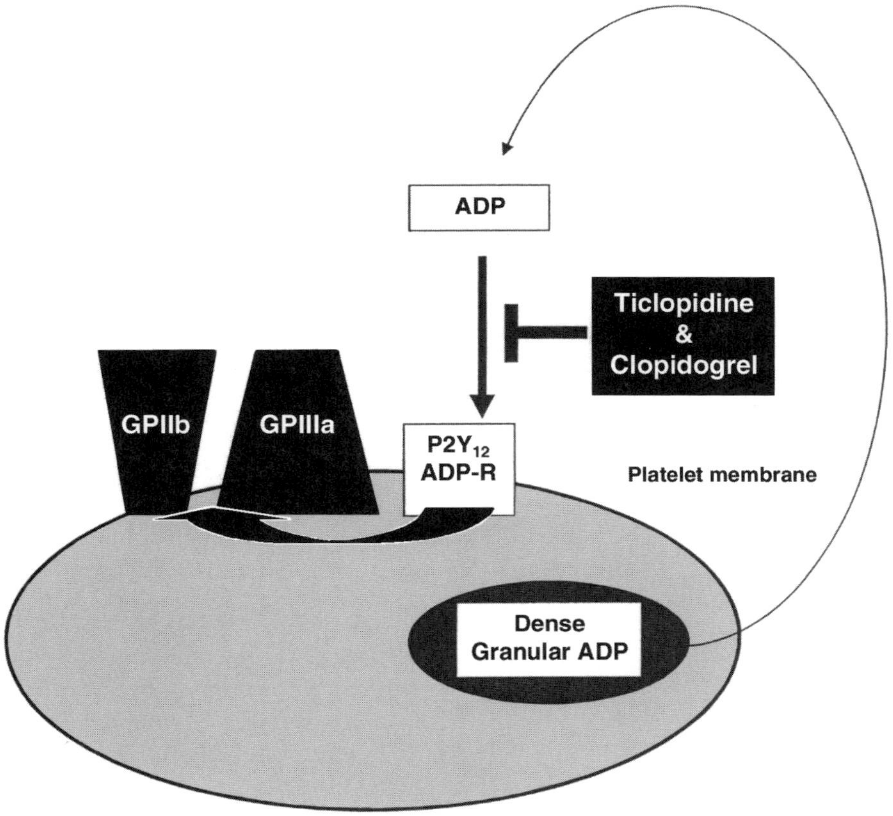

Fig 4. Mechanism of action of the thienopyridines ticlopidine and clopidogrel (ADP, adenosine diphosphate released from platelets and erythrocytes; GpIIb/IIIa, glycoprotein IIb/IIIa platelet receptor; $P2Y_{12}$ ADP-R, $P2Y_{12}$ ADP platelet receptor).

presumed cardiac embolism) in the preceding 3 months *(48)*. Ticlopidine significantly reduced the 3-year risk of recurrent stroke by 21% compared with aspirin. However, adverse events were common in the ticlopidine group. Diarrhea occurred in 20% of patients, requiring discontinuation of the drug in 6%. Gastritis and GI hemorrhage were more common in the aspirin group, but "all-site" hemorrhage was equally common with ticlopidine (9%) and aspirin (10%). Neutropenia occurred in 2.3% of patients on ticlopidine and was severe in 0.9%, requiring regular hematological monitoring of patients. In most cases, neutropenia was first noted between 1 and 3 months after commencing treatment and resolved within 3 weeks of cessation of the drug. Ticlopidine treatment was associated with the development of hypercholesterolemia (mean increase in total cholesterol of 9 ± 20%), although the long-term implications of this finding are unknown.

A rare, but important, adverse effect associated with ticlopidine therapy is thrombotic thrombocytopenic purpura (TTP). Ticlopidine-associated TTP has an estimated incidence of between 1 in 1600 to 1 in 5000 *(49)* and a mortality rate of up to 21%. Ticlopidine is now rarely used for secondary stroke prevention because of the more favorable side effect profile associated with its chemically related compound, clopidogrel.

Clopidogrel

Clopidogrel is a newer thienopyridine derivative, chemically related to ticlopidine, but with antithrombotic activity greater than ticlopidine in animal models *(50)*. Clopidogrel is also inactive in its native form, but it is metabolized in the liver to form an active thiol derivative that covalently binds to the $P2Y_{12}$ receptor in vivo *(46,51)*. Although the antiplatelet effects of clopidogrel have been reported to be maximal after 3 to 5 days of therapy *(45)*, use of a loading dose (150 to 300 mg) produces a more rapid and stable inhibitory effect than that seen with 75 mg daily *(52)*.

A modest clinical benefit of clopidogrel over aspirin has been demonstrated in the Clopidogrel Versus Aspirin in Patients at Risk of Ischemic Events (CAPRIE) trial *(50)*. In this trial, 19,185 patients with recent ischemic stroke, MI, or symptomatic peripheral atherosclerotic disease were randomly assigned to receive clopidogrel (75 mg daily) or aspirin (325 mg daily). The relative risk reduction in the average annual incidence of ischemic stroke, MI, or vascular death was 8.7% with clopidogrel compared with aspirin (absolute RR of 0.51%, $p = 0.04$) (Fig. 5).

The trend toward a reduction in the relative risk of subsequent events with clopidogrel compared with aspirin in the subgroup of patients presenting with stroke was not statistically significant (7.3%, $p = 0.26$). However, the study was not adequately powered to detect treatment effects in different subgroups. In comparison with aspirin, severe rash (0.3%) and diarrhea (4.5%) occurred more commonly with clopidogrel, but there was no excess of neutropenia (0.1%) or hypercholesterolemia. GI hemorrhage was less common with clopidogrel than aspirin (1.99 vs 2.66%, $p < 0.05$), and there was a nonsignificant trend toward a lower rate of intracranial hemorrhage with clopidogrel (0.35 vs 0.49%, $p = 0.23$). There have been reports of TTP associated with clopidogrel *(49)* with an estimated incidence of approx 1 in 15,000 users *(53)*. The majority of cases occurred with 2 weeks of initiation of treatment, although some of the reported cases were also receiving other drugs that may have contributed to the development of the syndrome *(49,54)*.

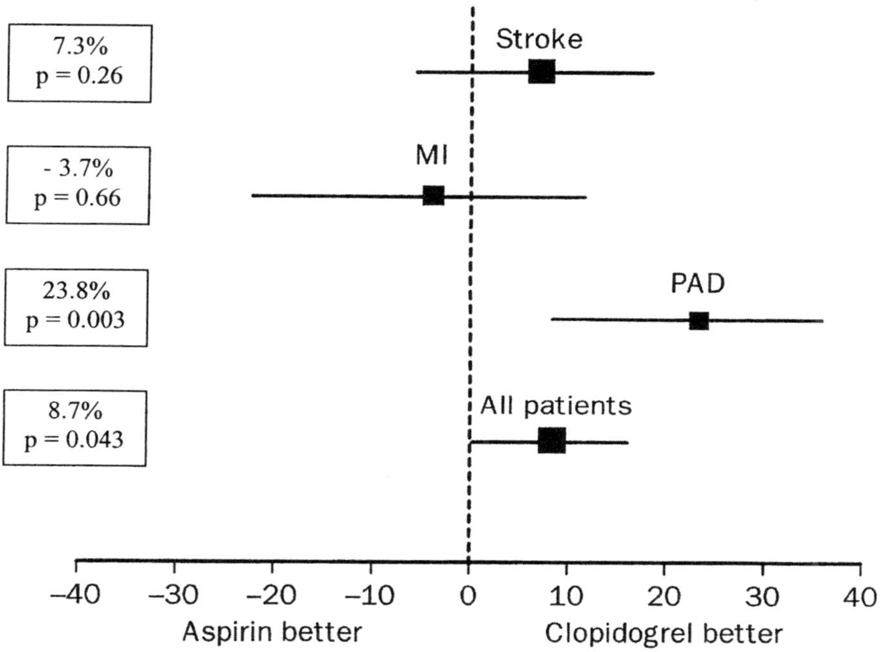

Fig. 5. Percentage relative risk reduction in the primary outcome of ischemic stroke, MI, or vascular death in the subgroups of patients presenting with stroke, MI, or peripheral arterial disease (PAD) in the CAPRIE Trial. (Data redrawn from ref. *50*.)

The mortality rate among patients with clopidogrel-associated TTP who were treated with plasma exchange was 9% in one series *(49)*. It has been suggested that weekly blood counts be performed in the first few weeks of initiating therapy *(53)*.

The MATCH (Management of Atherothrombosis With Clopidogrel in High Risk Patients With Recent TIA or Stroke) trial is compared the safety and efficacy of combination therapy with aspirin and clopidogrel with clopidogrel alone in high-risk patients with ischemic stroke or TIA. Recruitment was completed in 2002, and the results are pending.

GLYCOPROTEIN IIB/IIIA ANTAGONISTS

Platelet-to-platelet aggregation is ultimately mediated by ligand binding to the glycoprotein IIb/IIIa (GpIIb/IIIa) receptor *(55)*. Platelet activation leads to a conformational change in this receptor that facilitates ligand binding, and this change is the final common pathway in platelet aggregation *(56)*. GpIIb/IIIa antagonists bind to this receptor on both resting and activated platelets. Intravenous preparations have improved outcome in acute coronary syndromes and in patients undergoing percutaneous coronary interventional procedures *(57)*.

The results of the first randomized, placebo-controlled, dose-escalation trial of an intravenous GpIIb/IIIa antagonist (abciximab) in acute ischemic stroke have been published *(58)*. In this trial, 54 patients were randomly assigned to receive one of four doses of abciximab, and 20 patients were randomly assigned to receive placebo within 24 hours of onset of CT-proven ischemic stroke. Subsequent CT scans were obtained 24 to 36 hours after administration of the study agent and thereafter at the discretion of the treating physician. The patients were followed up for 3 months. There was a trend toward a lower rate of stroke recurrence (2 vs 5%) and a higher rate of functional recovery at 3 months with abciximab compared with placebo. The rate of asymptomatic hemorrhagic transformation of the original infarct noted on CT was much higher with abciximab therapy (19 vs 5%). However, no clinical deterioration was associated with this hemorrhagic change. Seven percent of patients treated with abciximab had moderate thrombocytopenia during the first 5 days of treatment, but the rates of extracranial or intracranial hemorrhage were not increased.

Trials of oral GpIIb/IIIa antagonists in patients with ischemic heart disease have shown little benefit to date *(59)*. The Blockade of the glycoprotein IIb/IIIa Receptor to Avoid Vascular Occlusion (BRAVO) trial was the first study to examine an oral GpIIb/IIIa antagonist (lotrafiban) for the secondary prevention of vascular events in patients with cerebrovascular disease *(60)*. The study included patients with recent ischemic stroke or TIA, recent acute myocardial infarction or unstable angina, or peripheral vascular disease in association with either cerebrovascular or ischemic heart disease (double bed vascular disease). Overall, 41% of subjects had cerebrovascular disease at study entry. Patients were randomly assigned to receive lotrafiban (n = 4600) or matching placebo (n = 4590), and were concomitantly treated with aspirin (75 to 325 mg daily), with the prescribed dose left to the discretion of the treating physician. The trial was prematurely discontinued after a median follow-up period of 366 days because of a higher mortality rate with lotrafiban than placebo (3 vs 2.3%), with this difference primarily accounted for by an excess of vascular deaths with lotrafiban (n = 107) compared with placebo (n = 78). The rate of stroke during follow-up was similar with lotrafiban and placebo (2.1 vs 2.4%, $p = 0.35$), and the lotrafiban group did not have an increased risk of hemorrhagic stroke or hemorrhagic infarct transformation. However, significant thrombocytopenia and other serious bleeding complications were more common with lotrafiban ($p = 0.001$) *(60)*.

Therefore, there is currently insufficient evidence to support the routine use of intravenous GpIIb/IIIa antagonists for early secondary prevention, and there is no evidence to support the use of oral GpIIb/IIIa antagonists for long-term secondary prevention after ischemic stroke or TIA.

SUMMARY

Table 3 presents recommendations for use of antiplatelet agents in clinical practice.

Table 3
Recommendations for Use of Antiplatelet Agents in Clinical Practice

Aspirin
Early secondary prevention: Within 48 hours of onset of ischemic stroke in patients in whom intracranial hemorrhage has been excluded by urgent CT or magnetic resonance imaging, assuming no contraindication to therapy exists (aspirin intolerance or allergy, other antithrombotic medications, significant thrombocytopenia, bleeding disorder, active peptic ulcer or gastritis). (Based on IST/CAST *[13,14]*, data and American Heart Association *[34a]* recommendations.)

Late secondary prevention: Because aspirin has proven benefit in the long-term secondary prevention of stroke and other vascular events, it is reasonable to continue treatment indefinitely unless a clear contraindication to therapy develops. (From ref. *26*.)

Dose: The optimal dose of aspirin is unclear. Because at least 160 mg (and perhaps 300 mg) daily is required for days to 2 weeks for maximal inhibition of TXA_2 biosynthesis, initial treatment with 325 mg daily for 2 weeks is reasonable, although a lower dose (75–150 mg daily) may subsequently suffice. (From refs. *26* and *61*.).

Dipyridamole
Late secondary prevention: Combination therapy with aspirin (25 mg twice daily) and dipyridamole (200 mg modified-release formulation twice daily) was superior to aspirin 25 mg twice daily in the secondary prevention of stroke or the combined outcome of stroke or death, but not MI, in the ESPS-2 trial. Based on these data, it is reasonable to use a combination of aspirin and dipyridamole as initial therapy for long-term secondary prevention of stroke or death.

Because the main evidence for the use of combination therapy with aspirin and dipyridamole is based on a single trial, it is also reasonable to reserve this regimen for patients who have a further event on aspirin monotherapy, pending confirmation of benefit in further trials. (From American Heart Association guidelines.)

(continued)

Table 3 (Continued)

Clopidogrel
Based on the CAPRIE study, it is reasonable to reserve clopidogrel for the following indications: patients with ischemic stroke or TIA who are intolerant of, or allergic to, aspirin or dipyridamole; to replace aspirin or aspirin and dipyridamole in patients who have a further vascular event on these agents, especially in patients with a history of ischemic heart disease. Although substantial variation in physician practice exists, some physicians use clopidogrel in conditions in which shear-induced platelet activation is likely to be present (e.g., in patients with severe carotid stenosis waiting for carotid endarterectomy or endovascular treatment and following carotid angioplasty or stenting). Use of clopidogrel in these situations is empiric because insufficient trial data are available to make an evidence-based recommendation.

REFERENCES

1. Warlow CP, Dennis MS, van Gijn J, et al. What pathological type of stroke is it? In: Warlow CP, Dennis MS, van Gijn J, et al., eds. Stroke. A Practical Guide to Management. Oxford, UK: Blackwell Science, 1996:146–189.
2. Burn J, Dennis M, Bamford J, Sandercock P, Wade D, Warlow C. Long-term risk of recurrent stroke after a first-ever stroke. The Oxfordshire Community Stroke Project. Stroke 1994;25:333–337.
3. Warlow CP, Dennis MS, van Gijn J, et al. A practical approach to the management of stroke patients. In: Warlow CP, Dennis MS, van Gijn J, et al., eds. Stroke. A Practical Guide to Management. Oxford, UK: Blackwell Science, 1996:360–384.
4. Warlow CP. Epidemiology of stroke. Lancet 1998;352(Suppl 3):1–4.
5. McCabe DJH, Brown MM. Early prevention of stroke recurrence. In: Bogousslavsky J, ed. Drug Therapy for Stroke Prevention. London: Taylor and Francis, 2001:168–188.
6. Grau AJ, Ruf A, Vogt A, et al. Increased fraction of circulating activated platelets in acute and previous cerebrovascular ischemia. Thromb Haemost 1998;80:298–301.
7. Meiklejohn DJ, Vickers MA, Morrison ER, et al. In vivo platelet activation in atherothrombotic stroke is not determined by polymorphisms of human platelet glycoprotein IIIa or Ib. Br J Haematol 2001;112:621–631.
8. Yamazaki M, Uchiyama S, Iwata M. Measurement of platelet fibrinogen binding and p-selectin expression by flow cytometry in patients with cerebral infarction. Thromb Res 2001;104:197–205.
9. Roth GJ, Calverley DC. Aspirin, platelets, and thrombosis: theory and practice. Blood 1994;83:885–898.
10. Weber AA, Zimmermann KC, Meyer-Kirchrath J, Schror K. Cyclooxygenase-2 in human platelets as a possible factor in aspirin resistance. Lancet 1999;353:900.
11. FitzGerald GA, Patrono C. The coxibs, selective inhibitors of cyclooxygenase-2. N Engl J Med 2001;345:433–442.
12. Harker LA. Therapeutic inhibition of platelet function in stroke. Cerebrovasc Dis 1998;8(Suppl 5):8–18.

13. International Stroke Trial Collaborative Group. The International Stroke Trial (IST): a randomized trial of aspirin, subcutaneous heparin, both, or neither among 19435 patients with acute ischemic stroke. International Stroke Trial Collaborative Group. Lancet 1997;349:1569–1581.
14. CAST (Chinese Acute Stroke Trial) Collaborative Group. CAST: randomized placebo-controlled trial of early aspirin use in 20,000 patients with acute ischemic stroke. Lancet 1997;349:1641–1649.
15. Multicenter Acute Stroke Trial—Italy (MAST-I) Group. Randomized controlled trial of streptokinase, aspirin, and combination of both in treatment of acute ischemic stroke. Lancet 1995;346:1509–1514.
16. Gruppo Italiano per lo Studio della Sopravvivenza nell'Infarto Miocardico. GISSI-2: a factorial randomized trial of alteplase vs streptokinase and heparin vs no heparin among 12,490 patients with acute myocardial infarction. Lancet 1990;336:65–71.
17. ISIS-3 (Third International Study of Infarct Survival) Collaborative Group. ISIS-3: a randomized comparison of streptokinase vs tissue plasminogen activator vs anistreplase and of aspirin plus heparin vs aspirin alone among 41,299 cases of suspected acute myocardial infarction. Lancet 1992;339:753–770.
18. Farrell B, Godwin J, Richards S, Warlow C. The United Kingdom Transient Ischemic Attack (UK-TIA) aspirin trial: final results. J Neurol Neurosurg Psychiatry 1991; 54:1044–1054.
19. The SALT Collaborative Group. Swedish Aspirin Low-Dose Trial (SALT) of 75 mg aspirin as secondary prophylaxis after cerebrovascular ischemic events. Lancet 1991;338:1345–1349.
20. The Dutch TIA Trial Study Group. A comparison of two doses of aspirin (30 mg vs 283 mg a day) in patients after a transient ischemic attack or minor ischemic stroke. N Engl J Med 1991;325:1261–1266.
21. Diener HC, Cunha L, Forbes C, Sivenius J, Smets P, Lowenthal A. European Stroke Prevention Study. 2. Dipyridamole and acetylsalicylic acid in the secondary prevention of stroke. J Neurol Sci 1996;143:1–13.
22. Algra A, van Gijn J. Aspirin at any dose above 30 mg offers only modest protection after cerebral ischemia. J Neurol Neurosurg Psychiatry 1996;60:197–199.
23. Johnson ES, Lanes SF., Wentworth CE III, Satterfield MH, Abebe BL, Dicker LW. A metaregression analysis of the dose-response effect of aspirin on stroke. Arch Intern Med 1999;159:1248–1253.
24. Antithrombotic Trialists' Collaboration. Collaborative meta-analysis of randomized trials of antiplatelet therapy for prevention of death, myocardial infarction, and stroke in high risk patients. BMJ 2002;324:71–86.
25. Warlow C. Aspirin should be first-line antiplatelet therapy in the secondary prevention of stroke. Stroke 2002;33:2137–2138.
26. Antiplatelet Trialists' Collaboration. Collaborative overview of randomized trials of antiplatelet therapy—I: Prevention of death, myocardial infarction, and stroke by prolonged antiplatelet therapy in various categories of patients. BMJ 1994;308: 81–106.
27. European Carotid Surgery Trialists' Collaborative Group. Randomized trial of endarterectomy for recently symptomatic carotid stenosis: final results of the MRC European Carotid Surgery Trial (ECST). Lancet 1998;351:1379–1387.

28. North American Symptomatic Carotid Endarterectomy Trial Collaborators. Beneficial effect of carotid endarterectomy in symptomatic patients with high-grade carotid stenosis. N Engl J Med 1991;325:445–453.
29. Kroll MH, Hellums JD, McIntire LV, Schafer AI, Moake JL. Platelets and shear stress. Blood 1996;88:1525–1541.
30. Uchiyama S, Yamazaki M, Maruyama S, et al. Shear-induced platelet aggregation in cerebral ischemia. Stroke 1994;25:1547–1551.
31. Taylor DW, Barnett HJ, Haynes RB, et al. Low-dose and high-dose acetylsalicylic acid for patients undergoing carotid endarterectomy: a randomized controlled trial. ASA and Carotid Endarterectomy (ACE) Trial Collaborators. Lancet 1999;353: 2179–2184.
32. EAFT (European Atrial Fibrillation Trial) Study Group. Secondary prevention in non-rheumatic atrial fibrillation after transient ischemic attack or minor stroke. Lancet 1993;342:1255–1262.
33. Chen ZM, Sandercock P, Pan HC, et al. Indications for early aspirin use in acute ischemic stroke: a combined analysis of 40,000 randomized patients from the Chinese Acute Stroke Trial and the International Stroke Trial. On behalf of the CAST and IST collaborative groups. Stroke 2000;31:1240–1249.
34. Coté R, Battista RN, Abrahamowicz M, Langlois Y, Bourque F, Mackey A. Lack of effect of aspirin in asymptomatic patients with carotid bruits and substantial carotid narrowing. The Asymptomatic Cervical Bruit Study Group. Ann Intern Med 1995;123:649–655.
34a. Wolf PA, Clagett P, Easton JD, et al. Preventing stroke in patients with prior stroke and transient ischemic attack. Stroke 1999;30:1991–1994.
35. FitzGerald G.A. Dipyridamole. N Engl J Med 1987;316:1247–1257.
36. Eisert WG. Near-field amplification of antithrombotic effects of dipyridamole through vessel wall cells. Neurology 2001;57:S20–S23.
37. Diener HC. Antiplatelet drugs in secondary prevention of stroke. Int J Clin Pract 1998;52:91–97.
38. ESPS Group. European Stroke Prevention Study. Stroke 1990;21:1122–1130.
39. Wilterdink JL, Easton JD. Dipyridamole plus aspirin in cerebrovascular disease. Arch Neurol 1999;56:1087–1092.
40. ESPRIT investigators. Anticoagulants vs aspirin and the combination of aspirin and dipyridamole vs aspirin only in patients with transient ischemic attacks or nondisabling ischemic stroke: ESPRIT (European and Australian Stroke Prevention in Reversible Ischemia Trial). Major ongoing stroke trials [abstract]. Stroke 1999;30: 1301.
41. Daniel JL, Dangelmaier C, Jin J, Ashby B, Smith JB, Kunapuli SP. Molecular basis for ADP-induced platelet activation. I. Evidence for three distinct ADP receptors on human platelets. J Biol Chem 1998;273:2024–2029.
42. Jin J, Daniel JL, Kunapuli SP. Molecular basis for ADP-induced platelet activation. II. The P2Y1 receptor mediates ADP-induced intracellular calcium mobilization and shape change in platelets. J Biol Chem 1998;273:2030–2034.
43. Hollopeter G, Jantzen HM, Vincent D, et al. Identification of the platelet ADP receptor targeted by antithrombotic drugs. Nature 2001;409:202–207.
44. Schršr K. The basic pharmacology of ticlopidine and clopidogel. Platelets 1993;4: 252–261.

45. Quinn MJ, Fitzgerald DJ. Ticlopidine and clopidogrel. Circulation 1999;100:1667–1672.
46. Gachet C. ADP receptors of platelets and their inhibition. Thromb Haemost 2001; 86:222–232.
47. Gent M, Blakely JA, Easton JD, et al. The Canadian American Ticlopidine Study (CATS) in thromboembolic stroke. Lancet 1989;1:1215–1220.
48. Hass WK, Easton JD, Adams HP Jr, et al. A randomized trial comparing ticlopidine hydrochloride with aspirin for the prevention of stroke in high-risk patients. Ticlopidine Aspirin Stroke Study Group. N Engl J Med 1989;321:501–507.
49. Bennett CL, Connors JM,Carwile JM, et al. Thrombotic thrombocytopenic purpura associated with clopidogrel. N Engl J Med 2000;342:1773–1777.
50. CAPRIE Steering Committee. A randomized, blinded, trial of Clopidogrel Versus Aspirin in Patients at Risk of Ischemic Events (CAPRIE). Lancet 1996;348:1329–1339.
51. Savi P, Pereillo JM, Uzabiaga MF, et al. Identification and biological activity of the active metabolite of clopidogrel. Thromb Haemost 2000;84:891–896.
52. Savcic M, Hauert J, Bachmann F, Wyld PJ, Geudelin B, Cariou R. Clopidogrel loading dose regimens: kinetic profile of pharmacodynamic response in healthy subjects. Semin Thromb Hemost 1999;25(Suppl 2):15–19.
53. Bennett CL, Connors JM, Moake JL. Clopidogrel and thrombotic thrombocytopenic purpura [letter (response)]. N Engl J Med 2000;343:1193–1194.
54. Cheung RT. Clopidogrel and thrombotic thrombocytopenic purpura. N Engl J Med 2000;343:1192–1194.
55. Wagner CL, Mascelli MA, Neblock DS, Weisman HF, Coller BS, Jordan RE. (1996) Analysis of GPIIb/IIIa receptor number by quantification of 7E3 binding to human platelets. Blood 88, 907–914.
56. Moran N, FitzGerald GA. Mechanisms of action of antiplatelet drugs. In: Colman RW, Hirsh J, Marder VJ, Salzman EW, eds. Haemostasis and Thrombosis: Basic Principles and Clinical Practice. Philadelphia: J. B. Lippincott, 1994:1623–1637.
57. Topol EJ, Byzova TV, Plow EF. Platelet GPIIb-IIIa blockers. Lancet 1999;353: 227–231.
58. The Abciximab in Ischemic Stroke Investigators. Abciximab in acute ischemic stroke: a randomized, double-blind, placebo-controlled, dose-escalation study. Stroke 2000;31:601–609.
59. Coller BS. Anti-GPIIb/IIIa drugs: current strategies and future directions. Thromb Haemost 2001;86:427–443.
60. Topol EJ, Easton D, Harrington RA, et al. Randomized, double-blind, placebo-controlled international trial of oral IIb/IIIa antagonist lotrafiban in coronary and cerebrovascular disease. Circulation 2003;108:399–406.
61. Sandercock P. Antiplatelet therapy with aspirin in acute ischemic stroke. Thromb Haemost 1997;78:180–182.

9
Hormonal Therapy

MingMing Ning, Karen L. Furie, Jan L. Shifren, and J. Philip Kistler

Premenopausal women have fewer strokes than similarly aged men, an observation that prompted speculation that there might be a protective effect of the female hormones estrogen and progesterone. Observational studies suggested that this benefit might be potentiated through hormone therapy (HT) in later life. However, this has been extremely controversial, as recent studies have shown that HT actually increases the risk of heart disease and stroke. The risk–benefit profile of HT has changed rapidly with the results of large, randomized, controlled trials.

Paradoxically, although HT in late life was believed to have cardiovascular protective properties, it has long been established that these hormones were prothrombotic when administered in supraphysiological doses in oral contraceptive pills (OCPs). The risk of stroke with OCP use, especially when combined with factors such as smoking, hypertension, genetic predisposition to thromboembolism, and migraine, needs to be considered carefully before these medications are prescribed. More than 150 million women worldwide use OCPs. In the United States, approximately one-third of women of child-bearing age use an OCP *(1)*. Therefore, the prothrombotic risk of OCP is of public health concern.

HORMONE REPLACEMENT THERAPY AND STROKE

Over the last decade, estrogen and progestin combination therapy has been commonly prescribed to relieve postmenopausal symptoms, to reduce osteoporosis, and possibly to increase quality of life. These hormones were initially thought to improve the vascular risk profile through a variety of factors, including lowering low-density lipoprotein, reducing lipoprotein(a), increasing high-density lipoprotein, reducing platelet aggregation, and increasing fibrinolysis *(1–3)*. However, the use of unopposed estrogen increases the risk of endometrial cancer more than 10-fold *(4)*, so it is not recommended that patients with an intact uterus take estrogen alone. Progestin is usually used as a protective

From: *Current Clinical Neurology: Handbook of Stroke Prevention in Clinical Practice*
Edited by: K. L. Furie and P. J. Kelly © Humana Press Inc., Totowa, NJ

agent in conjunction with estrogen to reduce the endometrial cancer risk. By negatively impacting levels of low-density and high-density lipoproteins, the addition of progestin has been postulated to negate the vascular benefits of estrogen.

Although early observational studies and angiographic data suggested anti-atherogenic effects of estrogen *(5)*, the most recent randomized trials (Table 1) do not support the use of HT for the prevention of initial or recurrent stroke or heart disease. Recent meta-analysis also suggests that the perceived protective effects of HT in early observational studies may have been related to confounding by socioeconomic status and healthy user bias *(6)*. In addition, early adverse events often are not detected in observational studies.

A brief review of three major randomized clinical trials, using combined estrogen and progestin or estradiol alone, for the primary and secondary prevention of stroke follows.

First, the Woman's Health Initiative (WHI) study was a primary prevention trial involving healthy, postmenopausal women in the United States *(7,8)*. Women were randomized to oral-conjungated equine estrogens (CEE) (0.625 mg/day), a mixture of estrogens, in combination with medroxyprogestin (MPA) (2.5 mg/day). The oral CEE plus MPA portion of the trial was stopped prematurely at 5.2 years because of a 26% increased risk of invasive breast cancer (38 vs 30 per 10,000 person-years, hazard ratio [HR] 1.26, 95% confidence interval [CI] 0.83–1.92). This large randomized study (N = 16,000) reported an increased risk of stroke for patients on HT (HR 1.31, 95% CI 1.02–1.68). Nonfatal coronary events increased by 29% (37 vs 30 per 10,000 person-years). Among stroke subtypes, there was a relatively higher risk of ischemic stroke (HR 1.44, 95% CI 1.09–1.9), particularly strokes of undetermined and small-vessel subtypes, than of hemorrhagic stroke (HR 0.82, 95% CI 0.43–1.56). The higher risk was present regardless of the status of other known risk factors and could not be explained by effects on inflammatory or coagulation biomarkers. A significant disparity in stroke events was apparent as early as the end of the first year of therapy. The other arm of this trial, estrogen alone for the prevention of coronary heart disease (CHD) in 10,739 patients without a uterus, is ongoing and has a projected report date of 2005 *(7,8)*. The WHI follow-up study also showed no benefit to mild cognitive impairment or improvement in health-related quality of life *(9–11)*. An increased risk of probable dementia was seen in HT users in the WHI Memory Study (WHIMS) trial, a substudy of older women enrolled in the WHI *(10)*.

Second, the Heart and Estrogen–Progestin Replacement Study (HERS), was a large secondary prevention trial that enrolled older women with a history of heart disease *(12)*. HERS concluded that there was no risk or benefit for combined cerebrovascular events (transient ischemic attack or stroke) in

Table 1
Summary of Major HT Studies With Focus on Data of Stroke Risk

Trial name	Outcome	Stroke subtype	*N*	Duration
WHI: Primary prevention *(5)*	Nonfatal RR 1.5 (95% CI 0.83–2.7) Fatal RR 1.2 (95% CI 0.32–4.49)		16,608	5.2 years
Stroke follow-up data *(5a)*	Ischemic RR 1.44 (95% CI 1.09–1.9) Hemorrhagic RR 0.82 (95% CI 0.43–1.56)	Ischemic vs hemorrhagic (more than 39% of undetermined mechanism)	16,608	5.6 years
HERS: Secondary prevention *(6)*	Overall RR 1.09 (95% CI 0.84–1.43) Nonfatal RR 1.18 (95% CI 0.83–1.66) Fatal RR 1.61 (95% CI 0.73–3.55)	85% ischemic, 8% hemorrhagic, 6% unknown	2,763	4.1 years 6.8 years (HERS II)
WEST: Secondary prevention *(7)*	Any stroke RR 1.1 (95% CI 0.8–1.6) Nonfatal RR 1.1 (95% CI 0.7–1.4) Fatal RR 2.9 (95% CI 0.9–9)		664	2.8 years
Nelson et al. meta-analysis: All English-language literature since 1966, including WHI and HERS *(4)*	Incidence: Overall RR 1.12 (95% CI 1.01–1.23)	Ischemic thromboembolic RR 1.20 (95% CI 1.01–1.40) Subarachnoid hemorrhage RR 0.8 (95% CI 0.57–1.04) Intracerebral hemorrhage RR 0.71 (95% CI 0.25–1.29)	Meta-analysis	36 years

RR, relative risk.

patients taking HT (relative risk 1.09, 95% CI 0.84–1.43), although a significant increase in cardiovascular events was seen in the first year of use. The risk of cardiovascular events was highest in the first 6 months of HT. HERS confirmed modifiable risk factors such as hypertension, atrial fibrillation, diabetes, and smoking as important contributors to stroke in women and black women had approximately twice the risk of stroke as white women regardless of treatment assignment.

Third, Women's Estrogen for Stroke Trial (WEST) was a smaller secondary prevention trial, also using oral estradiol without progestin, in patients with recent ischemic stroke or transient ischemic attack; these individuals were followed on average for 2.8 years *(13,14)*. There was no significant difference in the overall risk of strokes for patients on estradiol, but among stroke victims, the estradiol group had poorer functional outcome and a higher risk of death *(14)*.

Hormone Therapy Preparations

In the WHI and HERS trials, patients were given conjungated equine estrogen (0.625 mg/day), a mixture of estrogens, in combination with medroxyprogestin (2.5 mg/day) to protect against endometrial hyperplasia. In the WEST trial, patients were given unopposed 17-β®-estradiol, with frequent endometrial sampling *(15,16)*. It has been suggested that 17-β®-estradiol may be more efficacious in decreasing the risk of atherosclerosis because of its readily bioavailable form *(17)*, but this advantage may be curtailed when it is used in conjunction with progestin. Further studies are needed to clarify whether different forms of oral estrogen or transdermal estrogen may have different risk and benefit profiles. For patients who have had a hysterectomy, the result of estrogen monotherapy is still pending from the WHI study.

Duration of Treatment

The WHI data showed an increase in stroke after only 1 year of HT use, and the stroke follow-up showed no relationship between stroke, age, or time from menopause. Invasive breast cancer, the reason for the early termination of the WHI trial, showed a significant increased risk after 4 years of therapy. This may give a small window of opportunity allowing safe treatment of women with menopausal symptoms for short periods. Other risks, however, such as venous thromboembolism and CHD, showed steady increases from the initiation of HT. On the other hand, some benefits of HT, such as for colorectal cancer, were only obvious after 3 years.

Conclusions

The WHI, HERS, and WEST investigations demonstrated no protective effect of HT on stroke or cardiovascular risk. The American Heart Association and North American Menopause Society (NAMS) currently recommend that estrogen–progestin therapy not be used for primary or secondary prevention of CHD, and that HT be permanently discontinued after an acute CHD event. It should be noted, however, that the absolute risk for adverse events on HT is low. For example, in WHI for 10,000 patients using HT, compared to non-users, in 1 year, there may be 8 more nonfatal strokes, 8 more invasive breast cancer, 8 more cases of pulmonary embolism, and 7 more CAD, but 6 fewer cases of colorectal cancer and 5 fewer cases of hip fracture. The estimation that there will be more adverse events overall (19 events per 10,000 individuals per year) has driven the recommendations for restraint.

The current studies do not preclude patients from taking short-term HT for other proven benefits, such as intractable menopausal symptoms and bone health, but the results of these recent trials indicate the need for greater education of patients on the risks and benefits of HT. Taking into account that short-term therapy yields fewer adverse effects, the challenge now is to provide a way of stratifying women with higher risks of cardiovascular events or other major morbidity on HT before the initiation of therapy.

Summary and Recommendations

1. HT is not recommended for the primary or secondary prevention of stroke.
2. Risk of stroke is increased after 1 year of therapy according to WHI data.
3. For patients with hysterectomy, the study of estrogen alone for the prevention of CHD in 10,739 women is still ongoing, with uncertain overall risk–benefit profile. Planned termination and data reporting is expected in 2005.

ORAL CONTRACEPTIVE PILLS AND STROKE

OCP preparations have been evolving since the 1960s. They contain estrogen and progestin, which inhibit the gonadotropin surge (luteinizing hormone/follicle-stimulating hormone) involved in follicular maturation and prevent ovulation by inducing a hyperestrogenic state that mimics pregnancy *(18)*.

Preparations with a high estrogen content (150 μg) have been associated with both arterial and venous thromboembolism. For the newer, low-dose, second-generation preparations (ranging from 20 to 50 μg estrogen, with the most common dosage 30–35 μg), the effect on stroke risk is less clear. Several studies of such low-estrogen preparations reported a low (2 to 11 per 100,000 per year) or nonexistent increased risk of stroke *(19–21)*. However, the newest, low-estrogen third-generation OCP, containing gesteogene or desogestrel, has been associated with an increased risk of venous thromboembolic disease *(22)*. Some studies reported the risks of aneurysmal bleeding and hemorrhagic stroke were higher in users of the low-dose estrogen and norgestrel or levonorgestrel combination *(22,23)*.

The most recent meta-analysis found that, in women without other risk factors, the addition of OCP raised the annual stroke incidence from 4.4 to 8.5 per 100,000 person-years *(21)*. This risk is nearly 20 times smaller than the 8 per 10,000 person-years risk of stroke associated with postmenopausal HT *(7)*. According to the low risk profile reported in recent studies, it is postulated that the treatment of 24,000 women will result in 1 additional ischemic stroke per year *(17)*.

OCP preparations have been associated with a reversible mild increase in blood pressure *(24)*. Less frequently, they may cause hypertension, which is known to increase the risk of stroke and myocardial infarction *(24)*. Furthermore, smoking and medical comorbidities that increase with age, such as hypertension, raise stroke risk dramatically. Therefore, in heavy smokers over the age of 35 years and in women with previous thromboembolic events, OCPs are contraindicated. Novel risk factors, particularly genetic markers of risk, may help stratify patients prior to initiation of therapy.

Widespread screening for thrombophilias is not cost-effective, but patients with factor V Leiden, prothrombin gene mutation, deficiencies in protein S or C or antithrombin III, and hyperhomocysteinemia are at significantly increased risk for cerebral vein thrombosis (CVT). However, the timing and interpretation of the hypercoagulable panel are essential in obtaining accurate and clinically useful results. Clinicians should note that warfarin reduces the functional activity of protein C and protein S, and elevates antithrombin III levels. Heparin can decrease antithrombin III concentration. Any acute thrombosis can transiently reduce antithrombin III, and to a lesser extent, protein C and S concentration.

In patients with hypercoagulable states who take OCPs, the risk of CVT is multiplicative for each independent risk factor *(25)*. Because the morbidity of CVT can be quite high, screening patients with a family history of prothrombotic states, late and recurrent miscarriage, or past thrombotic events with neurological symptoms such as headache, blurry vision, or focal neurological findings is reasonable.

Hormones and Migraine

Migraine with aura has been shown to be an independent risk factor for stroke *(26–31)*. It is still unclear whether this is a causal relationship or merely an association with other stroke risk factors. For example, congenital heart defects, such as patent foramen ovale (PFO), have been associated with symptoms of migraine, and closure of PFO decreases the frequency of migraines. It is unclear whether the presence of PFO, potentially generating microemboli, induces vascular reactivity and causes migraine. Similarly, patients with cerebral autosomal dominant arteriopathy with subcortical infarcts and leukoencephalopathy (CADASIL), a hereditary microangiopathy caused by mutation in the Notch3 gene, also have migraine. These patients are prone to stroke from progressive small-vessel occlusion.

Although migraine may be a result of a heterogeneous group of underlying causes, the presence of migraine with aura is strongly associated with an increased incidence of strokes *(28–30)*. The symptom of aura with migraine corresponds to a six- to eightfold increased risk of stroke for patients under the age of 45 years, but a less significant increase for older patients.

Recommendations

In younger women, the risks of stroke associated with OCP, migraine, and inherited thrombophilic disease are important topics for patient counseling. They are significant both because of the multiplicative nature of the independent stroke risk factors and because OCP and migraine are both very common. Although migraine with aura is not an absolute contraindication for the initiation of OCP, closer follow-up, monitoring the change in migraine symptoms, and the development of or change in aura should suggest the discontinuation of OCP.

Although the risk of stroke is low in healthy, young women, those women with migraine history, history of miscarriage, and thrombotic phenomena in the family (mostly an autosomal dominant pattern) should have seritological testing for evidence of hypercoagulability prior to the initiation of OCP use (Table 2).

REFERENCES

1. Cauley JA, Seeley DG, Browner WS, et al. Estrogen replacement therapy and mortality among older women. The study of osteoporotic fractures. Arch Intern Med 1997;157:2181–2187.
2. Binder EF, Williams DB, Schechtman KB, et al. Effects of HT on serum lipids in elderly women. A randomized, placebo-controlled trial. Ann Intern Med 2001; 134:754–760.
3. Darling GM, Johns JA, McCloud PI, Davis SR. Estrogen and progestin compared with simvastatin for hypercholesterolemia in postmenopausal women. N Engl J Med 1997;337:595–601.
4. Chu J, Wchwid AI, Wiss NS. Survival among women with endometrial cancer: a comparison of estrogen users and nonusers. Am J Obstet Gynecol 1982;143: 569–573.
5. Grodstein F, Stampfer MJ, Manson JE, et al. Postmenopausal estrogen and progestin use and the risk of cardiovascular disease. N Engl J Med 1996;335:453–461.
6. Nelson HD, Humphrey LL, Nygren P, Teutsch SM, Allan JD. Postmenopausal hormone replacement therapy: scientific review. JAMA 2002;288:872–881.

Table 2
Coagulation Screening in Moderate- to High-Risk Patients Prior to OCP Initiation

Thrombophilic disease	Epidemiology	Presentation	Diagnosis
Factor V Leiden: mutated gene product; more potent in activating the conversion of prothrombin to thrombin	Most common: 5.27% white population; 40–50% all hereditary thrombophilia	Deep vein thrombosis, with or without pulmonary embolism; increased CVT in women on OCP or peripartum; late fetal loss	aPTT as screen; serum APC resistance using coagulation assay; serum polymerase chain reaction analysis of A to G at nucleotide 1691
Prothrombin gene G 20210: point mutation G>A at nucleotide 20210; vitamin K-dependent precursor of thrombin	Hispanic/white population, 0.7 to 6.5%	Venous (deep vein thrombosis, CVT) >> arterial; late fetal loss	Serum polymerase chain reaction DNA (deoxyribo-nucleic acid) genomic analysis
Antithrombin (AT) (also known as antithrombin III): Vitamin K-dependent glycoprotein inhibits thrombin and other serine proteases	All: 0.2–0.5% adults Type I: Reduced synthesis of normal AT Type II: defect in AT molecule	Severe thrombotic disease in types I and II, with defects in thrombin-binding domain; venous >>>>>>arterial	Type I: antigenic and functional activity both reduced Type II: antigenic AT normal and functional activity markedly reduced

Protein C: Vitamin K-dependent protein inactivates coagulation factors Va and VIIIa	0.2–0.5% healthy adults; mostly autosomal dominant Type I: Reduced synthesis of normal protein Type II: Decreased activity	Similar to antithrombin III; venous >>> arterial; late fetal loss; can be acquired in septic shock and infection	Serum functional assays for screening, then immunologic (antigenic) assays to detect quantitative deficiencies
Protein S: Cofactor of protein C (S stands for Seattle, where it was initially isolated)	Predominantly autosomal dominant	Venous >>> arterial (arterial by case reports only); same as protein C	Same as protein C (important to measure free protein S levels; total level maybe falsely normal)
Antiphospholipid antibodies: Antibody against phospholipids or plasma protein bound to them		Venous > arterial; recurrent miscarriages; associated with other autoimmune disorders such as systemic lupus erythematosus	Both clinical and laboratory abnormality (need two or more positive results repeated in 6-week interval); aPTT prolonged; anticardiolipin immunoglobulin G or M in medium or high titer; lupus anticoagulant
Hyperhomocysteinemia: Intermediary amino acid from the conversion of methionine to cysteine; hereditary autosomal recessive is rare	5–7% of general population	Arterial > venous	Fasting serum level; vitamin B_{12}, folate, B_6; genetic testing for methylene tetrahydrofolate reductase deficiency, cystathionine synthase activity deficiency

7. Rossouw JE, Anderson GL, Prentice RL, et al. Risks and benefits of estrogen plus progestin in healthy post-menopausal women. Principal results from the Women's Health Initiative randomized controlled trial. JAMA 2002;288:321–333.
8. Wassertheil-Smoller S, Hendrix SL, Limacher M, et al. Effect of estrogen plus progestin on stroke in postmenopausal women. The Women's Health Initiative: a randomized trial. JAMA 2003;289:2673–2684.
9. Rapp SR. Espeland MA, Shumaker SA, et al. Effect of estrogen plus progestin on global cognitive function in postmenopausal women: the Women's Health Initiative Memory Study: a randomized controlled trial. JAMA 2003;289:2663–2672.
10. Shumaker SA, Legault C, Thal L, et al. Estrogen plus progestin and the incidence of dementia and mild cognitive impairment in postmenopausal women: the Women's Health Initiative Memory Study: a randomized controlled trial. JAMA 2003;289:2651–2662.
11. Hays J, Ockene JK, Brunner RL, et al. Effects of estrogen plus progestin on health-related quality of life. N Engl J Med 2003;348:1839–1854.
12. Simon JA, Hsia J, Cauley J, et al. Postmenopausal hormone therapy and the risk of stroke: the Heart and Estrogen–Progestin Replacement Study (HERS). Circulation 2001;103:638–642.
13. Viscoli CM, Brass LM, Kernan WN, Sarrel PM, Suissa S, Horwitz RI. A clinical trial of estrogen replacement therapy after ischemic stroke. N Engl J Med 2001;345: 1243–1249.
14. Mosca L, Collins P, Herrington DM, et al. Hormone replacement therapy and cardiovascular disease: a statement for healthcare professionals from the American Heart Association. Circulation 2001;104:499–503.
15. Angerer P, Stork S, Kothny W, Schmitt P, von Schacky C. Effect of oral postmenopausal hormone replacement on progression of atherosclerosis: a randomized, controlled trial. Arterioscler Thromb Vasc Biol 2001;21:262–268.
16. Hodis HN, Mack, WJ, Lobo RA, et al. Estrogen in the prevention of atherosclerosis. A randomized double-blind, placebo-controlled trial. Ann Intern Med 2001; 135:939–953.
17. Martin KA, Daouglas PS. Risks and side effects associated with oral contraceptives. Up To Date 2002.
18. Beckmann CRB, Ling FW, Herbert WNP, et al. Obstetrics and Gynecology. Baltimore, MD: Williams and Wilkins, 1998.
19. Heinemann LA, Lewis MA, Thorogood M, et al. Case–control study of oral contraceptives and risk of thromboembolic stroke: results from international study on oral contraceptives and health of young women. BMJ 1997;315:1502–1504.
20. Petitti DB, Sidney S, Bernstein A, et al. Stroke in users of low dose oral contraceptives. N Engl J Med 1996;335:8–15.
21. Gillium AL, Mamidipudi SK, Johnston SC. Ischemic stroke risk with oral contraceptives: a meta-analysis. JAMA 2000;284:72–78.
22. WHO Collaborative Study of Cardiovascular Disease and Steroid Hormone Contraception. Effect of different progestagens in low estrogen oral contraceptives on venous thromboembolic disease. Lancet 1995;346:1582–1588.
23. Schwartz SM, Siscovick DS, Longstreth WT Jr, et al. Use of low-dose oral contraceptives and stroke in young women. Ann Intern Med 1997;127:596–603.

24. Chasan-Taber L, Willet WC, Manson WC, et al. Prospective study of oral contraceptives and hypertension among women in the United States. Circulation 1996;94: 483–489.
25. de Bruijn SF, Stam J, Koopman MM, et al. Case–control study of risk of cerebral sinus thrombosis in oral contraceptive users who are carriers of hereditary prothrombotic conditions. BMJ 1998;316:589–592.
26. Lidegaardd O. Oral contraceptives, pregnancy and the risk of cerebral thromboembolism: the influence of diabetes, hypertension, migraine and previous thrombotic disease. Br J Obstet Gynaecol 1995;102:153–159.
27. Musolino, R, La Spina P, Granata A, et al. Ischaemic stroke in young people: a prospective and long-term follow-up study. Cerebrovasc Dis 2003;15:121–128.
28. Tzourio C, Tehindrazanarivelo A, Iglesias S, et al. Case-control study of migraine and risk of ischaemic stroke in young women. BMJ 1995;310:830–833.
29. Carolei A, Marini C, De Matteis G, and the Italian National Research Council Study Group on Stroke on the Young. History of migraine and risk of cerebral ischaemia in young adults. Lancet 1996;347:1503–1506.
30. Henrich JB, Horwitz RI. A controlled study of ischemic stroke risk in migraine patients. J Clin Epidemiol 1989;42:773–780.
31. Merikanga KR, Fenton BT, Cheng SH, Stolar MJ, Risch N. Association between migraine and stroke in a large-scale epidemiological study of the United States. Arch Neurol 1997;54:362–368.

10
Stroke Due to Large Artery Atherosclerosis

Karen L. Furie, Stelios M. Smirnakis, Walter J. Koroshetz, and J. Philip Kistler

EXTRACRANIAL CAROTID ATHEROSCLEROSIS

Chiari recognized atherosclerotic disease of the internal carotid artery (ICA) as a cause of stroke as early as 1905. In 1937, Moniz described four cases of carotid occlusion with transient ischemic attack (TIA) preceding stroke. In the 1950s, Miller Fisher described the clinical syndrome of transient deficits preceding stroke above an occluded carotid. Carotid atherosclerosis is associated with conventional vascular risk factors: hypertension, hyperlipidemia, diabetes, and smoking *(1–5)*.

Carotid and coronary heart disease are often coexistent *(6)*. The extent of plaque, as measured by the degree of stenosis, correlates with risk of stroke and cardiac events *(7)*. In addition, the earliest stages of atherosclerotic disease in the ICA, intimal medial thickening (IMT), has been associated with risk of stroke, myocardial infarction, and death *(8)*. The nature of the plaque itself is receiving increased attention. Elements of plaque vulnerability (features that make a plaque more likely to progress, rupture, and cause symptoms) include a thin fibrous cap, high lipid content, intraplaque hemorrhage, and inflammation *(9–16)*.

Mechanism of Ischemic Symptoms

Determination of how carotid atherosclerosis contributes to ischemic symptoms is important for management. Carotid atherosclerosis causes symptoms through two mechanisms: artery-to-artery embolism and low flow *(16–19)*. Low-flow symptoms are typically brief and stereotyped and generally (>70%) are associated with stenoses. Embolism of atheroma and superimposed thrombus is believe to be the more common pathophysiology, although in cases of high-grade stenoses, it can be difficult to discriminate between the two with absolute certainty.

From: *Current Clinical Neurology: Handbook of Stroke Prevention in Clinical Practice*
Edited by: K. L. Furie and P. J. Kelly © Humana Press Inc., Totowa, NJ

The targeted therapy for acute, and in some cases chronic, low-flow symptoms, is improving blood flow across the stenotic lesion. Transcranial Doppler (TCD), an ultrasound examination of the intracranial vessels, can provide direct evidence of the homodynamic significance of a carotid lesion. Alternatively, a perfusion study, using computed tomography (CT), magnetic resonance imaging (MRI), or positron emission tomography, can provide support for the determination of a flow-limiting lesion. If the mechanism of ischemia is related to artery-to-artery embolism, therapies that stabilize plaque and inhibit thrombus formation are most likely to reduce risk of recurrence. In both cases, the risks and benefits of definitively treating the plaque with either carotid endarterectomy (CEA) or stenting should be considered.

Symptomatic vs Asymptomatic Carotid Disease

Carotid artery stenosis is classified as either asymptomatic or symptomatic based on whether there are symptoms or signs of carotid territory ischemia in the ipsilateral eye or hemisphere. In the CEA clinical trials, symptomatic carotid disease was defined as the presence of transient monocular blindness (TMB), TIA, or stroke. Silent infarcts on CT or MRI were not considered symptomatic. Detection of infarctions within the distribution of a stenotic carotid artery on neuroimaging, even without a corresponding history, may suggest a higher risk of future stroke, but this has not been proven.

Symptoms or findings suggestive of a carotid atheroma include carotid bruit, transient or fixed neurological symptoms referable to the internal carotid distribution (homonymous hemianopia, hemisensory deficit, hemimotor deficit, hemisensorimotor deficit, aphasia, neglect, apraxia, dysarthria), or TMB. Additionally, patients with multiple vascular risk factors, coronary heart disease, or peripheral vascular disease should be considered high risk.

TIAs can be the result of large-artery atherosclerosis, cardioembolism, or small-vessel lacunar disease, but they are most characteristic of large-vessel atherosclerotic disease. TMB and stereotyped TIAs are classic symptoms of high-grade carotid stenosis. Symptoms lasting longer than 1 hour are likely to be caused by infarction *(20)*. CT scanning or MRI is useful for evaluating possible infarctions in the ICA territory. Infarctions can be small-vessel/lacunar involving the deep structures, in subcortical white matter cortex, or a combination. There may be a single lesion or multiple infarcts in the ICA distribution. Although carotid stenosis may appear the "smoking gun" in cases of anterior circulation ischemia, it is always important to consider other mechanisms of stroke because there are often competing risk factors, such as a high-risk cardioembolic source or small-vessel disease, that could have an impact on management decisions.

Table 1
Clinical Risk Factors Affecting Risk of Stroke After Transient Monocular Blindness

Risk factors	
>75 years of age	
• Male sex	
• History of hemispheric TIA or stroke or intermittent claudication	
• Carotid artery stenosis of 80–94%	
• Absence of collateral flow	
3-year stroke risk	
0–1 risk factors	1.8%
2 risk factors	12.3
>3 risk factors	24.2%

Source: From ref. *20*.

A TIA in association with large-artery disease carries a more ominous prognosis regarding recurrence than transient symptoms because of other mechanisms of stroke. In patients with more than 50% stenosis enrolled in the North American Symptomatic Carotid Endarterectomy Trial (NASCET), a hemispheric TIA at entry conveyed a higher risk of ipsilateral stroke than TMB or completed stroke at entry. At 2 days, there was a 5.5% rate of stroke in the TIA group, and none in the stroke group. At 90 days, the risk after TIA was 10 times that of stroke, 20.1 vs 2.3% *(21)*. A TIA should be considered a medical emergency given the high risk of 90-day morbidity and mortality *(22)*. In a study of patients seen in an emergency department for TIA, 25.1% had a stroke or other adverse event within 90 days. Half the strokes occurred within 2 days of the TIA *(23)*.

TMB, also called amaurosis fugax, can be caused by low flow or a small artery-to-artery embolus from the ICA to the ophthalmic artery. TMB is less often caused by a cardioembolic source *(24)*. Clinical features shown in Table 1 are useful in predicting risk of stroke after an episode of TMB *(21)*.

Evaluation of the Carotid Arteries

Ultrasound

Carotid duplex ultrasound (CDUS) is a safe, sensitive (81–77%), specific (82–89%), and relatively inexpensive technique for evaluating the carotid arteries *(25,26)*. Although the wide availability of CDUS is an advantage, it is critical that individual laboratories adhere to strict quality assurance guidelines to ensure valid results. Pathological specimens have been used to establish Doppler criteria for residual lumen diameter, and using receiver–operator curves, the thresholds for interpreting the carotid artery velocities can be adjusted to optimize the study *(27,28)*. CDUS is also highly sensitive and specific for diagnosing carotid occlusion, although a trace amount of residual flow can be missed *(29,30)*. CDUS provides data on plaque composition, which may affect the risk of embolism and have an impact on prognosis *(9–14)*. TCD, ultrasound of the intracranial vessels, is often used in conjunction with CDUS to evaluate the hemodynamic significance of ICA stenosis and improve the sensitivity and specificity of CDUS in diagnosing a potentially surgical lesion *(31)*.

MRA

An advantage of obtaining magnetic resonance angiography (MRA) of the head and neck is that it allows simultaneous evaluation of the brain parenchyma. Access and expense are limiting factors with MRA. Additionally, a significant proportion of patients are unable to undergo an MRI because of contraindications such as metal implants, pacemakers, claustrophobia, or an inability to remain still throughout the period of image acquisition *(32)*. For detecting high-grade carotid stenosis, MRA images the carotid bifurcation with high sensitivity (73–100%) and specificity (59–99%), which may be improved with the newer techniques using gadolinium *(33–38)*. MRA, like CDUS, is imperfect in distinguishing between a hairline residual lumen and complete occlusion *(39)*.

CTA

Computed tomographic angiography (CTA) is able to identify large- or medium-size vessel stenosis or occlusion. The main disadvantage is the need for intravenous contrast, which is contraindicated in patients with renal insufficiency, congestive heart failure, contrast allergy, or pregnancy. A review described a prospective study of 21 patients with acute nonhemorrhagic stroke imaged with both CTA and digital subtraction angiography. Two raters correctly assessed all trunk occlusions of the basilar artery, ICA, and middle cerebral artery (MCA), although assessment of more distal MCA branch occlusions was less reliable. In addition, there was an 88% agreement rate in judging the degree of collateral vessels and 62% accurate prediction of hemispheric infarct size *(40)*.

In a separate study of 145 patients with symptoms of acute stroke, arterial stenoses or occlusions were present on 43% of CTAs. When both CTA and MRA were obtained, findings were in agreement for 98% of the vessels, and agreement was 99% for the 28 cases for which both CTA and digital subtraction angiography were acquired *(41)*.

Therefore, current data attest to the accuracy of CTA in detecting lesions in large intracranial vessels. CT perfusion techniques also offer the opportunity to obtain quantitative blood volume maps. By tracing the first pass of contrast through the brain, maps of relative cerebral blood flow, mean transit time, and cerebral blood volume can be constructed.

Angiography

Cerebral angiography is the gold standard for imaging the carotid arteries, but it is less commonly performed because of the associated stroke risk, 1% on average, and the availability of safer, less-expensive noninvasive alternatives *(42)*. NASCET developed a method to calculate the percentage stenosis: The residual lumen diameter at the point of maximal stenosis is divided by the lumen diameter in the distal, normal caliber, ICA *(43)*. In contrast, the European Carotid Surgery Trial (ECST) measured the lumen diameter at the point of maximal stenosis divided by the estimated original diameter of the carotid bulb *(44)*.

We recommend that patients with suspected carotid stenosis undergo CDUS as an initial screening test. If there is 50% or less stenosis, aggressive medical intervention for risk factor modification and initiation of an antiplatelet agent are recommended. The stenosis should be followed with serial examinations, usually on an annual basis, to determine if there is progression. If there is 50% or greater stenosis, TCD and either CTA or MRA should be performed. CTA is performed in lieu of MRA if there is a contraindication to MRI and when the duplex ultrasound and MRA do not agree. Combined testing with noninvasive imaging modalities has largely replaced conventional transfemoral angiography. The advantage of combining CDUS and TCD with either CTA or MRA is the complementary nature of the angiographic and physiological blood flow data. In addition, the combined testing improves accuracy in selecting patients for invasive procedures *(45,46)*. Conventional angiography could be considered in patients unable to have an MRA and in whom the risk of dye is sufficient to warrant bypassing CTA or if there is a suspicion of nonatherosclerotic disease (e.g., dissection, vasculitis).

Management of Carotid Atherosclerosis

The utility of CEA in symptomatic and asymptomatic carotid stenosis was demonstrated in the clinical trials presented in Table 2. There is a clear benefit to CEA in cases of high-grade (>70%) symptomatic carotid stenosis. The benefits are less clear for moderate (50–69%) and asymptomatic disease. There are several important caveats to consider. The first is that these trials excluded patients with high-risk cardioembolic sources and other medical conditions that put them at high risk for surgery. In addition, the surgeons in these trials performed a high volume of CEAs and may have had complication rates below those in the general community. Higher rates of operative morbidity would reduce or nullify the benefits, depending on the clinical scenario. Finally, it must be appreciated that the timing of stroke in surgi-

Table 2
Clinical Trials Showing Beneficial Effects of CEA

Study	Stenosis (%)	Number enrolled (surgical or medical)	Follow-up	End point	End point event rate in surgical arm (%)	End point event rate in medical arm (%)
Symptomatic						
European Carotid Surgery Trial (ECST)	0–19	78/62	3 years	Major stroke or death	35.9	25.8
	20–29	162/117			37	33.3
	30–39	200/139			39	33.1
	40–49	190/122			34.2	26.2
	50–59	350/240			36	35.8
	60–69	232/137			35.3	35
	70–79	231/170			38.5	40.6
	80–89	251/159			39	44.7
	90–99	104/60			37.5	51.7
NASCET I	>70	328/331	2 years	Fatal or nonfatal ipsilateral stroke	9	26
NASCET II	50-69	1108/1118	5 years	Fatal or nonfatal ipsilateral stroke	15.7	22.2
Asymptomatic						
Veterans Affairs Cooperative Asymptomatic Study	>50	221/233	4 years	(1) TIA or TMB or stroke	12.8	24.5
				(2) Stroke or death	41.2	44.2
Asymptomatic Carotid Artery Study (ACAS)	>60%	825/834	2.7 years extrapolated to 5 years	Ipsilateral stroke or any perioperative stroke or death	5.1	11

Source: From refs. *43, 44,* and *47–49.*

Table 3
Recommended Evaluation in Patients With Carotid Atherosclerosis

Lipid profile
Hemoglobin A1c
High-sensitivity C-reactive protein
Fasting homocysteine, vitamin B_{12}
Electrocardiogram
CDUS
TCD, MRI or MRA of the head and neck, or CT/CTA of the head and neck

cally treated patients is usually perioperative, as opposed to stroke in medically treated patients, which occurs over the course of years. Patients with significant medical comorbidities and limited life expectancy might enjoy a better quality of life without the attendant surgical risk, especially if the lesion is asymptomatic. Although they are still under investigation, carotid stents are used increasingly to manage carotid disease; these are discussed in Chapter 11.

In symptomatic patients, the bulk of the evidence suggests that it is safe to perform CEA early, as opposed to waiting 6–8 weeks, if there has not been a large infarction. In the NASCET patients, there was no difference in postoperative morbidity or 18-month stroke or death in patients undergoing early (within 3–30 days of symptoms) as opposed to late (33–117 days after symptoms) CEA *(50)*. Other studies have shown that CEA can be safely performed within 30 days of a nondisabling stroke *(51)*. Patients with TIA with no infarcted tissue at risk for reperfusion injury stand to derive the most benefit from early CEA.

Medical management should be a major focus of intervention in both surgical and nonsurgical cases. Performing the diagnostic assessments outlined in Table 3 will elucidate targets for medical intervention in addition to conventional risk factor modification of hypertension, hyperlipidemia, diabetes, smoking, and lifestyle factors outlined in the other chapters of this book. Antiplatelet options are discussed in Chapter 8.

Recommendations for surgical intervention based on the large CEA clinical trials are outlined in Table 4 *(43,44,47–49)*. Although these studies randomly assigned nonsurgical patients to "best" medical therapy, the standard has changed over time. It may be that more aggressive risk factor management and the newer therapies, such as 3-hydroxy-3-methyl-glutaryl-coenzyme A reductase inhibitors and newer antiplatelet regimens, could improve prognosis in medically treated patients. Alternatively, procedural advances such as the eversion technique for CEA or neurointerventional techniques

Table 4
Recommended Management Based on Degree of Carotid Stenosis

Asymptomatic	
<60%	Medical management of vascular risk factors (hypertension, diabetes, hypercholesterolemia, smoking, alcohol, lifestyle, hyperhomocysteinemia) and antiplatelet therapy
60–99%	Consider CEA if surgical risk deemed <3% and long-term prognosis favorable Postoperative medical management of vascular risk factors (hypertension, diabetes, hypercholesterolemia, smoking, alcohol, lifestyle, hyperhomocysteinemia) and antiplatelet therapy
Occluded	Medical management of vascular risk factors (hypertension, diabetes, hypercholesterolemia, smoking, alcohol, lifestyle, hyperhomocysteinemia) and antiplatelet therapy
Symptomatic	
<50% with TIA or stroke in ipsilateral internal carotid artery (ICA)	Medical management of vascular risk factors (hypertension, diabetes, hypercholesterolemia, smoking, alcohol, lifestyle, hyperhomocysteinemia) and antiplatelet therapy
50–69% with TIA or stroke in ipsilateral ICS territory	Consider CEA; weigh risks and benefits and consider perioperative risk Medical management of vascular risk factors (hypertension, diabetes, hypercholesterolemia, smoking, alcohol, lifestyle, hyperhomocysteinemia) and antiplatelet therapy
>70% with symptoms in the territory of the ICA	CEA unless medically contraindicated; postoperative medical management of vascular risk factors (hypertension, diabetes, hypercholesterolemia, smoking, alcohol, lifestyle, hyperhomocysteinemia) and antiplatelet therapy
Occluded	Medical management of vascular risk factors (hypertension, diabetes, hypercholesterolemia, smoking, alcohol, lifestyle, hyperhomocysteinemia) and antiplatelet therapy; consider anticoagulation for 3–6 months with acute symptoms suggestive of stump embolus

could result in better outcomes in surgical patients. These hypotheses have not yet been tested in a randomized controlled trial. Future medical treatments will likely target the atherogenic process and have the potential for significant effect on the natural history of carotid disease.

INTRACRANIAL ATHEROSCLEROSIS

Risk of Stroke Associated With Intracranial Atherosclerosis

Intracranial atherosclerosis is an important cause of stroke. Data suggest that acute cerebral ischemia from intracranial MCA stenosis is most often caused by embolism rather than thrombosis *in situ* from unstable atherosclerotic plaque *(52)*. Atherosclerosis primarily affects large- or medium-size arteries, with a predilection for branching sites in the arterial tree. Intracranial sites most frequently affected are the basilar artery, the stem (M1) portion of the MCA, the intracranial portion of the ICA, the anterior cerebral artery, and the posterior cerebral artery. The incidence of focal intracranial arterial stenoses were estimated as 22–24% in a cohort of patients presenting with cerebral ischemia, although these were considered the cause of the event in only 8% of cases *(53)*.

In the Northern Manhattan Stroke Study, Sacco et al. estimated that of the 17% of all strokes categorized as large artery, 9% were caused by extracranial atherosclerosis and 8% by intracranial atherosclerosis *(54)*. This pattern may vary by racial or ethnic background. For example, data indicate that Chinese adults have more severe and frequent intracranial than extracranial atherosclerotic disease *(55)*.

Uncontrolled studies suggested that patients with intracranial atherosclerosis and stroke are at risk for recurrent ischemic events despite appropriate medical therapy. Petty and coworkers reported on a population-based cohort of patients with ischemic stroke that included 74 patients whose cause of stroke was intracranial or extracranial artery atherosclerosis *(56)*. They estimated the 30-day recurrence rate as 18.5% (including iatrogenic events) and 5-year death rates as 32.2%. Other studies reported somewhat lower recurrent stroke rates in patients with intracranial atherosclerosis, with recurrences ranging from 4 to 12% per year for disease involving the anterior circulation and from 2.5 to 15% per year for posterior circulation disease *(57)*.

Chimowitz and colleagues conducted a retrospective study examining recurrent stroke rates in patients treated with warfarin and aspirin for symptomatic intracranial stenosis *(58)*. Of 151 enrolled patients, 88 received warfarin and 63 aspirin according to the local physician preference. The recurrent stroke rate was 10.4 (per 100 patient-years) in the aspirin group, compared with only 3.6 for warfarin *(58)*.

Thijs and Albers followed 52 patients with symptomatic intracranial atherosclerosis. Over half (55.6%) had their initial event while on therapy (55% on an antiplatelet agent, 31% on warfarin, and 14% on heparin) *(57)*. Fewer patients had their first event on warfarin compared to antiplatelet therapy.

The incidence of recurrent ischemic events was high irrespective of medical therapy. The median time of recurrence was only 36 days. This suggests that patients with symptomatic intracranial atherosclerosis who failed antithrombotic therapy are at a particularly high risk for recurrence, and may benefit from other interventions.

Prevention of Early and Late Recurrent Stroke in Patients With Intracranial Atherosclerosis

Because the natural course of intracranial atherosclerosis is one of progressive increase in the severity of arterial narrowing, preventive measures should be instituted once the patient has moved from the acute to the chronic phase. Modifiable risk factors for atherosclerosis such as hypercholesterolemia, hyperhomocysteinemia, smoking, diabetes, and hypertension should be identified and treated *(59–66)*. No reliable data from randomized trials currently exist on the optimal use of antithrombotic therapy.

In the acute phase, proactive management of severe symptomatic intracranial atherosclerosis is warranted given the high risk of early stroke recurrence reported in uncontrolled studies. Although trial data specific to intracranial disease are unavailable, current treatment options include (1) anticoagulation; (2) antiplatelet therapy with oral (aspirin, clopidogrel, dipyridamole, or combination therapy) or intravenous (glycoprotein IIb/IIIa inhibitors) agents; (3) measures to increase cerebral perfusion pressure for carefully selected patients (induced hypertension, hydration, and fluid expansion with mineralocorticoid analogues); and (4) endovascular intervention (balloon angioplasty and stenting).

For highly selected patients with severe symptomatic intracranial stenosis, measures to improve perfusion distal to the stenosed vessel may be beneficial. These measures include hypertensive therapy with volume expansion and infusions of pressor agents and use of mineralocorticoid drugs. In general, this approach should be reserved for patients who have recurrent or progressive symptoms despite antithrombotic therapy and other supportive measures, have a small volume of infarcted tissue, and have clear clinical improvement in response to a brief therapeutic trial. The approach should be restricted to centers experienced in the management of acute stroke and performed in an intensive care setting, with continuous monitoring of blood pressure. Early uncontrolled studies have indicated that this strategy is safe and may be beneficial for carefully selected patients *(67,68)*.

Imaging modalities used to assess the degree of hemodynamic compromise may be helpful in deciding the management strategy. TCD studies can increase diagnostic sensitivity and specificity and provide an easy and accurate means of longitudinal follow-up *(69)*. Although unproven at present, MRI or CTA perfusion studies may have a future role in the selection of patients for hypertensive or endovascular therapy because they may demonstrate oligemic cerebral tissue at risk of infarction, which may not always correlate well with clinical findings. Further data from prospective studies are needed to clarify these issues.

Endovascular therapy may also have a role in the acute treatment of highly selected patients with intracranial atherosclerosis who fail to respond to more conservative measures. In a study of 15 patients with intracranial stenosis who failed medical therapy and underwent angioplasty and stenting, Ramee et al. reported a 100% acute successful recanalization rate and 93.5% 1-year rate of freedom from stroke or death, suggesting that this approach can be effective in experienced centers *(70,71)*.

Marks et al. reported 23 patients with symptomatic intracranial atherosclerosis treated with angioplasty and reported a low annual risk (4.8%) of recurrent stroke. However, there was a substantial risk of periprocedural stroke or death (8.7%), including a fatal balloon-induced vessel rupture *(72)*.

These data highlight the need for extreme care when selecting patients for endovascular interventions. Particular care should be taken in those with vertebrobasilar disease, in whom angioplasty has been associated with a higher complication rate *(73)*.

REFERENCES

1. Crouse JR, Toole JF, McKinney WM, et al. Risk factors for extracranial carotid artery atherosclerosis. Stroke 1987;18:990–996.
2. Duncan GW, Lees RS, Ojemann RG, David SS. Concomitants of atherosclerotic carotid artery stenosis. Stroke 1977;8:665–669.
3. Bogousslavsky J, Regli F, Van Melle G. Risk factors and concomitants of internal carotid artery occlusion or stenosis. A controlled study of 159 cases. Arch Neurol 1985;42:864–867.
4. Harrison MJ, Wilson LA. Effect of blood pressure on prevalence of carotid atheroma. Stroke 1983;14:550–551.
5. Ford CS, Crouse JR 3rd, Howard G, Toole JF, Ball MR, Frye J. The role of plasma lipids in carotid bifurcation atherosclerosis. Ann Neurol 1985;17:301–303.
6. Wilterdink JL, Furie KL, Easton JD. Cardiac evaluation of stroke patients. Neurology 1998;51(3 Suppl 3):S23–S26.
7. Chambers BR, Norris JW. Outcome in patients with asymptomatic neck bruits. N Engl J Med 1986;315:860–865.
8. O'Leary DH, Polak JF, Kronmal RA, Manolio TA, Burke GL, Wolfson SK Jr. Carotid-artery intima and media thickness as a risk factor for myocardial infarction and stroke in older adults. Cardiovascular Health Study Collaborative Research Group. N Engl J Med 1999;340:14–22.
9. Edwards JH, Kricheff II, Riles T, Imparrato A. Angiographically undetected ulceration of the carotid bifurcation as a cause of embolic stroke. Radiology 1979;132: 369–373.

10. Ammar AD, Mullins JR. Incidence of bilateral intraplaque hemorrhage in carotid artery disease. Cardiovasc Surg 1993;1:717–719.
11. Langsfeld M, Gray-Weale AC, Lusby RJ. The role of plaque morphology and diameter reduction in the development of new symptoms in asymptomatic carotid arteries. J Vasc Surg 1989;9:548–557.
12. O'Donnell TF Jr, Erdoes L, Mackey WC, et al. Correlation of B-mode ultrasound imaging and arteriography with pathologic findings at carotid endarterectomy. Arch Surg 1985;120:443–449.
13. Mathiesen EB, Bonaa KH, Joakimsen O. Echolucent plaques are associated with high risk of ischemic cerebrovascular events in carotid stenosis: the Tromso study. Circulation 2001;103:2171–2175.
14. Fayad ZA, Fuster V. Clinical imaging of the high-risk or vulnerable atherosclerotic plaque. Circ Res 2001;89:305–316.
15. Yuan C, Mitsumori LM, Beach KW, Maravilla KR. Carotid atherosclerotic plaque: noninvasive MR characterization and identification of vulnerable lesions. Radiology 2001;221:285–299.
16. Fisher CM, Ojemann RG. A clinico-pathologic study of carotid endarterectomy plaques. Rev Neurol (Paris) 1986;142:573–3589.
17. Beal MF, Williams RS, Richardson EP Jr, Fisher CM. Cholesterol embolism as a cause of transient ischemic attacks and cerebral infarction. Neurology 1981;31:860–865.
18. Pessin MS, Hinton RC, Davis KR, et al. Mechanisms of acute carotid stroke. Ann Neurol 1979;6:245–252.
19. Fisher CM, Pearlman A. The nonsudden onset of cerebral embolism. Neurology 1967;17:1025–1032.
20. Albers GW, Caplan LR, Easton JD, et al. Transient ischemic attack—proposal for a new definition. N Engl J Med 2002;347:1713–1716.
21. Benavente O, Eliaszin M, Streifler JY, Fox AJ, Barnett HJ, Meldrum H. Prognosis after transient monocular blindness associated with carotid-artery stenosis. N Engl J Med 2001;345:1084–1090.
22. Johnston SC. Clinical practice. Transient ischemic attack. N Engl J Med 2002;347:1687–1692.
23. Johnston SC, Gress DR, Browner WS, Sidney S. Short-term prognosis after emergency department diagnosis of TIA. JAMA 2000;284:2901–2906.
24. Anderson DC, Kappelle LJ, Eliaszin M, Babikian VL, Pearce LA, Barnett HJ. Occurrence of hemispheric and retinal ischemia in atrial fibrillation compared with carotid stenosis. Stroke 2002;33:1963–1967.
25. Zwiebel WJ. Duplex sonography of the cerebral arteries: efficacy, limitations, and indications. AJR Am J Roentgenol 1992;158:29–36.
26. Nederkoorn PJ, van der Graaf Y, Hunink MG. Duplex ultrasound and magnetic resonance angiography compared with digital subtraction angiography in carotid artery stenosis: a systematic review. Stroke 2003;34:1324–1332.
27. Wilterdink JL, Feldman E, Easton JD, Ward R. Performance of carotid ultrasound in evaluating candidates for carotid endarterectomy is optimized by an approach based on clinical outcome rather than accuracy. Stroke 1996;27:1094–1098.
28. Suwanwela N, Can U, Furie KL, et al. Carotid Doppler ultrasound criteria for internal carotid artery stenosis based on residual lumen diameter calculated from en bloc carotid endarterectomy specimens. Stroke 1996;27:1965–1969.

29. Dawson DL, Zierler RE, Strandness DE Jr, Clowes AW, Kohler TR. The role of duplex scanning and arteriography before carotid endarterectomy: a prospective study. J Vasc Surg 1993;18:673–680; discussion 680–683.
30. Furst G, Saleh A, Wenserski F, et al. Reliability and validity of noninvasive imaging of internal carotid artery pseudo-occlusion. Stroke 1999;30:1444–1449.
31. Can U, Furie KL, Suwarmela N, et al. Transcranial Doppler ultrasound criteria for hemodynamically significant internal carotid artery stenosis based on residual lumen diameter calculated from en bloc endarterectomy specimens. Stroke 1997;28: 1966–1971.
32. Sitzer M, Fwist G, Fisher H, et al. Between-method correlation in quantifying internal carotid stenosis. Stroke 1993;24:1513–1518.
33. Johnston DC, Goldstein LB. Clinical carotid endarterectomy decision making: noninvasive vascular imaging vs angiography. Neurology 2001;56:1009–1015.
34. Heiserman JE, Drayer BD, Fram EK, et al. Carotid artery stenosis: clinical efficacy of two-dimensional time-of-flight MR angiography. Radiology 1992;182:761–768.
35. Huston J 3rd, Lewis BD, Wiebers DO, Meyer FB, Riederer SJ, Weaver AL. Carotid artery: prospective blinded comparison of two-dimensional time-of-flight MR angiography with conventional angiography and duplex US. Radiology 1993; 186:339–344.
36. Mattle HP, Kent KC, Edelman RR, Atkinson DJ, Skillman JJ. Evaluation of the extracranial carotid arteries: correlation of magnetic resonance angiography, duplex ultrasonography, and conventional angiography. J Vasc Surg 1991;13:838–844; discussion 844–845.
37. Polak JF, Bajakian RL, O'Leary DH, Anderson MR, Donaldson MC, Jolesz FA. Detection of internal carotid artery stenosis: comparison of MR angiography, color Doppler sonography, and arteriography. Radiology 1992;182:35–40.
38. Wardlaw JM, Lewis SC, Humphrey P, Young G, Collie D, Warlow CP. How does the degree of carotid stenosis affect the accuracy and interobserver variability of magnetic resonance angiography? J Neurol Neurosurg Psychiatry 2001;71:155–160.
39. Riles TS, Eidelman EM, Litt AW, Pinto RS, Oldford F, Schwartzenberg GW. Comparison of magnetic resonance angiography, conventional angiography, and duplex scanning. Stroke 1992;23:341–346.
40. Knauth M, von Kummer R, Jansen O, Hahnel S, Dorfler A, Sartor K. Potential of CT angiography in acute ischemic stroke. AJNR Am J Neuroradiol 1997;18: 1001–1010.
41. Shrier DA, Tanaka H, Numaguchi Y, Konno S, Patel U, Shibata D. CT angiography in the evaluation of acute stroke. AJNR Am J Neuroradiol 1997;18:1011–1020.
42. Hankey GJ, Warlow CP, Sellar RJ. Cerebral angiographic risk in mild cerebrovascular disease. Stroke 1990;21:209–222.
43. Beneficial effect of carotid endarterectomy in symptomatic patients with high-grade carotid stenosis. North American Symptomatic Carotid Endarterectomy Trial Collaborators. N Engl J Med 1991;325:445–453.
44. Randomised trial of endarterectomy for recently symptomatic carotid stenosis: final results of the MRC European Carotid Surgery Trial (ECST). Lancet 1998;351: 1379–1387.
45. Kent KC, Kuntz KM, Patel MR, et al. Perioperative imaging strategies for carotid endarterectomy. An analysis of morbidity and cost-effectiveness in symptomatic patients. JAMA 1995;274:888–893.

46. Young GR, Sandercock PA, Slattery J, Humphrey PR, Smith ET, Brock L. Observer variation in the interpretation of intra-arterial angiograms and the risk of inappropriate decisions about carotid endarterectomy. J Neurol Neurosurg Psychiatry 1996; 60:152–157.
47. Endarterectomy for asymptomatic carotid artery stenosis. Executive Committee for the Asymptomatic Carotid Atherosclerosis Study. JAMA 1995;273:1421–1428.
48. Hobson RW 2nd, Weiss DG, Fields WS, et al. Efficacy of carotid endarterectomy for asymptomatic carotid stenosis. The Veterans Affairs Cooperative Study Group. N Engl J Med 1993;328:221–227.
49. Barnett HJ, Taylor DW, Eliasziw M, et al. Benefit of carotid endarterectomy in patients with symptomatic moderate or severe stenosis. North American Symptomatic Carotid Endarterectomy Trial Collaborators. N Engl J Med 1998;339:1415–1425.
50. Gasecki AP, Ferguson GG, EliasziwM, et al. Early endarterectomy for severe carotid artery stenosis after a nondisabling stroke: results from the North American Symptomatic Carotid Endarterectomy Trial. J Vasc Surg 1994;20:288–295.
51. Ballotta E, Da Giau G, Barracchini C, Abbruzzese E, Saladini M, Meneghetti G. Early vs delayed carotid endarterectomy after a nondisabling ischemic stroke: a prospective randomized study. Surgery 2002;131:287–293.
52. Lammie GA, Sandercock PA, Dennis MS. Recently occluded intracranial and extracranial carotid arteries. Relevance of the unstable atherosclerotic plaque. Stroke 1999;30:1319–1325.
53. Wityk RJ, Lehman D, Klag M, Coresh J, Ahn H, Litt B. Race and sex differences in the distribution of cerebral atherosclerosis. Stroke 1996;27:1974–1980.
54. Sacco RL, Kargman, DE, Gu Q, Zamanillo MC. Race–ethnicity and determinants of intracranial atherosclerotic cerebral infarction. The Northern Manhattan Stroke Study. Stroke 1995;26:14–20.
55. Leung SY, Nq TH, Yuen ST, Lauder IJ, Ho FC. Pattern of cerebral atherosclerosis in Hong Kong Chinese. Severity in intracranial and extracranial vessels. Stroke 1993; 24:779–786.
56. Petty GW, Brown RD Jr, Whisnant JP, Sicks JD, O'Fallon WM, Wiebers DO. Ischemic stroke subtypes: a population-based study of functional outcome, survival, and recurrence. Stroke 2000;31:1062–1068.
57. Thijs VN, Albers GW. Symptomatic intracranial atherosclerosis: outcome of patients who fail antithrombotic therapy. Neurology 2000;55:490–497.
58. Chimowitz MI, Kokkinos J, Strong J, et al. The Warfarin–Aspirin Symptomatic Intracranial Disease Study. Neurology 1995;45:1488–1493.
59. Akins PT, Pilgrim TK, Cross DT 3rd, Moran CJ. Natural history of stenosis from intracranial atherosclerosis by serial angiography. Stroke 1998;29:433–438.
60. Yasaka M, Yamaguchi T, Shichiri M. Distribution of atherosclerosis and risk factors in atherothrombotic occlusion. Stroke 1993;24:206–211.
61. Postiglione A, Napoli C. Hyperlipidaemia and atherosclerotic cerebrovascular disease. Curr Opin Lipidol 1995;6:236–242.
62. Vaverkova H, Novotny D, Ficker L, Viachova I, Chudackova J. Lipoprotein(a): a genetic risk factor for early ischemic cerebrovascular stroke [in Czech]. Vnitr Lek 1993;39:979–987.
63. Yoo JH, Chung CS, Kang SS. Relation of plasma homocyst(e)ine to cerebral infarction and cerebral atherosclerosis. Stroke 1998;29:2478–2483.

64. Tan NC, Venketasubramanian N, Saw SM, Tjia HT. Hyperhomocyst(e)inemia and risk of ischemic stroke among young Asian adults. Stroke 2002;33:1956–1962.
65. Caplan LR. Diabetes and brain ischemia. Diabetes 1996;45(Suppl 3):S95–S97.
66. Reed DM, Resch JA, Hayashi T, MacLean C, Yano K. A prospective study of cerebral artery atherosclerosis. Stroke 1988;19:820–825.
67. Rordorf G, Cramer SC, Efird JT, Schwamm LH, Buonanno F, Koroshetz WJ. Pharmacological elevation of blood pressure in acute stroke. Clinical effects and safety. Stroke 1997;28:2133–2138.
68. Rordorf G, Koroshetz WJ, Ezzeddine MA, Segal AZ, Buonanno FS. A pilot study of drug-induced hypertension for treatment of acute stroke. Neurology 2001;56: 1210–1213.
69. Wijman CA, McBee NA, Keyl PM, et al. Diagnostic impact of early transcranial Doppler ultrasonography on the TOAST classification subtype in acute cerebral ischemia. Cerebrovasc Dis 2001;11:317–323.
70. Ramee SR, Dawson R, McKinley KL, et al. Provisional stenting for symptomatic intracranial stenosis using a multidisciplinary approach: acute results, unexpected benefit, and 1-year outcome. Catheter Cardiovasc Interv 2001;52:457–467.
71. Chaloupka JC, Weigele JB, Mangla S, Lesley WS. Cerebrovascular angioplasty and stenting for the prevention of stroke. Curr Neurol Neurosci Rep 2001;1:39–53.
72. Marks MP, Marcellus M, Norbash AM, Steinberg GK, Tong D, Albers GW. Outcome of angioplasty for atherosclerotic intracranial stenosis. Stroke 1999;30:1065–1069.
73. Rasmussen PA, Perl J 2nd, Barr JD, et al. Stent-assisted angioplasty of intracranial vertebrobasilar atherosclerosis: an initial experience. J Neurosurg 2000;92:771–778.

11

Craniocervical Endovascular Stenting and Angioplasty

Cenk Ayata and Guy Rordorf

OVERVIEW OF ENDOVASCULAR THERAPY FOR CRANIOCERVICAL DISEASE

Following successful treatment of coronary and peripheral vascular stenoses, balloon angioplasty of the extracranial cervical vessels was introduced in the late 1970s. It was initially used on an investigative basis for medically refractory, surgically inaccessible lesions in the vertebrobasilar system *(1,2)* and for multiple or tandem vascular stenoses, such as in Takayasu's arteritis and in fibromuscular dysplasia *(3–6)*. In recent years, many uncontrolled case series and some registry data have reported reasonable technical success rates and variable efficacy for stroke prevention. Angioplasty and stent placement have been advocated as viable alternatives to surgery in patients with stenosis of the common and internal carotid arteries who are at high risk of perioperative medical and surgical complications and in other patients for whom endarterectomy may be technically difficult *(7–10)*.

Most data on the safety and benefit of carotid angioplasty and stenting comes from anecdotal reports and observational studies. These data do not substitute for well-conducted, large, randomized trials *(11)*. Reports of outcomes of small series from individual centers are subject to biased assessment by the interventionalists, who are usually not blinded. Patients may be preferentially selected, both for the procedure itself and for inclusion in the published report. Conflicts of interest, overt or covert, may exist. Such reports often compare outcomes to historical controls or data from previous trials. This approach is not sufficiently rigorous to make valid conclusions of efficacy because of advances in medical management and differences in case mix and selection criteria between studies.

Endovascular therapy for craniocervical stenosis has inherent attractions. General anesthesia is not required, which may translate into reduced morbidity, particularly in patients with severe cardiac or respiratory disease. It does

From: *Current Clinical Neurology: Handbook of Stroke Prevention in Clinical Practice*
Edited by: K. L. Furie and P. J. Kelly © Humana Press Inc., Totowa, NJ

not involve a cervical incision, thus eliminating morbidity caused by cervical hematoma and postoperative cranial neuropathies. It may have advantages compared to medical therapy for surgically inaccessible lesions in the distal cervical or intracranial carotid or vertebral arteries, for postsurgical restenosis, or for selected technically difficult cases (e.g., radiation stenosis or long stenoses).

However, despite the enthusiasm for endovascular therapy displayed by some advocates, important issues remain to be resolved regarding safety, efficacy, and indications for treatment. An expert committee from the American Heart Association *(12)* emphasized several of these. First, an established therapy exists for treatment of severe symptomatic internal carotid artery stenosis. This has considerable benefit (absolute stroke reduction of almost 5% annually) and relatively low complication rates in experienced hands. To prove benefit, endovascular approaches must demonstrate at least equivalent efficacy and risk to endarterectomy in large randomized trials of symptomatic patients with severe stenosis.

Second, the risk of stroke associated with diagnostic catheterization of the carotid artery is not trivial (1–3%) and is close to the risk of endarterectomy in some centers. This risk is likely to be higher following manipulation of the plaque.

Third, endovascular therapy has other acute and long-term complications, including bradycardia, cardiac arrest, hypotension, cerebral hyperperfusion injury, and restenosis. The morbidity associated with these problems requires direct comparison with that related to endarterectomy.

Fourth, acute stent thrombosis is not amenable to surgical correction (unlike coronary or limb angioplasty) and is often irreversible despite the use of thrombolytics and glycoprotein IIb/IIIa inhibitors. Also, poststent restenosis may be difficult or impossible to repair by conventional endarterectomy because of the presence of the stent.

Fifth, local or regional anesthesia is increasingly used for carotid endarterectomy (CEA), and the length of hospital stay is usually not more than 2 days. Therefore, some apparent attractions of endovascular treatment, such as lack of general anesthesia, shorter duration of stay, and lower cost may be more apparent than real.

Finally, few reliable long-term data exist on the efficacy of carotid endovascular intervention for stroke prevention.

To date, only one relatively small randomized trial comparing CEA with angioplasty has been completed. Other trials were discontinued prematurely because of higher morbidity in the angioplasty group. At the time of writing, other trials are under way in Europe and the United States. Until these data are available, there is no reliable evidence supporting the routine use of endovascular stenting for treatment of stenosis of the common or internal carotid artery outside the setting of a clinical trial. For very carefully selected patients (e.g., those with symptomatic carotid disease with a need for coronary revascularization, symptomatic restenosis after CEA or neck irradiation, symptomatic vertebral or intracranial carotid stenosis refractory to maximal medical therapy), an endovascular approach may be considered in some centers with experienced operators, providing informed consent is obtained.

UNCONTROLLED STUDIES OF ENDOVASCULAR INTERVENTION FOR CAROTID DISEASE

Most available safety and efficacy data on carotid angioplasty derive from uncontrolled series of patients with extracranial carotid stenosis. In different case series, the incidence of 30-day periprocedural stroke (minor and major) or death has varied from 0 to 9.7% *(13–24)*. In symptomatic patients with high-grade stenosis (≥90%), the risk of stroke or death has been 4.4–10.8% within 30 days and 6.8–12.7% over 6–23 months of follow-up. Lower rates have been reported in smaller series *(25)*. In a global carotid stent registry involving more than 5000 patients from 36 centers worldwide, the 30-day stroke and procedure-related death rate was 5.07% *(26)*. Although the risk of all in-hospital medical complications was higher than in the North American Symptomatic Carotid Endarterectomy Trial (NASCET), the rates of wound-related complications and perioperative cranial nerve injury were lower.

Reported early technical success rates have been 86–100% (98.4% in the global registry), and the degree of residual stenosis has been reported as minimal across the studies. Acute stent thrombosis, all asymptomatic, occurred in 2.5% of patients within the first 2 days in one series *(15)*. The duration of hospital stay was usually less than 2 days *(14)*. Ambulatory carotid stenting has also been reported to be safe *(27)*. The incidence of stroke or death during follow-up (up to 6 years) varied from 0 to 6.9% in two series *(15,22)*.

In a series of more than 500 patients considered high risk for CEA in the opinion of the investigators (71% coronary artery disease, 10% contralateral carotid occlusion, and 83% NASCET ineligible), the technical success rate was 98%, the 30-day rate of stroke or death was 8.1%, and the rate of major stroke or death was 2.6% *(28)*. Symptomatic and asymptomatic patients had similar 30-day outcomes. However, patients 80 years of age or older had significantly higher stroke or death rates. This study suggested that the majority of strokes related to carotid angioplasty and stenting take place within the first 30 days, and there is a long-lasting benefit. The incidence of late stroke (after 30 days, up to 3 years; average 17 months) was 3.2%, only 0.4% of which were major ipsilateral strokes. Although a direct comparison is not possible, these results are in the range reported by NASCET, despite the individuals being considered high risk and NASCET ineligible by the authors *(28)*.

Jordan and coworkers retrospectively compared the risks of stroke and death between endarterectomy and endovascular approaches, both under regional anesthesia, and found that angioplasty and stenting had a significantly higher stroke or death risk (9.7%) compared to endarterectomy (0.9%). However, the unusually low risk with endarterectomy in their series, likely related to the use of regional instead of general anesthesia, makes generalization difficult *(18)*.

RANDOMIZED CONTROLLED TRIALS OF ENDOVASCULAR THERAPY FOR CAROTID DISEASE

Two early trials comparing endovascular intervention with CEA were stopped prematurely because of excessive morbidity in the endovascular arm. One of these was discontinued after only 23 patients had been enrolled. In the other trial (WALLSTENT), among 219 patients with symptomatic carotid disease (60–90%), 12.2% of those randomized to the stent group had an ipsilateral stroke at 1 year compared to 3.6% of the group who underwent CEA ($p = 0.02$).

The Carotid and Vertebral Artery Transluminal Angioplasty Study (CAVATAS) trial randomly assigned 504 patients with symptomatic and asymptomatic stenoses of the common or internal carotid artery who required intervention in the opinion of the treating physician *(29)*. The degree of stenosis, calculated by the common carotid method, was greater than 70% in most patients. In an accompanying editorial, Spence and Eliasziw *(30)* estimated that this corresponded to more than 50% stenosis by the NASCET method, and more than 75% by the European Carotid Surgery Trial (ECST) method. If these estimates are accurate, the CAVATAS patients comprised a group of symptomatic (96%, about 90% with symptoms in the previous 6 months) and asymptomatic (4%) patients with moderate-to-severe stenosis by the NASCET criteria (mean stenosis 75% by NASCET).

At 30 days, the rates of stroke (>7 days) or death were 10% in the endovascular group and 9.9% in the CEA group. Rates of disabling stroke or death were also similar (6.4% in the endovascular and 5.9% in the CEA group). Although the numbers were small (only 93 followed for 3 years), no difference in stroke rates was detected between groups on follow-up. Severe (>70%) ipsilateral stenosis was more common in the endovascular group at 1 year (14 vs 4%, $p < 0.001$). However, angioplasty had a much lower rate of cranial neuropathy or hematoma formation.

Table 1
Indirect Comparisons of Major Endarterectomy Trials with CAVATAS

	3-Year stroke or death risk if medically treated (%)	3-Year stroke or death risk of intervention (%)	Risk difference (%)	Number needed to treat	30-Day periprocedural stroke or death (%)
Symptomatic severe NASCET (70–99%)	25.1	8.9	16.2	6	5.8
Symptomatic severe ECST (70–99%)	16.8	10.3	6.5	15	7.5
Symptomatic moderate NASCET (50–69%)	16.2	11.3	4.9	20	7.1
Asymptomatic moderate–severe ACAS (60–99%)	11	5.1	5.9	19	2.3
CAVATAS (CEA)	18.6[a]	13.9	4.7	21	9.9
CAVATAS (angioplasty or stent)	18.6[a]	14.4	4.2	24	10

Source: From data summarized in refs. *29* and *30*.

[a]No medical arm. Medical risk was calculated from a weighted average of medical arms from NASCET and ECST studies *(30)*.

ACAS, Asymptomatic Carotid Atherosclerosis Study.

Spence and Eliasziw compared these results to existing data from large trials that compared CEA to medical therapy (Table 1) *(30)*. Although indirect comparisons between studies must be interpreted with caution, they highlighted several points of concern. Most important was the fact that the rates of stroke and death at 30 days (about 10%) of both surgery and angioplasty or stenting were higher than those reported in the NASCET, ESCT, and Aspirin and Carotid Endarterectomy (ACE) trials (average 6.3%). Furthermore, all deaths (seven) in the endovascular group were caused by stroke (three hemorrhagic, four ischemic); only one death in the CEA group was stroke related. This suggests that angioplasty may have directly contributed to the fatal outcomes in this arm.

To benefit patients with moderate symptomatic or asymptomatic disease, intervention-related complication rates must be low (2.3% reported in ACAS). Based on the stroke or death rates of medically treated patients in these trials, neither endarterectomy nor endovascular therapy in CAVATAS was likely to have provided a meaningful benefit for patients with moderate symptomatic or asymptomatic disease. The 30-day rates of stroke (>7 days) or death in CAVATAS (10%) are almost identical to the rates at 3 years for medically treated asymptomatic patients (11%); there was no evidence to indicate benefit in this group. On the contrary, at 3 years more asymptomatic patients in CAVATAS had suffered stroke or death than similar medically treated patients in ACAS (14.4 vs 11%), suggesting that early events may have been precipitated as a result of the intervention. Comparing the rates of stroke (>7days) or death at 3 years in CAVATAS with those in NASCET for symptomatic patients with moderate stenosis, the benefit of angioplasty was negligible (absolute risk difference 1.8%, number needed to treat 56). Based on the clinical characteristics of subjects included in CAVATAS, it is unlikely that case mix accounts for these differences in outcome.

Other randomized, multicenter trials are ongoing. These include the International Carotid Stenting Study (ICSS) *(31)*, Carotid Revascularization–Endarterectomy vs Stent Trial (CREST) *(32)*, and Carotid Artery Revascularization With Endarterectomy or Stenting Systems (CARESS) *(33)*. It is anticipated that these studies will resolve some of the issues discussed here.

POTENTIAL INDICATIONS FOR CRANIOCERVICAL ANGIOPLASTY OR STENTING

Risk Stratification for CEA and Endovascular Therapy

A list of potential indications for craniocervical endovascular therapy is presented in Table 2 based on data from uncontrolled studies and the absence of safe alternative treatments *(12,34)*.

Several groups have examined potential predictors of adverse outcome after CEA and endovascular therapy. Mathur et al. *(35)* reported that age was associated with higher risk for neurological events associated with angioplasty and stenting; age older than 80 years had an overall stroke incidence of 19.2%. Long or multiple stenoses or severe lesions (>90% stenosis) carried a significantly higher risk for stroke in univariate analysis. In multivariate analysis, only age (odds ratio [OR] 1.1) and long and tandem stenoses (OR 5.1) were significantly associated with a higher risk of periprocedural stroke. Qureshi and colleagues reported an increased the risk of neurological complications with symptomatic lesions (OR 8.3), with a stenosis longer than 11.1 mm (OR 5.3), and absence of hypercholesterolemia (OR 5.4) *(36)*.

Risk Prediction Based on Medical, Neurological, and Angiographic Factors

Sundt and coworkers proposed a grading system for risk stratification of CEA *(37)*. They defined potential medical risk factors as angina pectoris or recent (<6 months) myocardial infarction (MI), congestive heart failure, blood pressure exceeding 180/110, chronic obstructive lung disease, age older than

Table 2
Potential Indications for Craniocervical Endovascular Therapy

1. Patients at high risk for CEA with progressive/recurrent neurological symptoms and who are unresponsive to maximal medical therapy (e.g., unstable coronary disease, heart failure)
2. Restenosis after endarterectomy or angioplasty
3. Radiation-induced stenosis
4. Patients with surgically inaccessible lesions, with progressive or recurrent neurological symptoms, unresponsiveness to maximal medical therapy (high cervical, intracranial carotid, vertebrobasilar stenosis)

Source: From ref. *34*.

70 years, and severe obesity. Neurological risk factors were defined as progressing neurological deficit, stable recent deficit (<24 hours from onset), frequent daily transient deficits, and deficits secondary to multiple cerebral infarcts. Potential angiographic risk factors were defined as contralateral carotid occlusion, siphon stenosis, long diseased segment, high carotid bifurcation, and soft thrombus over the plaque.

In a retrospective analysis of a relatively small cohort who underwent CEA, neurologically stable patients with no medical comorbidity with (grade II) or without (grade I) angiographic risk factors had 1–2% risk of developing myocardial infarction or persistent postoperative neurologic deficits. Patients with medical comorbidities without neurological risk factors (grade III) had a 7% risk of developing myocardial infarction. Of those with neurological risk factors, regardless of their medical or angiographic risks (grade IV), 10% had stroke associated with CEA.

Sieber et al. reported that the total morbidity (MI, stroke) and mortality from CEA increased from about 2% for grade I, to 10% for grade II, 11% for grade III, and 18% for grade IV *(38)*. The incidence of MI was highest in group III. Stroke was more common in groups II and IV, with worse outcome in the latter group *(39)*. This study, therefore, suggested an association between angio-graphic risk factors and increased incidence of stroke.

In a large multicenter retrospective review *(39)*, the presence of two or more proposed Sundt predictors was associated with a 1.7 times higher risk of stroke, MI, or death and twice the risk of stroke or death.

There is yet no published randomized trial comparing CEA and endovascular approaches in high-risk patients. However, small uncontrolled series have suggested lower morbidity and mortality associated with angioplasty or stenting. For example, Al-Mubarak et al. reported a major stroke or death rate of 4.5% in 44 Sundt grade IV patients, with good intermediate-term arterial patency *(40)*. Similarly, in patients with high medical risks, the 30-day procedural risk of stroke or death was 2.9%. Of these, 76% were ineligible for CEA by NASCET criteria (53% < 80 years, 26% had left ventricular ejection fraction ≥30%, and 44% had moderate-to-severe angina) *(41)*. Combined carotid and coronary interventions have also been well tolerated *(41, 42)*. In patients with contralateral carotid occlusion the 30-day risk of stroke and death was zero after angioplasty and stenting in a small case series *(43)*, compared to 14.3 % after CEA in NASCET *(44)*.

Endovascular Approaches for Restenosis and Radiation-Induced Stenosis

Post-CEA restenosis renders repeat endarterectomy technically difficult because of scarring. Surgery for recurrent stenosis has been reported to carry a 10% risk of death or major neurologic complications *(45)*, the latter mostly in symptomatic patients who had intraluminal thrombus. The risk was 11% in those patients with medical risk factors and recurrent stenosis *(38)*. In a series of 22 patients who had angioplasty and stenting for recurrent stenosis after CEA, the procedure was successful in all, with only one minor procedural stroke. There were no ipsilateral neurological events over a mean follow-up of 8 months. None of the patients had angiographic restenosis of 50% or more at 6 months, and mean restenosis was 19% *(46)*. In another series of patients who had angioplasty with or without stenting for recurrent carotid stenosis following CEA, Lanzino et al. reported no major periprocedural stroke or death. Patients remained asymptomatic for a mean follow-up of 27 months. More than 50% restenosis developed in 60% of patients treated with angioplasty alone and in only 5.6% of the vessels treated by combined angioplasty and stent placement *(47)*. Finally, in a larger series of restenosis following endarterectomy, the 30-day stroke and death rate was 3.7% *(48)*.

Cervical irradiation predisposes the involved arteries to accelerated stenosis because of destruction of the internal elastic lamina and myointimal hyperplasia *(49)*. These stenoses have a predilection for the distal common carotid artery after cervical irradiation. Although patients are often younger compared to those with atherosclerotic stenosis, the lesions involve longer segments of the artery and often show circumferential narrowing of the lumen. In a series of 14 patients who had stent placement for radiation-induced carotid stenosis, only one minor stroke happened with full recovery; there was no restenosis of 50% or more at 6-month follow-up *(50)*. Others have reported similar results *(51)*.

Intracranial Anterior and Posterior Circulation Stenoses

Intracranial stenoses are estimated to account for 5–10% of all ischemic strokes and transient ischemic attacks *(52–57)*. The cavernous portion of the internal carotid artery is the most common location of anterior circulation stenosis, followed by the petrous and clinoid carotid *(55)* and the proximal middle cerebral artery. The recommended treatment strategy for symptomatic intracranial stenosis is antiplatelet therapy and other secondary prevention measures. Randomized trials are required to evaluate the role of angioplasty and stenting for symptomatic intracranial disease. In the absence of such trials, endovascular approaches may have a role for selected cases if recurrent or progressive neurological symptoms are occurring despite maximal medical measures.

Factors that should be considered when selecting such patients for intervention include (1) the accessibility, length, degree, and eccentricity of the stenosis; (2) the presence of other lesions (contralateral occlusion, tandem stenoses); (3) the intracranial hemodynamic status assessed by positron emission tomography or other techniques; and (4) the experience of the performing center.

COMPLICATIONS OF ANGIOPLASTY AND STENTING

Stent Thrombosis and Distal Embolization

Acute thrombosis and embolism to the brain is the most common cause of periprocedural neurologic morbidity. Severe dissection and acute closure of the artery carry the highest risk *(14)*. Predisposing factors for thromboembolic complications of angioplasty and stenting have not been defined. However, data from small case series suggest that pre- and poststent combination antiplatelet coverage reduces stent thrombosis *(58)*.

Platelet activation has been demonstrated in coronary stenting, in which, in addition to dual antiplatelet therapy with aspirin and either clopidogrel or ticlopidine *(59)*, periprocedural intravenous abciximab (a platelet glycoprotein IIb/IIIa receptor antagonist) reduces the rate of ischemic complications. In one small series of carotid stent placement, abciximab was associated with a lower rate of periprocedural stroke without an increase in the risk of intracranial hemorrhage compared to historical controls *(60)*. A few reports have described successful recanalization with intraarterial, followed by intravenous, abciximab following acute stent occlusion *(61)*. Therefore, abciximab appears to be a promising prophylactic as well as therapeutic agent against ischemic events during angioplasty and stenting when used in combination with heparin, low-dose thrombolytics, aspirin, and clopidogrel *(62,63)*.

Similarly, another glycoprotein IIb/IIIa receptor antagonist, eptifibatide (135 μg/kg bolus followed by infusion at 0.5 μg/kg per minute), has been shown to be safe during carotid angioplasty and stenting in a small phase I study *(64)*.

Balloon inflation times of 15–30 seconds during carotid angioplasty have been well tolerated *(14)*. Both CEA and angioplasty with stenting are associated with complete interruption of blood flow during shunt insertion or balloon inflation. The duration of blood flow reduction and ischemia appears to be shorter for angioplasty (less than 0.5 minutes) compared to endarterectomy (longer than 2.5 minutes) *(65,66)*. On the other hand, four to eight times more microembolic signals were observed during angioplasty compared to endarterectomy; the pre- and postdilation and stent deployment phases have been associated with high frequency of microembolic signals *(66–68)*. Some of the microembolic signals observed during angioplasty are likely to be microscopic air bubbles associated with contrast injection and therefore of little clinical significance. However, the majority of microemboli consist of cholesterol crystals, lipoid masses, and fibrin material, with sizes between 1 μm and 5 mm (mean about 300 μm) *(69–71)*.

There are conflicting data regarding the clinical importance of flow reduction during occlusion as well as the number of microembolic signals. In some studies, neither the duration of occlusion nor the number of microemboli have been related to either the periprocedural stroke risk or long-term neuropsychological outcome *(66,72–74)*. However, using transcranial Doppler (TCD) during occlusion, others have found an increased risk of periprocedural transient ischemic attack and stroke when the mean middle cerebral artery blood flow velocity is reduced by 50% or more *(75)*. Similarly, in a series of 84 patients for whom a distal filter protection device was used, there was only one minor (1.2%) and no major periprocedural neurological event or procedure-related death *(69)*. Distal balloon protection devices may reduce the number of microembolic signals on TCD by more than 50% *(68)*. These devices are rapidly gaining favor and appear to reduce the periprocedural neurologic event rate *(76,77)*. Again, randomized trials are required to determine their efficacy and safety.

Restenosis

Late restenosis has been a major concern following angioplasty. Although more widespread use of stenting has reduced the reported incidence of restenosis *(47)*, rates vary widely. Degrees of restenosis (>60–70%), mostly asymptomatic, were seen in 0–25% of patients on long-term follow-up after stent angioplasty in different series *(13–15,19,30,41)*. The average degree of restenosis was 12–18% at 6 months *(13,14,41)*. In CAVATAS, stenting did not appear to reduce restenosis (severe stenosis or occlusion was seen in 22% of patients who received a stent vs 17% of patients who had angioplasty alone), although the number of stented cases was low ($n = 41$) *(29)*.

About half of restenoses after angioplasty with or without stenting have been estimated as caused by recurrent atherosclerosis, one-fourth caused by neointimal hyperplasia, and the rest caused by the presence of organized thrombus *(45)*. Recurrent atherosclerosis is characterized by lipid deposits and lipid-laden macrophages (foam cells), whereas neointimal hyperplasia predominantly involves smooth muscle cell proliferation and migration. Neointimal hyperplasia after coronary angioplasty has been associated with a smooth plaque surface. Therefore, neointimal hyperplasia after carotid angioplasty may be less likely to cause artery-to-artery embolism. In these cases, symptoms may be primarily related to hemodynamic insufficiency *(78)*.

Mechanisms of restenosis and potential preventive measures have been subjects of intense investigation. Among the promising approaches, nitric oxide and cytostatic agents have attracted particular attention. Increased nitric oxide/cyclic guanosine 5'-monophosphate signaling by supplemental L-arginine or nitric oxide synthase gene transfer reduces neointima formation after stenting via a mechanism dependent on nitric oxide synthase *(79)*. Drugs that inhibit cell proliferation at different levels, such as paclitaxel (antimitotic), sirolimus (inhibits cell division between phases G1 and S1), cytochalasin D (inhibits actin filament formation), and phosphorothioate oligodeoxynucleotides have been shown to halt neointimal hyperplasia when delivered locally in experimental animals *(80–83)*. However, further work is needed before these approaches find clinical use in prevention of restenosis.

Hyperperfusion Syndrome

Hyperperfusion syndrome occurs in about 1% of patients after CEA *(84)*. A sudden increase in cerebral perfusion pressure to a previously ischemic vascular territory with impaired autoregulation predisposes to cerebral edema formation and intracerebral or subarachnoid hemorrhages. The usual presenting features are headache, vomiting, altered mental state, focal neurologic deficits, hypertension, and seizures. Hyperperfusion syndrome has been associated with internal carotid, vertebral, or middle cerebral artery angioplasty and stenting *(85–87)*. In one series, it was reported in 5% of patients following cerebral angioplasty or stenting *(88)*. This number is higher than that after endarterectomy and requires verification by other investigators.

Angioplasty and stenting of major cerebral arteries immediately augments angiographic cerebral blood flow *(89–92)* and normalizes oxygen extraction fraction *(92,93)* as well as cerebrovascular reactivity *(90,94)*. However, persistently increased cerebral blood flow above normal levels (likely because of failure of cerebral vasculature to autoregulate and buffer quickly the rise in perfusion pressure) may be a marker of hyperperfusion syndrome *(86,88)*. Reported predictors of hyperperfusion syndrome after CEA are high-grade stenosis (>80%) with significant pressure gradient, poor collateral flow or contralateral carotid occlusion, perioperative hypertension, and the use of anticoagulation or antiplatelet agents *(95–101)*. Although factors associated with hyperperfusion syndrome after angioplasty are unknown, a profile similar to CEA would be expected. Strict blood pressure control is the mainstay of management, and TCD monitoring of flow velocities and pulsatility index has been used to titrate the mean arterial pressure level *(102)*.

Hypotension and Bradycardia

The problems of hypotension and bradycardia are relatively common after carotid angioplasty or stenting involving the carotid sinus *(103)*. They can occur immediately after balloon inflation because of stimulation of carotid sinus baroreceptors, simulating a sudden increase in intraarterial pressure. This culminates in increased vagal output and reduced sympathetic tone and may persist for many hours after the procedure. In one series, 71% of patients had transient bradycardia during balloon inflation *(14)*. In another, 70% of patients developed bradycardia, 56% became hypotensive, and 27% had asystole *(13)*. In a retrospective analysis, patients who developed hypotension with bradycardia during the procedure were at higher risk for doing so after the procedure for up to 24 hours *(104)*. Furthermore, patients who had a history of myocardial infarction were also at higher risk for developing postprocedural hypotension. Angioplasty-induced bradycardia appears to be more prevalent in radiation-induced stenosis and with symptomatic lesions. The proper management requires prompt recognition, fluid resuscitation, pharmacological pressors, and temporary venous demand pacing *(105)*. Atropine (1 mg iv) can be administered as needed during balloon inflation.

Complications of Intracranial Angioplasty

Complications of intracranial angioplasty are similar to those encountered with endovascular intervention of the extracranial vessels and include arterial dissection, rupture, spasm, acute thrombosis, and distal embolization *(106, 107)*. The introduction of stents has reduced arterial dissection, spasm, and immediate elastic recoil *(108–111)*. Improved technical details such as slow balloon inflation and the use of balloons smaller than the normal diameter of the artery have reduced complications such as dissection and acute vessel closure *(112)*. Acute dissection of the artery during angioplasty can be treated with a stent in selected patients *(113,114)*, whereas arterial spasm often responds to intraarterial vasodilator infusions. Anticoagulation and platelet glycoprotein IIb/IIIa antagonists during and after the procedure reduce the incidence of distal embolization and thrombosis. One often feared complication of stenting has been the occlusion of penetrating arteries that take off from the main artery, either by the stent (so-called jailing) or by debris from the crushed atherosclerotic plaque during balloon inflation; however, this has not been a frequent complication in clinical studies to date *(115–117)*.

REFERENCES

1. Sundt TM, Smith HC, Campbell JK, Vlietstra RE, Cucchiara RF, Stanson AW. Transluminal angioplasty for basilar artery stenosis. Mayo Clin Proc 1980;55: 673–680.
2. Motarjeme A, Keifer JW, Zuska AJ. Percutaneous transluminal angioplasty of the vertebral arteries. Radiology 1981;139:715–717.
3. Hasso AN, Bird CR, Zinke DE, Thompson JR. Fibromuscular dysplasia of the internal carotid artery: percutaneous transluminal angioplasty. AJR Am J Roentgenol 1981;136:955–960.
4. Belan A, Vesela M, Vanek I, Weiss K, Peregrin JH. Percutaneous transluminal angioplasty of fibromuscular dysplasia of the internal carotid artery. Cardiovasc Interv Radiol 1982;5:79-81.
5. Dublin AB, Baltaxe HA, Cobb CA 3rd. Percutaneous transluminal carotid angioplasty in fibromuscular dysplasia. Case report. J Neurosurg 1983;59:162–165.
6. Wilms GE, Smits J, Baert AL, De Wolf L. Percutaneous transluminal angioplasty in fibromuscular dysplasia of the internal carotid artery: 1 year clinical and morphological follow-up. Cardiovasc Interv Radiol 1985;8:20–23.
7. Bockenheimer SA, Mathias K. Percutaneous transluminal angioplasty in arteriosclerotic internal carotid artery stenosis. AJNR Am J Neuroradiol 1983;4:791–792.
8. Wiggli U, Gratzl O. Transluminal angioplasty of stenotic carotid arteries: case reports and protocol. AJNR Am J Neuroradiol 1983;4:793–795.
9. Kachel R, Basche S, Heerklotz I, Grossmann K, Endler S. Percutaneous transluminal angioplasty (PTA) of supra-aortic arteries especially the internal carotid artery. Neuroradiology 1991;33:191–194.
10. Numaguchi Y, Puyau FA, Provenza LJ, Richardson DE. Percutaneous transluminal angioplasty of the carotid artery. Its application to post surgical stenosis. Neuroradiology 1984;26:527–530.
11. Brott TG. Angioplasty and stenting should be performed only in the setting of a clinical trial. Stroke 2002;33:2519–2520.
12. Bettmann MA, Katzen BT, Whisnant J, et al. Carotid stenting and angioplasty: a statement for healthcare professionals from the Councils on Cardiovascular Radiology, Stroke, Cardio-Thoracic and Vascular Surgery, Epidemiology and Prevention, and Clinical Cardiology, American Heart Association. Stroke 1998;29: 336–338.
13. Gil-Peralta A, Mayol A, Marcos JR, et al. Percutaneous transluminal angioplasty of the symptomatic atherosclerotic carotid arteries. Results, complications, and follow-up. Stroke 1996;27:2271–2273.

14. Yadav JS, Roubin GS, Iyer S, et al. Elective stenting of the extracranial carotid arteries. Circulation 1997;95:376–381.
15. Dietz A, Berkefeld J, Theron JG, et al. Endovascular treatment of symptomatic carotid stenosis using stent placement: long-term follow-up of patients with a balanced surgical risk/benefit ratio. Stroke 2001;32:1855–1859.
16. Diethrich EB, Ndiaye M, Reid DB. Stenting in the carotid artery: initial experience in 110 patients. J Endovascr Surg 1996;3:42–62.
17. Dietrhrich EB. Indications for carotid artery stenting: a preview of the potential derived from early clinical experiences. J Endovasc Surg 1996;3:132–139.
18. Jordan WD Jr, Voellinger DC, Fisher WS, Redden D, McDowell HA. A comparison of carotid angioplasty with stenting vs endarterectomy with regional anesthesia. J Vasc Surg 1998;28:397–402; discussion 402–403.
19. Malek AM, Higashida RT, Phatouros CC, et al. Stent angioplasty for cervical carotid artery stenosis in high-risk symptomatic NASCET-ineligible patients. Stroke 2000;31:3029–3033.
20. Henry M, Amor M, Masson I, et al. Angioplasty and stenting of the extracranial carotid arteries. J Endovasc Surg 1998;5:293–304.
21. Roubin GS, Yadav S, Iyer SS, Vitek J. Carotid stent-supported angioplasty: a neurovascular intervention to prevent stroke. Am J Cardiol 1996;78:8–12.
22. Pappada G, Marina R, Fiori L, et al. Stenting of atherosclerotic stenoses of the extracranial carotid artery. Acta Neurochir 2001;143:1005–1011.
23. White CJ, Gomez CR, Iyer SS, et al. Carotid stent placement for extracranial carotid artery disease: current state of the art. Catheterization & Cardiovascular Interventions 2000;51:339–346.
24. Rosenwasser RH, Shanno GB. Angioplasty and stenting for carotid atherosclerotic disease. Neurosurg Clin N Am 2000;11:323–330.
25. Guterman L, Hopkins N. Carotid Angioplasty and Stenting. Philadelphia: American Association of Neurological Surgeons, 1998.
26. Wholey MH, Wholey M, Mathias K, et al. Global experience in cervical carotid artery stent placement. Catheter Cardiovasc Interv 2000;50:160–167.
27. Al-Mubarak N, Roubin GS, Vitek JJ, New G, Iyer SS. Procedural safety and short-term outcome of ambulatory carotid stenting. Stroke 2001;32:2305–2309.
28. Roubin GS, New G, Iyer SS, et al. Immediate and late clinical outcomes of carotid artery stenting in patients with symptomatic and asymptomatic carotid artery stenosis: a 5-year prospective analysis. Circulation 2001;103:532–537.
29. CAVATAS investigators. Endovascular vs surgical treatment in patients with carotid stenosis in the Carotid and Vertebral Artery Transluminal Angioplasty Study (CAVATAS): a randomised trial. Lancet 2001;357:1729–1737.
30. Spence D, Eliasziw M. Endarterectomy or angioplasty for treatment of carotid stenosis. Lancet 2001;357:1722–1723.
31. Brown MM. Angioplasty and stenting. Adv Neurol 2003;92:335–345.
32. Hobson RW 2nd. Update on the Carotid Revascularization Endarterectomy vs Stent Trial (CREST) protocol. J Am Coll Surg 2002;194(1 Suppl):S9–S14.
33. Roubin GS, Hobson RW 2nd, White R, et al. CREST and CARESS to evaluate carotid stenting: time to get to work! J Endovasc Ther 2001;8:107–110.
34. Chaturvedi S, Ressler R. Angioplasty and stenting for stroke prevention. Neurology 2002;59:664–668.

35. Mathur A, Roubin GS, Iyer SS, et al. Predictors of stroke complicating carotid artery stenting. Circulation 1998;97:1239–1245.
36. Qureshi AI, Luft AR, Janardhan V, et al. Identification of patients at risk for periprocedural neurological deficits associated with carotid angioplasty and stenting. Stroke 2000;31:376–382.
37. Sundt TM, Sandok BA, Whisnant JP. Carotid endarterectomy. Complications and preoperative assessment of risk. Mayo Clin Proc 1975;50:301–306.
38. Sieber FE, Toung TJ, Diringer MN, Wang H, Long DM. Preoperative risks predict neurological outcome of carotid endarterectomy related stroke. Neurosurgery 1992; 30:847–854.
39. McCrory DC, Goldstein LB, Samsa GP, et al. Predicting complications of carotid endarterectomy. Stroke 1993;24:1285–1291.
40. Al-Mubarak N, Roubin GS, Gomez CR, et al. Carotid artery stenting in patients with high neurologic risks. Am J Cardiol 1999;83:1411–1413, A8–A9.
41. Shawl F, Kadro W, Domanski MJ, et al. Safety and efficacy of elective carotid artery stenting in high-risk patients. J Am Coll Cardiol 2000;35:1721–1728.
42. Al-Mubarak N, Roubin GS, Liu MW, et al. Early results of percutaneous intervention for severe coexisting carotid and coronary artery disease. Am J Cardiol 1999; 84:600–602, A9.
43. Mericle RA, Kim SH, Lanzino G, et al. Carotid artery angioplasty and use of stents in high-risk patients with contralateral occlusions. J Neurosurg 1999;90:1031–1036.
44. Gasecki AP, Eliasziw M, Ferguson GG, Hachinski V, Barnett HJ. Long-term prognosis and effect of endarterectomy in patients with symptomatic severe carotid stenosis and contralateral carotid stenosis or occlusion: results from NASCET. North American Symptomatic Carotid Endarterectomy Trial (NASCET) Group. J Neurosurg 1995;83:778–782.
45. Meyer FB, Piepgras DG, Fode NC. Surgical treatment of recurrent carotid artery stenosis. J Neurosurg 1994;80:781–787.
46. Yadav JS, Roubin GS, King P, Iyer S, Vitek J. Angioplasty and stenting for restenosis after carotid endarterectomy. Initial experience. Stroke 1996;27:2075–2079.
47. Lanzino G, Mericle RA, Lopes DK, Wakhloo AK, Guterman LR, Hopkins LN. Percutaneous transluminal angioplasty and stent placement for recurrent carotid artery stenosis. J Neurosurg 1999;90:688–694.
48. New G, Roubin GS, Iyer SS, et al. Safety, efficacy, and durability of carotid artery stenting for restenosis following carotid endarterectomy: a multicenter study. J Endovasc Ther 2000;7:345–352.
49. Loftus CM, Biller J, Hart MN, Cornell SH, Hiratzka LF. Management of radiation-induced accelerated carotid atherosclerosis. Arch Neurol 1987;44:711–714.
50. Al-Mubarak N, Roubin GS, Iyer SS, Gomez CR, Liu MW, Vitek JJ. Carotid stenting for severe radiation-induced extracranial carotid artery occlusive disease. J Endovasc Ther 2000;7:36–40.
51. Houdart E, Mounayer C, Chapot R, Saint-Maurice JP, Merland JJ. Carotid stenting for radiation-induced stenoses: a report of 7 cases. Stroke 2001;32:118–121.
52. Caplan L, Babikian V, Helgason C, et al. Occlusive disease of the middle cerebral artery. Neurology 1985;35:975–982.
53. Thijs VN, Albers GW. Symptomatic intracranial atherosclerosis: outcome of patients who fail antithrombotic therapy. Neurology 2000;55:490–497.

54. Bogousslavsky J, Barnett HJ, Fox AJ, Hachinski VC, Taylor W. Atherosclerotic disease of the middle cerebral artery. Stroke 1986;17:1112–1120.
55. Marzewski DJ, Furlan AJ, St Louis P, Little JR, Modic MT, Williams G. Intracranial internal carotid artery stenosis: longterm prognosis. Stroke 1982;13:821–824.
56. Chimowitz MI, Kokkinos J, Strong J, et al. The Warfarin-Aspirin Symptomatic Intracranial Disease Study. Neurology 1995;45:1488–1493.
57. Sacco RL, Kargman DE, Gu Q, Zamanillo MC. Race–ethnicity and determinants of intracranial atherosclerotic cerebral infarction. The Northern Manhattan Stroke Study. Stroke 1995;26:14–20.
58. Chaturvedi S, Sohrab S, Tselis A. Carotid stent thrombosis: report of two fatal cases. Stroke 2001;32:2700–2702.
59. Bhatt DL, Kapadia SR, Bajzer CT, et al. Dual antiplatelet therapy with clopidogrel and aspirin after carotid artery stenting. J Invasive Cardiol 2001;13:767–771.
60. Kapadia SR, Bajzer CT, Ziada KM, et al. Initial experience of platelet glycoprotein IIb/IIIa inhibition with abciximab during carotid stenting: a safe and effective adjunctive therapy. Stroke 2001;32:2328–2332.
61. Kittusamy PK, Koenigsberg RA, McCormick DJ. Abciximab for the treatment of acute distal embolization associated with internal carotid artery angioplasty. Catheter Cardiovasc Interv 2001;54:221–233.
62. Qureshi AI, Suri MF, Khan J, Fessler RD, Guterman LR, Hopkins LN. Abciximab as an adjunct to high-risk carotid or vertebrobasilar angioplasty: preliminary experience. Neurosurgery 2000;46:1316–1324; discussion 1324–1325.
63. Ho DS, Wang Y, Chui M, Wang Y, Ho SL, Cheung RT. Intracarotid abciximab injection to abort impending ischemic stroke during carotid angioplasty. Cerebrovasc Dis 2001;11:300–304.
64. Qureshi AI, Ali Z, Suri MF, et al. Open-label phase I clinical study to assess the safety of intravenous eptifibatide in patients undergoing internal carotid artery angioplasty and stent placement. Neurosurgery 2001;48:998–1004; discussion 1004–1005.
65. Brown MM, Crawley F, Clifton A, Buckenham T, Taylor R. Percutaneous transluminal angioplasty of the internal carotid artery. Br J Surg 1997;84:729–730.
66. Crawley F, Clifton A, Buckenham T, Loosemore T, Taylor RS, Brown MM. Comparison of hemodynamic cerebral ischemia and microembolic signals detected during carotid endarterectomy and carotid angioplasty. Stroke 1997;28:2460–2464.
67. Jordan WD Jr, Voellinger DC, Doblar DD, Plyushcheva NP, Fisher WS, McDowell HA. Microemboli detected by transcranial Doppler monitoring in patients during carotid angioplasty vs carotid endarterectomy. Cardiovasc Surg 1999;7:33–38.
68. Al-Mubarak N, Roubin GS, Vitek JJ, Iyer SS, New G, Leon MB. Effect of the distal-balloon protection system on microembolization during carotid stenting. Circulation 2001;104:1999–2002.
69. Reimers B, Corvaja N, Moshiri S, et al. Cerebral protection with filter devices during carotid artery stenting. Circulation 2001;104:12–15.
70. Martin JB, Pache JC, Treggiari-Venzi M, et al. Role of the distal balloon protection technique in the prevention of cerebral embolic events during carotid stent placement. Stroke 2001;32:479–484.
71. Angelini A, Reimers B, Della Barbera M, et al. Cerebral protection during carotid artery stenting: collection and histopathologic analysis of embolized debris. Stroke 2002;33:456–461.

72. Markus HS, Clifton A, Buckenham T, Brown MM. Carotid angioplasty. Detection of embolic signals during and after the procedure. Stroke 194;25:2403–2406.
73. Crawley F, Stygall J, Lunn S, Harrison M, Brown MM, Newman S. Comparison of microembolism detected by transcranial Doppler and neuropsychological sequelae of carotid surgery and percutaneous transluminal angioplasty. Stroke 2000;31: 1329–1334.
74. Sivaguru A, Gaines PA, Beard J, et al. Neuropsychological outcome after carotid angioplasty: a randomised controlled trial [abstract]. J Neurol Neurosurg Psychiatry 1999;66:262.
75. Eckert B, Thie A, Valdueza J, Zanella F, Zeumer H. Transcranial Doppler sonographic monitoring during percutaneous transluminal angioplasty of the internal carotid artery. Neuroradiology 1997;39:229–234.
76. Theron J, Courteoux P, Alachpar F, Bouvard G, Maiza D. New triple coaxial catheter system for carotid angioplasty with cerebral protection. AJNR Am J Neuroradiol 1990;11:869–874.
77. Theron JG, Payelle GG, Coskun O, Huet HF, Guimaraens L. Carotid artery stenosis: treatment with protected balloon angioplasty and stent placement. Radiology 1996;201:627–636.
78. Crawley F, Clifton A, Taylor RS, Brown MM. Symptomatic restenosis after carotid percutaneous transluminal angioplasty. Lancet 1998;352:708–709.
79. Vermeersch P, Nong Z, Stabile E, et al. L-Arginine administration reduces neointima formation after stent injury in rats by a nitric oxide-mediated mechanism. Arterioscler Thromb Vasc Biol 2002;21:1604–1609.
80. Oberhoff M, Kunert W, Herdeg C, et al. Inhibition of smooth muscle cell proliferation after local drug delivery of the antimitotic drug paclitaxel using a porous balloon catheter. Basic Res Cardiol 2001;96:275–282.
81. Rensing BJ, Vos J, Smits PC, et al. Coronary restenosis elimination with a sirolimus eluting stent; First European human experience with 6-month angiographic and intravascular ultrasonic follow-up. Eur Heart J 2001;22:2125–2130.
82. Bruijns RH, Bult H. Effects of local cytochalasin D delivery on smooth muscle cell migration and on collar-induced intimal hyperplasia in the rabbit carotid artery. Br J Pharmacol 2001;134:473–483.
83. Rabbani LE, Wang W. Phosphorothioate oligodeoxynucleotide inhibition of restenosis. J Thromb Thrombolysis 1998;5:125–128.
84. Breen JC, Caplan LR, DeWitt LD, Belkin M, Mackey WC, O'Donnell TP. Brain edema after carotid surgery. Neurology 1996;46:175–181.
85. Schoser BG, Heesen C, Eckert B, Thie A. Cerebral hyperperfusion injury after percutaneous transluminal angioplasty of extracranial arteries. J Neurol 1997;244: 101–104.
86. McCabe DJ, Brown MM, Clifton A. Fatal cerebral reperfusion hemorrhage after carotid stenting. Stroke 1999;30:2483–2486.
87. Liu AY, Do HM, Albers GW, Lopez JR, Steinberg GK, Marks MP. Hyperperfusion syndrome with hemorrhage after angioplasty for middle cerebral artery stenosis. AJNR Am J Neuroradiol 2001;22:1597–1601.
88. Meyers PM, Higashida RT, Phatouros CC, et al. Cerebral hyperperfusion syndrome after percutaneous transluminal stenting of the craniocervical arteries. Neurosurgery 2000;47:335–343; discussion 343–345.

89. Purdy PD, Devous MD Sr, Unwin DH, Giller CA, Batjer HH. Angioplasty of an atherosclerotic middle cerebral artery associated with improvement in regional cerebral blood flow. AJNR Am J Neuroradiol 1990;11:878–880.
90. Touho H. Percutaneous transluminal angioplasty in the treatment of atherosclerotic disease of the anterior cerebral circulation and hemodynamic evaluation. J Neurosurg 1995;82:953–960.
91. Luft AR, Qureshi AI, Suri MF, Janardhan V, Guterman LR, Hopkins LN. Frequency and predictors for angiographically improved inflow of contrast medium after carotid angioplasty and stenting. Neuroradiology 2001;43:877–883.
92. Derdeyn CP, Cross DT 3rd, Moran CJ, Dacey RG Jr. Reversal of focal misery perfusion after intracranial angioplasty: case report. Neurosurgery 2001;48:436–439; discussion 439–440.
93. Uchiyama N, Kida S, Watanabe T, Yamashita J, Matsui O. Improved cerebral perfusion and metabolism after stenting for basilar artery stenosis: technical case report. Neurosurgery 2001;48:1386–1391; discussion 1391–1392.
94. Markus HS, Clifton A, Buckenham T, Taylor R, Brown MM. Improvement in cerebral hemodynamics after carotid angioplasty. Stroke 1996;27:612–616.
95. Solomon RA, Loftus CM, Quest DO, Correll JW. Incidence and etiology of intracerebral hemorrhage following carotid endarterectomy. J Neurosurg 1986;64:29–34.
96. Reigel MM, Hollier LH, Sundt TM Jr, Piepgras DG, Sharbrough FW, Cherry KJ. Cerebral hyperperfusion syndrome: a cause of neurologic dysfunction after carotid endarterectomy. J Vasc Surg 1987;5:628–634.
97. Hafner DH, Smith RB 3rd, King OW, et al. Massive intracerebral hemorrhage following carotid endarterectomy. Arch Surg 1987;122:305–307.
98. Schroeder T, Sillesen H, Sorensen O, Engell HC. Cerebral hyperperfusion following carotid endarterectomy. J Neurosurg 1987;66:824–829.
99. Schroeder T, Sillesen H, Boesen J, Laursen H, Sorensen P. Intracerebral haemorrhage after carotid endarterectomy. Eur J Vasc Surg 1987;1:51–60.
100. Piepgras DG, Morgan MK, Sundt TM Jr, Yanagihara T, Mussman LM. Intracerebral hemorrhage after carotid endarterectomy. J Neurosurg 1988;68:532–536.
101. Penn AA, Schomer DF, Steinberg GK. Imaging studies of cerebral hyperperfusion after carotid endarterectomy. Case report. J Neurosurg 1995;83:133–137.
102. Jorgensen LG, Schroeder TV. Defective cerebrovascular autoregulation after carotid endarterectomy. Eur J Vasc Surg 1993;7:370–379.
103. Qureshi AI, Luft AR, Lopes DK, et al. Postoperative hypotension after carotid angioplasty and stenting: report of three cases. Neurosurgery 1999;44:1320–1323.
104. Qureshi AI, Luft AR, Sharma M, et al. Frequency and determinants of postprocedural hemodynamic instability after carotid angioplasty and stenting. Stroke 1999; 30:2086–2093.
105. Harrop JS, Sharan AD, Benitez RP, Armonda R, Thomas J, Rosenwasser RH. Prevention of carotid angioplasty-induced bradycardia and hypotension with temporary venous pacemakers. Neurosurgery 2001;49:814–820; discussion 820–822.
106. Takis C, Kwan ES, Pessin MS, Jacobs DH, Caplan LR. Intracranial angioplasty: experience and complications. AJNR Am J Neuroradiol 1997;18:1661–1668.
107. Levy EI, Horowitz MB, Koebbe CJ, et al. Transluminal stent-assisted angioplasty of the intracranial vertebrobasilar system for medically refractory, posterior circulation ischemia: early results. Neurosurgery 2001;48:1215–1221; discussion 1221–1223.

108. Mori T, Kazita K, Chokyu K, Mima T, Mori K. Short-term arteriographic and clinical outcome after cerebral angioplasty and stenting for intracranial vertebrobasilar and carotid atherosclerotic occlusive disease. AJNR Am J Neuroradiol 2000; 21:249–254.
109. Gomez CR, Misra VK, Liu MW, et al. Elective stenting of symptomatic basilar artery stenosis. Stroke 2000;31:95–99.
110. Rasmussen PA, Perl J 2nd, Barr JD, et al. Stent-assisted angioplasty of intracranial vertebrobasilar atherosclerosis: an initial experience. J Neurosurg 2000;92: 771–778.
111. Ramee SR, Dawson R, McKinley KL, et al. Provisional stenting for symptomatic intracranial stenosis using a multidisciplinary approach: acute results, unexpected benefit, and 1-year outcome. Cathet Cardiovasc Interv 2001;52:457–467.
112. Connors JJ 3rd, Wojak JC. Percutaneous transluminal angioplasty for intracranial atherosclerotic lesions: evolution of technique and short-term results. J Neurosurg 1999;91:415–423.
113. Malek AM, Higashida RT, Phatouros CC, et al. Endovascular management of extracranial carotid artery dissection achieved using stent angioplasty. AJNR Am J Neuroradiol 2000;21:1280–1292.
114. Dorros G, Cohn JM, Palmer LE. Stent deployment resolves a petrous carotid artery angioplasty dissection. AJNR Am J Neuroradiol 1998;19:392–394.
115. Lanzino G, Wakhloo AK, Fessler RD, Hartney ML, Guterman LR, Hopkins LN. Efficacy and current limitations of intravascular stents for intracranial internal carotid, vertebral, and basilar artery aneurysms. J Neurosurg 1999;91:538–546.
116. Gomez CR, Misra VK, Campbell MS, Soto RD. Elective stenting of symptomatic middle cerebral artery stenosis. AJNR Am J Neuroradiol 2000;21:971–973.
117. Horowitz MB, Pride GL, Graybeal DF, Purdy PD. Percutaneous transluminal angioplasty and stenting of midbasilar stenoses: three technical case reports and literature review. Neurosurgery 1999;45:925–930; discussion 930–931.

12
Cardiac Embolism

**Karen L. Furie,
Aneesh B. Singhal, and J. Philip Kistler**

Cardioembolism, most often caused by atrial fibrillation (AF), is a major mechanism of stroke across a broad range of age groups in the developed world (Table 1) *(1–3)*. Identifying a potential cardioembolic mechanism has important implications for both management and outcome (Table 2). The prognosis after a cardioembolic stroke is poor, with high rates of recurrent stroke and mortality *(4–6)*. Therefore, when cardioembolism is suspected, there should be a rapid diagnostic assessment and initiation of targeted therapy.

The classic clinical features associated with embolic stroke are presented in Table 3 *(7,8)*. Transient ischemic attacks (TIAs) and transient monocular blindness (TMB) are unusual in embolic stroke, in which the onset is usually sudden *(9–17)*. Symptoms caused by cerebral embolism may have a stuttering course as the embolus propagates, lyses, or migrates *(18,19)*. Although any large- or medium-size artery intracranial occlusion should raise concern of cardioembolism, these emboli account for most posterior circulation infarcts *(20,21)*. Up to 18% of patients with symptoms and signs of lacunar syndrome harbor a cardioembolic source, raising an alternative embolic mechanism of small-vessel occlusion *(22,23)*.

DIAGNOSTIC STUDIES

Cardiac assessment of stroke and TIA patient should first exclude AF and structural cardiac disease:

- Standard 12-lead electrocardiogram
- 24- to 48-hour portable cardiac monitor if the electrocardiogram fails to reveal AF; may be repeated *(24)*
- Transthoracic echocardiography (TTE) evaluates cardiac function and can identify cardiomyopathy, segmental wall motion abnormalities, mitral annular calcification and other valvular pathology, left atrial dilation, intraventricular thrombus, and (if performed with agitated saline injection) patent foramen ovale

From: *Current Clinical Neurology: Handbook of Stroke Prevention in Clinical Practice*
Edited by: K. L. Furie and P. J. Kelly © Humana Press Inc., Totowa, NJ

Table 1
Cardiac Conditions Associated with Cerebral Emboli

Source	Percentage of all cardiogenic emboli
Nonvalvular atrial fibrillation	45
Acute MI	15
Ventricular aneurysm	10
Rheumatic heart disease	10
Prosthetic cardiac valve	10
Other	10

Source: From ref. *7*.

Table 2
Classification of Cardioembolic Cerebral Ischemic Events

A. Antithrombotic therapy considered the standard of practice
  1. Left ventricular (LV) thrombus/LV aneurysm
  2. Left atrial thrombus
  3. Recent transmural anterior myocardial infarction (MI)
  4. Rheumatic valvular disease
  5. Mechanical prosthetic valve
  6. Atrial fibrillation/flutter (if >65 years, with vascular risk factors)

B. Antithrombotic therapy may be of value
  1. Nonbacterial thrombotic endocarditis
  2. Sick sinus syndrome
  3. LV dysfunction (cardiomyopathy of EF < 30%)
  4. Papillary fibroelastoma
  5. Patent foramen ovale ± atrial septal aneurysm
  6. Chronic MI with reduced cardiac function

C. Antithrombotic therapy contraindicated
  1. Bacterial endocarditis
  2. Atrial myxoma

- Transesophageal echocardiography provides better resolution of the left atrium and left atrial appendage, atrial septum, mitral valve, and aortic arch, but is costly and carries a small risk of serious complications; it should be performed when cardioembolism is suspected, but cardiac monitoring and TTE fail to reveal a source, and results are expected to affect outcome (e.g., anticoagulation or invasive cardiac procedures would be considerations) *(25–27)*

More exploratory, but potentially useful studies include the following:

- Transcranial Doppler embolus detection can identify microemboli that manifest high-intensity transient signals *(28,29)*.
- Diffusion-weighted magnetic resonance imaging to identify potentially silent infarcts in multiple vascular territories that would be indicative of cardioembolism *(30)*.

Table 3
Clinical Characteristics of Cardioembolic Stroke

Neurological history and examination
Sudden onset
Isolated focal deficit
Seizure at onset
Loss of consciousness at onset
Peak of deficit at onset
Involvement of more than one vascular territory
Evidence of systemic embolization
Neuroimaging
Multiple infarcts in more than one vascular territory
Deep and/or superficial infarctions
Hemorrhagic conversion
Absence of large-artery stenosis or occlusion in parent vessels
Rapid recanalization of intracranial vessels by transcranial Doppler

ARRHYTHMIAS: AF, ATRIAL FLUTTER, SICK SINUS SYNDROME

The prevalence of AF is increasing in the United States as the population lives longer *(31)*. The prevalence of AF increases with age *(32–34)*. The overall risk of stroke in AF is approx 3–5% per year, but is significantly higher in AF related to rheumatic heart disease *(33)*. The rates of stroke associated with sustained AF and paroxysmal AF are similar. AF is the only cardioembolic source of stroke that has been subjected to randomized clinical trials comparing antithrombotic and antiplatelet therapies for stroke prevention *(35–43)*. Younger patients free of cardiac disease, diabetes, or hypertension have an extremely low rate of stroke despite AF, 1.3% over 15 years *(44)*.

Clinical risk factors associated with risk of stroke in AF include age older than 65 years, previous history of stroke or TIA, hypertension, and diabetes mellitus. Impaired left ventricular function was identified as an additional risk factor in the Stroke Prevention in Atrial Fibrillation (SPAF) population (Fig. 1) AF patients with no clinical risk factors and a normal TTE have a low (<1% per year) risk of stroke *(45)*. Low-risk patients (age < 65, no clinical or echocardiographic cardiac disease, no history of stroke or TIA) can be considered for aspirin therapy. Aspirin (50–325 mg per day) conveys a 21% stroke risk reduction of stroke, mainly reducing rates of smaller noncardioembolic strokes *(46)*. The rate of intracerebral hemorrhage in the major trials was less than 1% per year *(35–43)*. Major bleeding complications tend to occur with international normalized ratios (INRs) of 4 or more *(47,48)*.

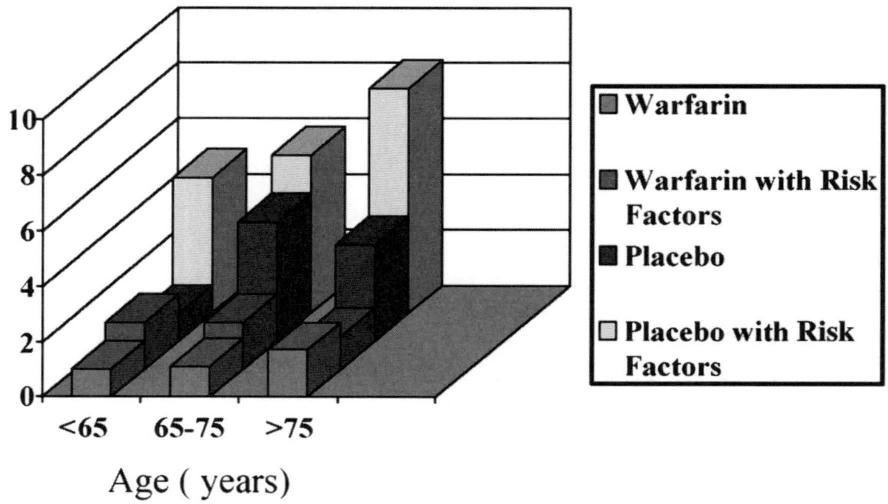

Fig. 1. Stroke risk in atrial fibrillation with risk factors hypertension, diabetes mellitus, prior stroke, or TIA.

Other vascular risk factors may also increase the risk of stroke caused by AF. Concomitant hypertension contributes to left ventricular dysfunction, left atrial enlargement, and hemostatic activation *(49–52)*. Hyperhomocysteinemia has also been reported to predispose to left atrial thrombus formation *(52)*. Treating these risk factors may enhance the stroke-reducing effect of antithrombotic therapy. The predicted risk of stroke for an individual can be calculated using an algorithm designed by the Framingham Study investigators using clinical factors such as advancing age, female sex, increasing systolic blood pressure, prior stroke or TIA, and diabetes *(53)*.

Warfarin reduces risk of stroke in AF by 68% (95% CI, 50–79%) as compared to aspirin, which reduced the risk of ischemic stroke by 36% (95% CI, 4–57%) (Fig. 2). The optimal INR reduces risk of ischemic stroke without increasing the serious hemorrhagic complications. Hylek et al. have studied this issue of optimal INR range extensively. The risk of stroke increases at INRs below 2.0. At an INR of 1.7, the odds ratio for stroke, as compared to an INR of 2.0, was 2.0 (95% CI, 1.6–2.4%); at an INR of 1.5, it was 3.3 (95% CI, 2.4–4.6%); and at an INR of 1.3, it was 6.0 (95% CI, 3.6–9.8%) *(54)*. In addition, the level on warfarin intensity affects outcome from AF-related stroke. An INR of less than 2.0, compared with an INR of 2.0 or greater, increased the odds of a severe stroke (odds ratio, 1.9; 95% CI, 1.1–3.4%) and the risk of death within 30 days (hazard ratio, 3.4; 95% CI, 1.1–10.1%) *(55)*.

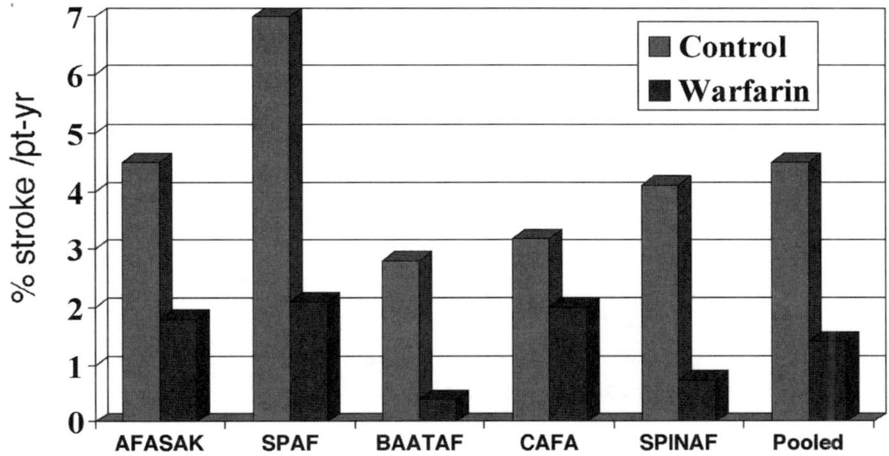

RRR 58% 67% 86% 42% 79% 68%

Fig. 2. Atrial fibrillation trials (AFASAK, Copenhagen Atrial Fibrillation Aspirin and Anticoagulation Trial; SPAF, Stroke Prevention in Atrial Fibrillation; BAATAF, Boston Area Anticoagulation Trial for Atrial Fibrillation; CAFA, Canadian Atrial Fibrillation Anticoagulation; SPINAF, Veterans Affairs Stroke Prevention in Atrial Fibrillation).

The use of low-dose or fixed mini-dose warfarin has been proposed to help simplify long-term warfarin management and reduce the risk of hemorrhagic complications. A recent meta-analysis of all randomized controlled trials evaluated low-dose or fixed mini-dose warfarin for prevention of thromboembolic events in AF. The relative risk was 0.46 (95%CI; 0.2–1.07%) for ischemic stroke. The lower warfarin dose did not statistically decrease the risk for major hemorrhage compared to adjusted-dose warfarin. Therefore, low- or mini-dose warfarin is not recommended. Conventional adjusted-dose warfarin should be used in patients with AF *(56)*.

Novel strategies for managing AF are being studied. Ximelagatran is a new oral direct thrombin inhibitor being studied as a therapy to prevent thromboembolism in patients with AF. Recent data from SPORTIF V, a double-blind study of 3922 patients comparing ximelagatran to warfarin in patients with AF recently reported comparable bleeding rates for the two therapies *(57, 58)*. Another innovative approach to reducing stroke as a result of AF is occlusion of the left atrial appendage (LAA), the primary source of thrombus in patients with AF. The Left Atrial Appendage Occlusion Study (LAAOS) is an ongoing randomized clinical trial designed to evaluate the safety and efficacy of this approach in high-risk patients undergoing coronary artery bypass grating *(59)*.

Many patients have a rhythm that varies between atrial flutter and AF. Atrial flutter is associated with a higher risk of stroke (relative risk 1.41), but that risk is lower than with AF (relative risk 1.64) *(60)*. Given that the concordance of the two rhythms is high, anticoagulation in patients with atrial flutter and coexisting cardiac pathology predisposing to left atrial thrombus should be considered *(61)*. Similarly, patients with sick sinus syndrome (SSS) often manifest atrial flutter and AF *(62)*. SSS has been associated with a higher risk of stroke *(63,64)*. There has not been a trial of antithrombotic agents for stroke prevention in SSS alone, and the main intervention is usually pacemaker placement *(65)*.

STRUCTURAL CARDIAC DISEASE: ACUTE MI, CARDIOMYOPATHY, VALVULAR DISEASE

Two to three percent of acute MIs are complicated by stroke within the first 4 weeks, increasing to 8.1% within 5 years *(66–69)*. Peri-MI stroke is more common in anterior wall MI (12%) compared to inferior wall infarction (1%), occurring in 4–12 and 1%, respectively *(66,67)*. Left ventricular thrombus can develop as an early or late complication in up to 40% of patients with an anterior wall MI *(66,67,70)*. A recent randomized 4-year trial compared warfarin (target international normalized ratio range 2.8–4.2) (n = 1216) to aspirin 160 mg per day (n = 1206) or combination therapy (n =1208) with an international normalized ratio range of 2.0 to 2.5 for the primary end point of death, nonfatal reinfarction, or thromboembolic cerebral stroke *(71)*. End point events occurred in 241 (20%) of aspirin-treated patients, 203 (16.7%) of warfarin-treated patients, and 181 (15%) of patients on combined therapy. The difference between the two groups receiving warfarin was not statistically significant. Major, nonfatal bleeding was more common in the warfarin arms, 0.62% with warfarin vs 0.17% with aspirin.

Patients with ischemic and idiopathic cardiomyopathy have an annual stroke rate of 1.3 to 3.5% *(7,34,69,72–76)*. The risk of stroke is inversely related to the ejection fraction (EF) *(69,77)*. In the Survival and Ventricular Enlargement (SAVE) study, patients with an EF of 29–35% had a stroke rate of 0.8% per year compared to 2.5% per year in those with an EF of 28% or less *(69)*. There are conflicting data about the safety and efficacy of warfarin for stroke prevention in this situation *(78–80)*. An ongoing study (Warfarin Aspirin Reduced Cardiac Ejection Fraction study) is comparing warfarin to aspirin for the pre-vention of first and recurrent stroke in patients with an EF below 30% *(74)*.

Mitral stenosis is associated with left atrial thrombus and AF and conveys a 2% per year risk of stroke *(81,82)*. The annual rate of embolism with mechanical or bioprosthetic valves is higher in the mitral (3–4%) than aortic (1.3–3.2%) position *(83–85)*. Patients with bioprosthetic valves should be anticoagulated for the first 3 months and continued on warfarin if there is evidence of AF, left atrial thrombus, or previous emboli *(86,87)*. Patients with mechanical valves and high-risk bioprosthetics have lower annual rates of vascular mortality and systemic embolism and no increased bleeding with combination aspirin and warfarin (1.9%) compared to warfarin alone (8.5%) *(88)*.

Fever, a new murmur, and an elevated erythrocyte sedimentation rate are hallmarks of infective endocarditis. The diagnosis can usually be made with serial blood cultures, a transthoracic echocardiogram, or a transesophageal echocardiogram. Stroke is an early (within 48 hours) complication of infective endocarditis in 15–20% of cases. Initiation of appropriate antibiotic therapy significantly reduces the risk of stroke *(89,90)*. Because of an associated risk of mycotic aneurysms and subarachnoid hemorrhage, patients with suspected infective endocarditis should not receive anticoagulation.

Nonbacterial thrombotic endocarditis, or marantic endocarditis, is associated with malignancy and autoimmune disorders such as systemic lupus erythematosis and with a systemic hypercoagulable state *(91)*. Transthoracic and transesophageal echocardiography are useful for defining the valvular lesion *(92)*. It is unclear whether a particular form of antithrombotic therapy (low-molecular-weight heparin, warfarin, or antiplatelet agent) is more efficacious for preventing cardioembolism. Anticoagulation would be indicated if Trousseau's syndrome is suspected.

REFERENCES

1. Sacco RL, Ellenberg JH, Mohr JP, et al. Infarcts of undetermined cause: the NINCDS Stroke Data Bank. Ann Neurol 1989;25:382–390.
2. Kittner SJ, Stein BJ, Wozniak M, et al. Cerebral infarction in young adults: the Baltimore–Washington Cooperative Young Stroke Study. Neurology 1998;50:890–894.
3. Adams HP Jr, Butler MJ, Biller J, Toffel GJ. Nonhemorrhagic cerebral infarction in young adults. Arch Neurol 1986;43:793–796.
4. Arboix A, Vericat MC, Pujades R, Massons J, Garcia-Eroles L, Oliveres M. Cardioembolic infarction in the Sagrat Cor-Alianza Hospital of Barcelona Stroke Registry. Acta Neurol Scand 1997;96:407–412.
5. Petty GW, Brown RD Jr, Whisnant JP, Sicks JD, O'Fallon WM, Wiebers DO. Ischemic stroke subtypes: a population-based study of functional outcome, survival, and recurrence. Stroke 2000;31:1062–1068.
6. Cisternino MD, Giaquinto S, Maiolo I, Palma E, Valeriani M, Vittoria E. On the outcome in stroke patients one year later: the role of atrial fibrillation. Eur J Neurol 2003;10:67–70.

7. Cardiogenic brain embolism. Cerebral Embolism Task Force. Arch Neurol 1986; 43:71–84.
8. Cardiogenic brain embolism. The second report of the Cerebral Embolism Task Force. Arch Neurol 1989;46:727–743.
9. Ramirez-Lassepas M, Cipolle RJ, Bjork RJ, et al. Can embolic stroke be diagnosed on the basis of neurologic clinical criteria? Arch Neurol 1987;44:87–89.
10. Caplan LR, Hier DB, D'Cruz I. Cerebral embolism in the Michael Reese Stroke Registry. Stroke 1983;14:530–536.
11. Foulkes MA, Wolf PA, Price TR, Mohr JP. Hier DB. The Stroke Data Bank: design, methods, and baseline characteristics. Stroke 1988;19:547–554.
12. Bogousslavsky J, Cachin C, Regli F, Despland PA, Van Melle G, Kappenberger L. Cardiac sources of embolism and cerebral infarction—clinical consequences and vascular concomitants: the Lausanne Stroke Registry. Neurology 1991;41:855–859.
13. Appen RE, Wray SH, Cogan DH. Central retinal artery occlusion. Am J Ophthalmol 1975;79:374–381.
14. Babikian VL, Wijman CA, Hyde C, et al. Cerebral microembolism and early recurrent cerebral or retinal ischemic events. Stroke 1997;28:1314–1318.
15. Hankey GJ, Slattery JM, Warlow CP. Prognosis and prognostic factors of retinal infarction: a prospective cohort study. BMJ 1991;302:499–504.
16. Babikian VL, Hyde C, Pochay V, Winter MR. Clinical correlates of high-intensity transient signals detected on transcranial Doppler sonography in patients with cerebrovascular disease. Stroke 1994;25:1570–1573.
17. Murkin JM. Etiology and incidence of brain dysfunction after cardiac surgery. J Cardiothorac Vasc Anesth 1999;13(4 Suppl 1):12–17; discussion 36–37.
18. Fisher CM, Pearlman A. The nonsudden onset of cerebral embolism. Neurology 1967;17:1025–1032.
19. Minematsu K, Yamaguchi T, Omae T. "Spectacular shrinking deficit": rapid recovery from a major hemispheric syndrome by migration of an embolus. Neurology 1992;42:157–162.
20. Yamamoto Y, Georgiadis AL, Cgang HM, Caplan LR. Posterior cerebral artery territory infarcts in the New England Medical Center Posterior Circulation Registry. Arch Neurol 1999;56:824–832.
21. Pessin MS, Lathi ES, Cohen MB, Kwan ES, Hedges TR 3rd, Caplan LR. Clinical features and mechanism of occipital infarction. Ann Neurol 1987;21:290–299.
22. Horowitz DR, Turhim S, Weinberger JM, Rudolph SH. Mechanisms in lacunar infarction. Stroke 1992;23:325–327.
23. Staaf G, Samuelsson M, Lindgren A, Norrving B. Sensorimotor stroke; clinical features, MRI findings, and cardiac and vascular concomitants in 32 patients. Acta Neurol Scand 1998;97:93–98.
24. Rem JA, Hachinski VC, Boughner DR, Barnett HJ. Value of cardiac monitoring and echocardiography in TIA and stroke patients. Stroke 1985;16:950–956.
25. Pop G, Sutherland GR, Koudstaal PJ, Sit TW, de Jong G, Roelandt JR. Transesophageal echocardiography in the detection of intracardiac embolic sources in patients with transient ischemic attacks. Stroke 1990;21:560–565.
26. Hata JS, Ayres RW, Biller J, et al. Impact of transesophageal echocardiography on the anticoagulation management of patients admitted with focal cerebral ischemia. Am J Cardiol 1993;72:707–710.

27. Pearson AC, Labovitz AJ, Tatineni S, Gomez CR. Superiority of transesophageal echocardiography in detecting cardiac source of embolism in patients with cerebral ischemia of uncertain etiology. J Am Coll Cardiol 1991;17:66–72.
28. Sliwka U, Job FP, Wissuwa D, et al. Occurrence of transcranial Doppler high-intensity transient signals in patients with potential cardiac sources of embolism. A prospective study. Stroke 1995;26:2067–2070.
29. Tong DC, Bolger A, and Albers GW. Incidence of transcranial Doppler-detected cerebral microemboli in patients referred for echocardiography. Stroke 1994;25: 2138–2141.
30. Ay H, Oliveira-Filho J, Buonanno FS, et al. Diffusion-weighted imaging identifies a subset of lacunar infarction associated with embolic source. Stroke 1999;30: 2644–2650.
31. Tsang TS, Petty GW, Barnes ME, et al. The prevalence of atrial fibrillation in incident stroke cases and matched population controls in Rochester, Minnesota: changes over three decades. J Am Coll Cardiol 2003;42:93–100.
32. Kannel WB, Wolf PA, Benjamin EJ, Levy D. Prevalence, incidence, prognosis, and predisposing conditions for atrial fibrillation: population-based estimates. Am J Cardiol 1998;82:2N–9N.
33. Wolf PA, Dawber TR, Thomas HE Jr., Kannel WB. Epidemiologic assessment of chronic atrial fibrillation and risk of stroke: the Framingham study. Neurology 1978; 28:973–977.
34. Wolf PA, Abbott RD, Kannel WB. Atrial fibrillation: a major contributor to stroke in the elderly. The Framingham Study. Arch Intern Med 1987;147:1561–1564.
35. The effect of low-dose warfarin on the risk of stroke in patients with nonrheumatic atrial fibrillation. The Boston Area Anticoagulation Trial for Atrial Fibrillation Investigators. N Engl J Med 1990;323:1505–1511.
36. Stroke Prevention in Atrial Fibrillation Study. Final results. Circulation 1991;84: 527–539.
37. Warfarin vs aspirin for prevention of thromboembolism in atrial fibrillation: Stroke Prevention in Atrial Fibrillation II Study. Lancet 1994;343:687–691.
38. Adjusted-dose warfarin vs low-intensity, fixed-dose warfarin plus aspirin for high-risk patients with atrial fibrillation: Stroke Prevention in Atrial Fibrillation III randomised clinical trial. Lancet 1996;348:633–638.
39. Ezekowitz MD, Bridgers SL, James KE, et al. Warfarin in the prevention of stroke associated with nonrheumatic atrial fibrillation. Veterans Affairs Stroke Prevention in Nonrheumatic Atrial Fibrillation Investigators. N Engl J Med 1992;327:1406–1412.
40. Kistler JP, Singer DE, Millenson MM, et al. Effect of low-intensity warfarin anticoagulation on level of activity of the hemostatic system in patients with atrial fibrillation. BAATAF Investigators. Stroke 1993;24:1360–1365.
41. Connolly SJ, Laupacis A, Gent M, Roberts RS, Cairns JA, Joyner C. Canadian Atrial Fibrillation Anticoagulation (CAFA) Study. J Am Coll Cardiol 1991;18:349–355.
42. Risk factors for stroke and efficacy of antithrombotic therapy in atrial fibrillation. Analysis of pooled data from five randomized controlled trials. Arch Intern Med 1994;154:1449–1457.
43. Petersen P, Boysen G, Godtfredsen J, Andersen ED, Andersen B. Placebo-controlled, randomised trial of warfarin and aspirin for prevention of thromboembolic complications in chronic atrial fibrillation. The Copenhagen AFASAK study. Lancet 1989;1:175–179.

44. Bogousslavsky,J, Adnet-Bonte C, Regli F, Van Melle G, Kappenberger L. Lone atrial fibrillation and stroke. Acta Neurol Scand 1990;82:143–146.
45. Predictors of thromboembolism in atrial fibrillation: II. Echocardiographic features of patients at risk. The Stroke Prevention in Atrial Fibrillation Investigators. Ann Intern Med 1992;116:6–12.
46. Hart RG, Pearce LA, Miller VT, Anderson DC, Rothrock JF, Albers GW, Nasco E. Cardioembolic vs. noncardioembolic strokes in atrial fibrillation: frequency and effect of antithrombotic agents in the stroke prevention in atrial fibrillation studies. Cerebrovasc Dis 2000;10:39–43.
47. The European Atrial Fibrillation Trial Study Group. Optimal oral anticoagulant therapy in patients with nonrheumatic atrial fibrillation and recent cerebral ischemia. The European Atrial Fibrillation Trial Study Group. N Engl J Med 1995;333: 5–10.
48. Hylek EM, Singer DE. Risk factors for intracranial hemorrhage in outpatients taking warfarin. Ann Intern Med 1994;120:897–902.
49. Healey JS, Connolly SJ. Atrial fibrillation: hypertension as a causative agent, risk factor for complications, and potential therapeutic target. Am J Cardiol 2003;91: 9G–14G.
50. Lip GY, Lowe GD, Rumley A, Dunn FG. Increased markers of thrombogenesis in chronic atrial fibrillation: effects of warfarin treatment. Br Heart J 1995;73:527–533.
51. Lip GY, Rumley A, Dunn FG, Lowe GD. Plasma fibrinogen and fibrin D-dimer in patients with atrial fibrillation: effects of cardioversion to sinus rhythm. Int J Cardiol 1995;51:245–251.
52. Ay H, Arsava EM, Tokgozoglu SL, Ozer N, Saribas O. Hyperhomocysteinemia is associated with the presence of left atrial thrombus in stroke patients with nonvalvular atrial fibrillation. Stroke 2003;34:909–912.
53. Wang TJ, Massaro JM, Levy D, et al. A risk score for predicting stroke or death in individuals with new-onset atrial fibrillation in the community. JAMA 2003;290: 1049–1056.
54. Hylek EM, Skates SJ, Sheehan MA, Singer DE. An analysis of the lowest effective intensity of prophylactic anticoagulation for patients with nonrheumatic atrial fibrillation. N Engl J Med 1996;335:540–546.
55. Hylek EM, Go AS, Chang Y, et al. Effect of intensity of oral anticoagulation on stroke severity and mortality in atrial fibrillation. N Engl J Med 2003;349:1019–1026.
56. Perret-Guillaume C, Wahl DG. Low-dose warfarin in atrial fibrillation leads to more thromboembolic events without reducing major bleeding when compared to adjusted-dose—A meta-analysis.Thromb Haemost 2004;91:394–402.
57. Halperin JL; Executive Steering Committee, SPORTIF III and V Study Investigators. Ximelagatran compared with warfarin for prevention of thromboembolism in patients with nonvalvular atrial fibrillation: rationale, objectives, and design of a pair of clinical studies and baseline patient characteristics (SPORTIF III and V). Am Heart J 2003;146:431–438.
58. Albers GW. On behalf of the SPORTIF V Investigators. Ximelagatran, an Oral Direct Thrombin Inhibitor, Compared With Dose-Adjusted Warfarin for Primary and Secondary Stroke Prevention in Patients With Atrial Fibrillation (SPORTIF V). Stroke 2004;1:242.

59. Crystal E, Lamy A, Connolly SJ, et al. Left Atrial Appendage Occlusion Study. Left Atrial Appendage Occlusion Study (LAAOS): a randomized clinical trial of left atrial appendage occlusion during routine coronary artery bypass graft surgery for long-term stroke prevention. Am Heart J 2003;146:E26.
60. Biblo LA, Yuan Z, Quan KJ, Mackall JA, Rimm AA. Risk of stroke in patients with atrial flutter. Am J Cardiol 2001;87:346–349, A9.
61. Stoddard MF. Risk of thromboembolism in acute atrial fibrillation or atrial flutter. Echocardiography 2000;17:393–405.
62. Rubenstein JJ, Schulman CL, Yurchak PM, DeSanctis RW. Clinical spectrum of the sick sinus syndrome. Circulation 1972;46:5–13.
63. Fairfax AJ, Lambert CD, and Leatham A. Systemic embolism in chronic sinoatrial disorder. N Engl J Med 1976;295:190–192.
64. Fairfax AJ, Lambert CD. Neurological aspects of sinoatrial heart block. J Neurol Neurosurg Psychiatry 1976;39:576–580.
65. Santini M, Alexidou G, Ansalone G, Cacciatore G, Cini R, Turitto G. Relation of prognosis in sick sinus syndrome to age, conduction defects and modes of permanent cardiac pacing. Am J Cardiol 1990;65:729–735.
66. Komrad MS, Coffey CE, Coffey KS, McKinnis R, Massey EW, Califf RM. Myocardial infarction and stroke. Neurology 1984;34:1403–1409.
67. Puletti M, Cusmano E, Testa MG, Borgia C, Fanari F, Curione M. Incidence of systemic thromboembolic lesions in acute myocardial infarction. Clin Cardiol 1986; 9:331–333.
68. Stratton JR, Resnick AD. Increased embolic risk in patients with left ventricular thrombi. Circulation 1987;75:1004–1011.
69. Loh E, Sutton MS, Wun CC, et al. Ventricular dysfunction and the risk of stroke after myocardial infarction. N Engl J Med 1997;336:251–257.
70. Asinger RW, Mikell FL, Elsperger J, Hodges M. Incidence of left-ventricular thrombosis after acute transmural myocardial infarction. Serial evaluation by two-dimensional echocardiography. N Engl J Med 1981;305:297–302.
71. Hurlen M, Abdelnoor M, Smith P, Erikssen J, Arnesen H. Warfarin, aspirin, or both after myocardial infarction. N Engl J Med 2002;347:969–974.
72. Katz SD, Marantz PR, Biasucci L, et al. Low incidence of stroke in ambulatory patients with heart failure: a prospective study. Am Heart J 1993;126:141–146.
73. Fuster V, Gersh BJ, Giuliani ER, Tajik AJ, Brandenburg RO, Frye RL. The natural history of idiopathic dilated cardiomyopathy. Am J Cardiol 1981;47:525–531.
74. Pullicino PM, Halperin JL, Thompson JL. Stroke in patients with heart failure and reduced left ventricular ejection fraction. Neurology 2000;54:288–294.
75. Cleland JG. Anticoagulant and antiplatelet therapy in heart failure. Curr Opin Cardiol 1997;12:276–287.
76. Kannel WB, Wolf PA, Verter J. Manifestations of coronary disease predisposing to stroke. The Framingham study. JAMA 1983;250:2942–2946.
77. Dries DL, Rosenberg YD, Waclawin MA, Domanski MJ. Ejection fraction and risk of thromboembolic events in patients with systolic dysfunction and sinus rhythm: evidence for gender differences in the studies of left ventricular dysfunction trials. J Am Coll Cardiol 1997;29:1074–1080.
78. Effect of long-term oral anticoagulant treatment on mortality and cardiovascular morbidity after myocardial infarction. Anticoagulants in the Secondary Prevention

of Events in Coronary Thrombosis (ASPECT) Research Group. Lancet 1994;343: 499–503.
79. Smith P, Arnesen H, Holme I. The effect of warfarin on mortality and reinfarction after myocardial infarction. N Engl J Med 1990;323:147–152.
80. A double-blind trial to assess long-term oral anticoagulant therapy in elderly patients after myocardial infarction. Report of the Sixty Plus Reinfarction Study Research Group. Lancet 1980;2:989–994.
81. Coulshed N, Epstein EJ, McKendrick CS, Galloway RW, Walker E. Systemic embolism in mitral valve disease. Br Heart J 1970;32:26–34.
82. Szekely P. Rheumatic heart disease in three decades (1942–1971). Singapore Med J 1973;14:417–419.
83. Chesebro JH, Adams PC, Fuster V. Antithrombotic therapy in patients with valvular heart disease and prosthetic heart valves. J Am Coll Cardiol 1986;8(6 Suppl B): 41B–56B.
84. Kuntze CE, Ebels T, Eijgelaar A, Homan van der Heide JN. Rates of thromboembolism with three different mechanical heart valve prostheses: randomised study. Lancet 1989;1:514–517.
85. Kuntze CE, Blackstone EH, Ebels T. Thromboembolism and mechanical heart valves: a randomized study revisited. Ann Thorac Surg 1998;66:101–107.
86. Olesen KH, Rygg IH, Wennevold A, Nyboe J. Long-term follow-up in 185 patients after mitral valve replacement with the Lillehei–Kaster prosthesis. Overall results and prosthesis-related complications. Eur Heart J 1987;8:680–688.
87. Olesen KH, Rygg IH, Wennevold A, Nyboe J. Long-term follow-up in 262 patients after aortic valve replacement with the Lillehei–Kaster prosthesis. Overall results and prosthesis-related complications. Eur Heart J 1986;7:808–816.
88. Turpie AG, Gent M, Laupacis A, et al. A comparison of aspirin with placebo in patients treated with warfarin after heart-valve replacement. N Engl J Med 1993; 329:524–529.
89. Salgado AV, Furlan AJ, Keys TF, Nichols TR, Beck GJ. Neurologic complications of endocarditis: a 12-year experience. Neurology 1989;39(2 pt 1):173–178.
90. Hart RG, Foster JW, Luther MF, Kanter MC. Stroke in infective endocarditis. Stroke 1990;21:695–700.
91. Lopez JA, Ross RS, Fishbein MC, Siegal RJ. Nonbacterial thrombotic endocarditis: a review. Am Heart J 1987;113:773–784.
92. Lopez JA, Fishbein MC, Siegel RJ. Echocardiographic features of nonbacterial thrombotic endocarditis. Am J Cardiol 1987;59:478–480.

13

Cryptogenic Emboli and Other Elusive Causes of Stroke

Stelios M. Smirnakis and Walter J. Koroshetz

In a significant proportion of stroke patients (20–40%), the exact cause of stroke cannot be clearly identified. In some, stroke risk factors are identified, but it is not possible to know definitively whether the risk factor is causally linked to the stroke. A large subgroup of patients with such "undetermined" stroke mechanisms has clinical syndromes and neuroimaging consistent with an embolic event.

In this chapter, we focus on the evaluation and management of cerebral infarction that results from presumed embolism from an unidentified source (cryptogenic embolism) and other elusive causes of ischemic stroke that are often difficult to ascribe for an individual patient. We discuss the evaluation and available treatment options for several of the most likely etiologies of cryptogenic infarction.

DETERMINING EMBOLIC ETIOLOGY

The first challenge the physician faces after the diagnosis of stroke has been established is to identify the underlying cause in order to institute appropriate management. Modern imaging modalities have helped define more precisely the characteristic pattern of various stroke syndromes (see Chapter 2 for a more detailed discussion of stroke subtypes). Brain computed tomography (CT) or magnetic resonance imaging (MRI) coupled with magnetic resonance angiography (MRA) or computed tomographic angiography (CTA) are the imaging modalities that provide the most useful information regarding the type of infarct and its probable etiology.

Embolic brain infarcts often produce a neurologic deficit of sudden onset and have a distinctive appearance on MRI. They appear as wedge-shaped areas of ischemic damage caused by the sudden occlusion of distal branches of the intracerebral arteries. Over time, a major proportion of vessels occluded

From: *Current Clinical Neurology: Handbook of Stroke Prevention in Clinical Practice*
Edited by: K. L. Furie and P. J. Kelly © Humana Press Inc., Totowa, NJ

by emboli recanalize. If multiple emboli entered the brain simultaneously, then there will be multiple such acute infarcts in different vascular territories. The embolic infarct's neuroradiological appearance depends on the size of the embolic particles and the affected vascular territory. Embolic infarcts can range from large territorial infarctions (as, for example, in the case of emboli large enough to occlude the stem of the middle cerebral artery, 2-mm diameter) to midsize, cortically based, wedge-shaped infarcts (usually due to occlusion of a higher order branch of the bifurcating intracranial arteries, <1-mm diameter), to considerably smaller, pinpoint cortical or subcortical infarcts resulting from occlusion of vessels whose size is on the order of a few hundred micrometers. The latter are occasionally located in "watershed" areas, between major vascular territories, as seen with infarcts caused by acute hypoperfusion. The brain is a sensitive reporter of particulate matter in the circulation. Particles too small to cause symptoms in any other organ cause neurologic deficits if they enter the brain circulation. Tracking the origin of such small particles can be very difficult.

When infarction occurs simultaneously in multiple vascular territories, the probability of a "shower" of emboli from the heart or a proximal common parent vessel is the most likely etiology. The identification of such an embolic source should be pursued proactively. Different vascular territories are subject to embolic infarction at different rates (see Table 1; *1–3*). Even small (<15 mm in size) lenticulostriate infarcts having the appearance of classic lacunes, which are generally caused by microvascular lipohyalanosis or atheroma, may be caused by embolism and should be thoroughly evaluated. This is particularly true in subjects without evidence of hypertension or other risk factors leading to microvascular pathology.

Gan et al., summarizing the lacunar experience from the Northern Manhattan Stroke Study *(4)*, found that patients presenting with a classical lacunar artery syndrome with a single, small, deep infarct on imaging still had a 25% chance to have the infarct as a result of an alternative etiology. Ay and colleagues found that 16% of patients with lacunar syndromes had evidence on diffusion-weighted imaging of multiple small simultaneous infarcts suggestive of emboli *(5)*. Striatocapsular infarcts, which are generally larger (>20–30 mm) and are thought to result from the occlusion of several lenticulostriate arteries simultaneously, are most frequently caused by embolus to the middle cerebral artery, either from the heart (37%) or from a parent artery (38%) *(2)*. If an obvious embolic etiology has been excluded, other possible etiologies that can mimic embolic infarction should be considered, including low-flow or venous infarction, vasculitis, radiation vasculopathy, mitochondrial disorders, or cerebral autosomal dominant arteriopathy with subcortical infarcts and leukoencephalopathy (CADASIL).

Table 1
Rates of Embolic Infarction Stratified by Vascular Territory

1. MCA (large) most often CE or CAE, <8% atherothrombosis
2. ACA most often CE, or CAE, possibly propagation of ICA clot
3. PCA 28–40% CE, 10–30% CPE, 16.5–50% PAD, 0–16% IPD
4. SCA 35–70% CE, 17–30% large artery
5. PICA 50% CE, 50% large-artery atherosclerosis
6. AICA usually basilar atherosclerosis, very rarely embolic
7. Basilar 43% LAD, 18% SAD, 19% CE, 20% AAE *(3)*
8. Vertebral 25% CE, 75% thrombotic (including dissection)
9. Anterior choroidal (large) 54% CE, 20% AAE
10. Striatocapsular (>20 mm) 37% CE, 38% CAE
11. Classical MCA lacunar (<15 mm) 12–20% CE
12. Brainstem/cerebellum (multifocal) 17% CE, 35% LAD
13. Brainstem/cerebellum (unifocal) 6% CE, 27% LAD

Source: From refs. *1* and *2*.

Note: The large-artery etiology includes low flow secondary to atherosclerosis as well as artery-to-artery embolus. AAE, artery-to-artery embolus; CAE, carotid artery embolus; CE, cardioembolic; CPE, cryptogenic embolus; IPD, intrinsic PCA disease; LAD, large-artery disease; PAD, proximal arterial disease; SAD, small-artery disease.

In cases of suspected embolic infarction, a thorough diagnostic evaluation should be undertaken to establish a firm diagnosis and to guide further management for prevention of future events. Common causes of embolic infarction include cardiac arrhythmia, valvular disease, myocardial infarction, paradoxical embolism from venous thrombosis through a patent foramen ovale (PFO) or pulmonary arteriovenous malformations, artery-to-artery embolism from a diseased parent vessel, or an underlying hypercoagulable state.

Given the broad differential diagnosis, a comprehensive evaluation may include brain CT or MRI, MRA or CTA of craniocervical vessels, transcranial Doppler or carotid Doppler ultrasound, 24- to 72-hour Holter monitoring, or transthoracic (TTE) or transesophageal echocardiogram (TEE) with agitated saline contrast injection to evaluate for intracardiac pathology, including PFO. Laboratory investigations may include a complete serum chemistry and hematologic panel, fasting lipid panel and homocysteine level, B_{12}, folate, prothrombin time, partial thromboplastin time, platelet count, antinuclear antibody, erythrocyte sedimentation rate, cardiac enzymes, and a hypercoagulability panel, including tests for lupus anticoagulant, anticardiolipin antibodies, proteins C and S, antithrombin III, or functional or genetic testing for activated protein C resistance because of the factor V Leiden mutation. These studies are aimed at identifying risk factors for stroke that have been identified in population studies. Sometimes, ascribing a specific stroke to one of these risk factors can be a difficult and inaccurate process.

Despite extensive investigation, the cause of ischemic stroke remains undefined (cryptogenic) in up to 40% of cases *(6)*. The Northern Manhattan Stroke Study estimated the 1-year cumulative rate of death or stroke recurrence for cryptogenic stroke as about 10% in an urban population *(7)*. This underscores the potential importance of effective prevention. The rates given in the Manhattan study do not take into account the potential etiology of the cryptogenic stroke or the effects of therapy. We discuss management recommendations in cases of cryptogenic stroke in the setting of (1) PFO, (2) aortic arch disease, and (3) hypercoagulable state, with particular focus on the antiphospholipid antibody syndrome (APS).

PATENT FORAMEN OVALE

Risk of Stroke Associated With PFO

Understanding whether a PFO is causally related to embolic stroke in a given individual is currently a major problem in the field. A PFO is a potential venous-to-arterial shunt through which embolic material originating in the leg or pelvic veins might cause stroke, so-called paradoxical embolus. Although the pressure on the left side of the heart is higher than on the right, jets of blood can cross from right to left through a PFO at rest and are more likely to do so when right-sided pressures increase, such as during the release from a Valsalva maneuver or after pulmonary embolism (PE).

Visualization of the movement of injected microbubbles from the right to the left side of the heart during a cardiac ultrasound is a sensitive means of detecting a right-to-left shunt. Once a PFO is identified, determining whether the right-to-left shunt was responsible for the embolic stroke remains a problem.

Prevalence

The prevalence of PFO is increased in young (<55 years old) patients with stroke, particularly in cryptogenic stroke *(8)*. Autopsy studies of unselected cases indicated that the prevalence of a PFO is approx 27–29% in the general population. Of these PFOs, 6% had maximal diameter greater than 6 mm *(9,10)*.

In a prospective study of 581 patients younger than 55 years with cryptogenic stroke, Lamy et al. found that 46% had a PFO *(11)*, an incidence considerably higher than the 27% expected in the general population. A number of other studies *(12–16)* confirmed the association of cryptogenic stroke and PFO in younger (less than 55–60 years old) patients, in whom the more common age-related stroke risk factors have not yet appeared.

In studies of older stroke populations, the association of PFO and stroke is not as well proven. This is likely because of the diluting effects of other, more powerful age-related stroke risk factors. In the cohort of somewhat older patients (mean age 59 years) enrolled in the Warfarin–Aspirin Recurrent Stroke Study (WARSS) and studied by TEE (PFO in Cryptogenic Stroke Study [PICSS], discussed later in this section), PFO incidence was 34%. In the subgroup with cryptogenic stroke, PFO was found in 39% of patients, compared to 29% for those with other defined causes of stroke ($p < 0.02$).

Recurrent Stroke

Estimates for the rate of annual stroke recurrence in cryptogenic stroke patients with PFO vary widely, ranging from 12% *(17)*, to 7–8% *(16)*, to 1.5–4% *(12,18–20)*, depending on the study population. Bogousslavsky and colleagues *(12)* studied stroke recurrence prospectively in 140 patients younger than 60 years old presenting with stroke and PFO. Only 16% of these individuals had an identifiable coexisting cause of stroke, mostly cardiac (8%). After 3 years of follow-up, the investigators reported a rate of 2.4% for recurrent stroke or death per year (3.8% when they included transient ischemic attacks [TIAs]). Interestingly, only 9.5% of the patients with stroke and PFO had a clinical history of deep venous thrombosis, 16% gave a history of Valsalva maneuver immediately preceding the stroke, and only 2% had a hypercoagulable state. Despite the absence of a clear embolic source in the majority of cases, the incidence of intracranial embolic occlusion by angiography was 86% in patients who underwent angiography within the first 12 hours, suggesting that the etiology of most strokes is embolic in stroke patients with PFO.

Several comorbidity factors have been reported to increase the probability of stroke recurrence in patients with cryptogenic stroke and PFO. A partial list includes (1) the presence of interatrial septal aneurysm (ISA) *(18,19,21)*, (2) a large right-to-left shunt *(20,22–26)*, (3) the presence of prior embolic infarcts as noted by MRI or history *(27)*, (4) the presence of hypercoagulable state or an embolic source in the form of a deep venous clot *(28)*, or (5) a history of Valsalva maneuver immediately prior to the stroke *(29)*.

A prospective French study examined recurrent stroke in patients (18–55 years of age) who had ischemic cryptogenic stroke and PFO on TEE and who were treated with 300 mg daily of aspirin *(19)*. On survival analysis, the rates of recurrent stroke after 4 years were 2.3% (PFO alone), 15.2% (ISA and PFO), and 4.2% (neither ISA nor PFO). These data suggest that PFO in combination with ISA was a significant stroke risk factor, but that PFO alone was not. The difference was statistically significant, suggesting that cryptogenic stroke patients with PFO and ISA are at increased risk for stroke recurrence despite antiplatelet therapy and therefore may benefit from other preventive strategies.

Although several other studies *(18,21,30)* found a similar relationship between ISA and recurrence, the data are not completely consistent. For example, in the Lausanne study *(12)*, ISA, defined as a larger than 1.5-cm bulge of the interatrial septum, was not associated with increased chance of stroke recurrence despite having a high prevalence (25%) in patients with stroke and PFO. The PICSS trial *(16)* also did not find an increase in the risk of stroke or death for PFOs associated with the presence of ISA. Because patients in the French study *(19)* received mostly aspirin as treatment, it is possible that the difference between the series can be explained by the different treatment regimens of the Lausanne and PICSS studies, which included anticoagulation (PICSS, Lausanne) and surgical repair (Lausanne).

Additional risk factors, such as PFO size or recurrent ischemic events, are likely to be predictors of increased risk and should be evaluated *(20,22,23)*. Assessment of PFO size can be made by echocardiography using agitated saline injection and counting the bubbles that appear in the left atrium within three heartbeats *(22)* after the injection. Valsalva or coughing should be performed during the test to increase sensitivity. Most studies define the size of the PFO by the number of bubbles seen across the atrial septum: large, more than 30 bubbles; moderate, 10–30 bubbles; and small, fewer than 10 bubbles. Alternatively, PFO size can be measured directly under TEE visualization of the fossa ovalis or by sizing the Doppler jet, but these methods are reported to be less sensitive *(31)*.

Multiple ischemic events in cryptogenic stroke patients with PFO are also associated with an increased rate of recurrence and argue for aggressive management. Nedeltchev et al. reported that the average annual recurrence of stroke or TIA after one ischemic event in patients treated with aspirin or warfarin is 4.8%, whereas the recurrence rate is as high as 9.9% after multiple ischemic events *(27)*.

Treatment Options for Stroke Associated With PFO

To date, only one large randomized trial has compared aspirin and low-intensity anticoagulation with warfarin for the prevention of recurrent stroke associated with PFO. More trials comparing medical therapies with each other or with surgical and endovascular closure are required. In the absence of such data, the current treatment choices available to the physician include (1) aspirin or other antiplatelet agents, (2) anticoagulation with warfarin, (3) percutaneous endovascular closure, or (4) surgical closure. The data supporting each of these management strategies are discussed next.

Medical Management

Both warfarin and aspirin have been studied for prevention of stroke recurrence in patients with PFO in a single randomized trial (PICSS), a subgroup of the WARSS trial *(16)*. In PICSS, 630 patients (203 [33.8%] with PFO) were randomly assigned to treatment with low-intensity warfarin (goal international normalized ratio [INR] 1.4–2.8; mean INR achieved 2.04) vs 325 mg aspirin and were followed for 2 years. Inclusion in PICSS was determined primarily by the willingness of WARSS participants to undergo TEE. Participants were 30–85 years old, had a stroke in the 30 days prior to enrollment, and their stroke etiology was other than atrial fibrillation (AF)AF or surgically treatable carotid stenosis. The rates of major hemorrhage were almost identical in both treatment groups, indicating that low-intensity anticoagulation was safe in this context.

Of the 630 patients enrolled in PICSS, 42% had cryptogenic stroke, with other defined stroke subtypes accounting for the remainder. No significant difference was detected for the primary end point of stroke recurrence or death in patients with PFO vs no PFO in either the aspirin or the warfarin treatment arms. This result remained valid even when the analysis was restricted to the cryptogenic stroke subgroup. This suggests that, for patients on medical therapy, the presence of a PFO does not imply an increased rate of recurrent stroke or death, at least for the first 2 years of follow-up.

When comparing the two treatment arms in the subgroup of patients with cryptogenic stroke and PFO, the recurrent stroke or death rate at 2 years was nearly twice as high in patients treated with aspirin compared to those treated with warfarin, suggesting a possible benefit for warfarin treatment. This result, however, did not reach statistical significance (17.9 vs 9.5%, $p = 0.28$). Moreover, the trend favoring warfarin persisted for the cryptogenic subgroup without a PFO, suggesting that the PFO may not have been causally related to the end point events. Although suggestive, the results of these post hoc analyses must be interpreted with caution because of the relatively small number of subjects in each subgroup. Moreover, the patients included in the PICSS study, at a mean age of 59 years, were older on average than those in most observational studies reporting an association between PFO and stroke, and they were followed for only 2 years. Therefore, caution is required when attempting to generalize the PICSS findings to younger adults with PFO and cryptogenic stroke.

Several other observational studies have examined recurrence rates associated with different treatment strategies. In the Lausanne study *(12)*, patients were followed for a mean of 3 years after being treated with anticoagulation (26% of enrollees), antiplatelet agents (66%), or surgical closure (8%). Factors associated with recurrence, in addition to ISA, included infarction in the territory of the posterior cerebral artery, recent migraine, and not surprisingly, a coexisting cause of stroke. Treatment modality, however, was not associated with the risk of recurrence. The coexistence of more than two of the risk factors mentioned above conferred a greater than 50% risk of recurrent stroke in the next 3 years despite treatment *(12)*. This observation suggests that there are subpopulations at very high risk for recurrence among patients with cryptogenic stroke and PFO. Cujec et al. analyzed retrospectively a cohort of 90 cryptogenic stroke patients younger than 60 years, 52 of whom had a PFO, and reported that warfarin was more effective than antiplatelet therapy in preventing stroke recurrence *(17)*.

Given these inconclusive data, no definitive recommendations can be formulated at present regarding the relative benefits of antiplatelet therapy vs warfarin for stroke prevention in patients with cryptogenic stroke and PFO. Carefully monitored low-intensity anticoagulation (INR ~ 2) and aspirin therapy are both safe and reasonable treatment options, and either may be used depending on clinical judgment after weighing the presence of additional risk factors and formulating a risk-and-benefit analysis individually for each patient.

If the clinical suspicion for paradoxical embolism is high (e.g., proven deep leg or pelvic venous thrombosis in the presence of a PFO) and there are no contraindications to anticoagulation, we typically initiate warfarin therapy with an INR goal of 2–3 and then consider switching to aspirin after a 6-month interval. Long-term treatment with warfarin or PFO closure may be considered when there are proven nonmodifiable risk factors for thrombosis (e.g., factor V Leiden mutation, etc.) or if recurrent embolism occurs while on antiplatelet therapy.

Surgical and Endovascular PFO Closure

Ruchat et al. attempted to establish criteria for surgical intervention by studying a series of patients with cryptogenic stroke and PFO *(29)*. In this series, 32 patients younger than 60 years were selected for surgery among a group of patients with cryptogenic embolism or TIAs and PFO. Inclusion was determined by the presence of at least two of the following criteria: history of Valsalva before stroke, multiple clinical events or multiple infarcts on MRI, atrial septal aneurysm, or large (>50 bubbles) right-to-left shunt. There were no major complications or recurrent vascular events for an average follow-up of 19 months, demonstrating that surgical closure of the PFO can be accomplished with very low morbidity and can successfully reduce the risk of recurrence. Devuyst et al. reported on 30 patients selected with identical criteria with similar results *(32)*.

Dearani et al. *(33)* retrospectively followed a cohort of 91 patients with PFO for a mean of 2 years following surgical PFO closure. Of these patients, 59 had presented with cryptogenic stroke and 32 with cryptogenic TIA. No major complications occurred during the follow-up period, and only 7 recurrent cryptogenic TIAs occurred, suggesting a benefit for surgical closure.

By contrast, Homma et al. reported an actuarial rate of recurrence of 19.5% at 13 months in 28 patients selected for surgical PFO closure after refusing or failing warfarin therapy; they concluded that surgical closure does not consistently prevent recurrence of ischemic events *(34)*. Three of the four recurrent events (one stroke, three TIAs) in the latter study occurred in older patients, who have higher *a priori* likelihood of coexisting stroke etiologies not addressed by PFO closure (the single stroke in this series occurred in a 62-year-old patient with renal cell carcinoma).

To make an informed decision about the risks and benefits of PFO closure, the surgical risk of atrial septal defect repair should be considered. This is low for young healthy patients, but increases as the clinical status of the patients deteriorates. Thus, for young healthy patients, the risk of complications is less than 1.6%, but can rise to 5% for patients in New York Heart Association classes III and IV heart failure *(35)*. This suggests that the surgical option should be exercised with caution. When surgical risks are carefully evaluated, this approach merits careful consideration, especially for young, otherwise healthy patients with cryptogenic stroke and PFO, for whom the lifetime rates of major hemorrhagic complications from long-term antiplatelet therapy or warfarin anticoagulation are considerable *(36)*. This is particularly true for patients meeting the criteria outlined in the studies of Ruchat and coworkers *(29)* and Devuyst and colleagues *(32)*, which are likely to confer an increased risk of stroke recurrence.

In centers with large interventional vascular practices, percutaneous closure of the PFO may present a viable alternative to medical or surgical management. Hung et al. followed for a mean of 2.6 years 63 patients who underwent percutaneous PFO closure with the Clamshell (Bard Clamshell Septal Umbrella, USC I Division, C.R. Bard, Billerica, MA), CardioSEAL (NMT Medical Inc., Boston, MA), or Buttoned device (Pediatric Cardiology and Custom Medical Devices, Amarillo, TX) *(37)*. There were four recurrent events (3.2% recurrence per year), two of which were associated with suboptimal device performance, and 14% of the patients had residual shunting after device placement (11% with 1- to 3-mm jet, 3% with larger than 3-mm jet). The patient series by Bridges et al. *(38)* and Windecker et al. *(39)* reported similar or higher degrees of recurrence or complications. Overall, percutaneous closure appears to have a lower success rate than surgery in eliminating the PFO and potentially higher risk for complications associated with the particular device deployed. However, this field is advancing quickly and is likely to replace surgical closure over time.

Randomized trials need to be performed as a matter of priority to evaluate these options objectively, particularly in young patients with cryptogenic stroke and PFO. Given the high prevalence of PFO in the population, the limited data on recurrence rates and causal role of PFO in stroke is currently problematic. Although substantial variation in physician practices currently exists, we generally reserve percutaneous closure as an option for otherwise healthy, young stroke patients without other stroke risk factors. A search is made for evidence of a deep vein thrombosis (DVT) or PE during the patient's admission. Decisions on closure are usually put off for 3 months after stroke while the patient is treated with warfarin. This allows time for other stroke risk factors to appear (AF, results of antiphospholipid antibody tests, etc.). Additionally, if the stroke was caused by a paradoxical embolus, then 3 months of warfarin is indicated for the presumed underlying DVT.

Summary

The current state of evidence on the optimal management of cryptogenic stroke with PFO does not allow definitive recommendations. The following are suggestions for management based on existing evidence and our clinical experience (Table 2):

1. It is important to stratify the risk for the individual patient by looking for coexisting factors that may influence the risk of recurrence. It is essential to perform a TEE with agitated saline contrast injection to assess the size of the PFO and the potential presence of an ISA. Evidence of prior strokes on MRI and potential history of a Valsalva maneuver preceding the acute event should be sought. We also recommend looking for sites of active thrombosis, performing a hypercoagulability panel (particularly in younger patients), and completing a thorough general stroke workup to exclude other potential etiologies for stroke. Workup for active thrombosis should include a lower extremity ultrasound to rule out DVT, the incidence of which is known to be high in patients with stroke and PFO (Lethen et al. reported a 9.5% incidence of DVT in a cohort of 53 patients with stroke or TIA and PFO, but without large-artery disease; *40*). Depending on clinical suspicion, a pelvic MR venogram could be considered to rule out pelvic vein thrombosis, as could a pulmonary CT angiogram to assess for PE.
2. For patients older than 60 years, in the absence of any contraindication, we generally empirically treat with a short (3- to 6-month) course of anticoagulation with warfarin (INR ~ 2–3), followed by aspirin. Data from PICSS provide some support for the safety and possible efficacy of this approach.
3. In the case of very young patients (younger than 40 years), for whom the lifetime risks of long-term antithrombotic therapy are considerable *(36)*, we generally advocate surgical or percutaneous repair of the PFO, depending on the estimated risk for recurrent embolism, degree of surgical risk, experience of the interventional team, and patient preference. A short course of anticoagulation followed by antiplatelet agents is also acceptable in patients with a clearly reversible thrombophilic risk factor.

Table 2
Summary of Recommendations for Management of Cryptogenic Stroke in Patients With PFO

We recommend taking into account the following criteria to facilitate decision making in cases of cryptogenic strokes with PFO:

a. Definite evidence of venous blood clot
b. Recurrent cryptogenic infarction, particularly when it indicates failure of antiplatelet agents
c. Presence of reversible hypercoagulable state
d. High risk for recurrence as assessed by satisfying one of the following criteria: (1) associated ISA > 15 mm, (2) large shunt (>30 bubbles), (3) high clinical suspicion, as determined, for example, by history of Valsalva immediately preceding the stroke

For patients who satisfy criterion (a), a 3- to 6-month period of anticoagulation is indicated, followed by antiplatelet agents, provided no irreversible thrombophilic risk factor is identified and criteria (b), (c), and (d) are not satisfied. For patients who satisfy criterion (b), (c), or (d), temporary anticoagulation followed by PFO closure could be a reasonable choice. We tend to favor closure of PFO in patients at risk younger than 40 years who do not have a clearly reversible thrombophilic risk factor. We recommend addressing the issue of closure case by case for older patients, taking into account the degree of clinical suspicion, risk of recurrence, and surgical or interventional risk (see also the section on hypercoagulability syndromes for further discussion).

4. Patients between 40 and 60 years old are generally managed with one of these approaches as assessed on a case-by-case basis.
5. Failure of medical therapy should prompt a search for an alternative cause of stroke; if no satisfactory explanation for the recurrence is found, we recommend closure of the PFO. Stroke recurrence after PFO closure should prompt reinvestigation with TEE to determine if closure was indeed successful. If so, warfarin anticoagulation should be considered, and an alternative etiology for the recurring strokes should be sought aggressively.

AORTIC ARCH ATHEROSCLEROSIS

Association Between Aortic Atherosclerosis and Stroke

Atherosclerotic disease of the aortic arch is highly prevalent in older patient populations. It is estimated that more than 60% of patients above 60 years old who have had brain infarction have evidence of coexisting aortic arch atherosclerosis *(41)*. Amarenco et al. *(42)* reported on 500 autopsies of patients with cerebrovascular or other neurological diseases and found that ulcerated aortic arch plaques were present in 26% of patients with cerebrovascular disease, as opposed to 5% of patients with other neurological diseases. In patients with cryptogenic stroke, ulcerated aortic plaque prevalence was 61%, compared to 22% in patients with other known cause of stroke. Several other studies also suggested that ulcerated aortic arch plaques, particularly large (>4 mm) protruding atherosclerotic lesions with mobile components because of superimposed thrombi, may be an important cause of embolic disease *(41–51)*.

The French Study of Aortic Plaques in Stroke Group *(41)* prospectively followed a cohort of 331 patients older than 60 years who were consecutively admitted with brain infarction to a tertiary care center; the investigators stratified the risk of stroke recurrence based on the TEE characteristics of atheromatous aortic arch plaques. Plaque thickness correlated strongly with recurrent brain infarction and other embolic vascular events during the follow-up period of 2–4 years. For plaque thickness larger than 4 mm, the rate of stroke recurrence was 12%, compared to 3.5% for plaque thickness 1–3.9 mm and 2.8% for plaques less than 1 mm (per 100 patient-years). Plaque size larger than 4 mm remained an independent predictor of recurrent stroke even after adjusting for other risk factors, such as carotid stenosis, peripheral vascular disease, and AF (relative risk factor 3.8). Among 102 patients with cryptogenic stroke, there was a 16.4% recurrence per 100 patient-years for plaque size larger than 4mm. Because most of the patients in this study were treated with antiplatelet agents or anticoagulation and statins, these numbers probably underestimate the rate of recurrence in untreated aortic disease. No statistical difference in the rate of recurrent stroke was observed in the group of patients treated with warfarin compared to those treated with aspirin, but the study lacked sufficient power to demonstrate small-to-moderate treatment differences between groups.

Management of Patients With Stroke and Aortic Atherosclerosis

The optimal management of patients with stroke and protruding aortic atheromas has not been studied in randomized trials. Measures for vascular risk prevention should be instituted in all patients with stroke and visible aortic plaque on TEE. These include addressing modifiable risk factors, such as smoking, hyperlipidemia, and hypertension *(52)*. Homocysteine level has been shown to predict independently the progression of aortic arch atherosclerosis *(53,54)*. Therefore, the homocysteine level should be determined and vitamin supplementation with folate and vitamins B_6 and B_{12} considered.

Apart from these general measures, a frequent clinical dilemma is the choice between antithrombotic therapy with antiplatelet agents and warfarin anticoagulation. Until randomized trial data become available, this decision may be better informed after stratifying the severity of aortic arch atherosclerosis with TEE *(55)*. Antiplatelet therapy remains the treatment of choice in most situations and may decrease the risk of vascular events by as much as 25% in patients with atherosclerosis *(56)*. Aspirin, dipyridamole, or clopidogrel are reasonable options *(57)*, although none has been studied specifically in trials of patients with aortic atherosclerosis. Further evidence is awaited from the Management of Atherothrombosis With Clopidogrel in High-Risk Patients with Recent Transient Ischaemic Attack or Ischaemic Stroke trial.

A reasonable approach based on existing data is to recommend low-intensity anticoagulation to patients with irregular aortic plaque with a mobile component, presumably because of attached thrombus. This rationale *(58)* is based on a number of small retrospective series, which suggested that (1) the mobile elements in a plaque often consist of thrombus *(59–61)*, and (2) the mobile elements appear to decrease in size with anticoagulation *(50,62,63)*.

Despite the rationale of this approach, the safety of warfarin for this indication is unclear. Of particular concern are case reports that describe hemorrhage into atherosclerotic plaque, leading to rupture and cholesterol embolization, which has been attributed to warfarin therapy *(64,65)*. We suggest that a reasonable strategy is to consider a short course of warfarin for patients with TEE evidence of adherent thrombus with mobile components, followed by repeat TEE in 2–3 months. At this time, antiplatelet therapy may be initiated if TEE data indicate that the mobile thrombus has resolved. Surgical removal of atheromas can also be considered in exceptional cases of patients with severe recurrent embolism, but this procedure carries considerable risk *(66)* and should be reserved for patients at very high risk who are excellent surgical candidates *(45)*.

Although a detailed discussion is beyond the scope of this chapter, aortic atherosclerosis is highly correlated with the risk of stroke during cardiac surgery involving aortic cannulation or manipulation *(50,67)*, particularly during aortic valve replacement. Intraoperative ultrasound has contributed to reducing the risk of this procedure by guiding the surgeon in selecting safer sites for aortic manipulation.

HYPERCOAGULABILITY SYNDROMES

Various coagulation disorders are associated with venous or arterial thrombosis and ischemic stroke *(68)*. Bushnell and Goldstein *(68)* estimated prevalence data for various thrombophilic states in patients presenting with ischemic stroke (Table 3). In one study of 36 patients (younger than 40 years) with cryptogenic stroke *(70,71)*, 9 (25%) had a deficiency of one natural anticoagulant, five had a deficiency of protein S, and one each had deficiencies of ATIII, protein C, and plasminogen. The authors concluded that a hypercoagulability workup should be pursued in all young patients with cryptogenic infarction. It is especially important to perform a complete hypercoagulability workup for children with ischemic stroke.

A recent series by Chan and deVeber *(72)* reported that the overall incidence of prothrombotic disorders in children with stroke ranges from 20 to 50%. Studies in older stroke patients have not confirmed a major role of the common disorders (prothrombin gene mutation, factor V Leiden mutation, protein C or S deficiency) in arterial occlusive disease, although they do contribute to venous thrombosis.

Insufficient data are currently available to estimate stroke risk reliably and make recommendations for primary prevention to patients with most nonmodifiable prothrombotic risk factors *(73)*. However, patients should be counseled to avoid smoking and oral contraceptive use and to receive antithrombotic prophylaxis during high-risk situations, such as prolonged immobility and surgery. Although the prevalence of having at least one of the known hypercoagulable disorders approaches 10–15% in the general population, routine screening is not recommended because of the prohibitive cost involved and the relatively low positive predictive value for thromboembolic events *(73)*. Stroke in children is a possible exception.

Clinical trials comparing antithrombotic therapies in these disorders have not been performed and are unlikely to be conducted soon because of the difficulties in recruiting adequate numbers of patients. In the absence of hard data, substantial variation in physician practices exists for secondary stroke prevention in patients with thrombophilic disorders following cryptogenic embolic stroke. One empiric approach, favored by many stroke specialists, is to treat with warfarin anticoagulation (INR 2–3) for 3–6 months in those with a nonmodifiable thrombophilic state and a second risk factor (e.g., surgery); the assumption is that undetected arterial or venous thrombosis may pose a higher risk of early recurrent embolism. At the end of the warfarin course, a transition to antiplatelet medications can be considered on a case-by-case basis. Factors that influence this decision include the nature of the coagulation abnormality (usually anticoagulation is continued for protein C, S, or ATIII deficiencies), the severity of the initial event, the presence of other nonmodifiable risk factors, the estimated risk of continued anticoagulation *(36,74)*, patient age, and patient preference. Patients should be instructed to seek prophylaxis for future surgical procedures or prolonged immobility and to avoid smoking and oral contraceptive use.

Table 3
Prevalence of Hereditary Hypercoagulable States in the General Population[a] and in Ischemic Stroke[b]

Thrombophilic disorder	Prevalence in general population	Prevalence in ischemic stroke	Relative risk for stroke
APL antibody	3–5% (30% RI, 18–86% SLE, 20–42% human immunodeficiency virus)	17% (21% for <50 years)	0.8–8.83
Lupus anticoagulant	?	3% (8% for <50 years)	?
APCR/FVL	3–5% (20% with history of DVT)	7% (11% for <50 years)	1.0–2.75
Prothrombin G20120A	0–4.4% (5–10% with history of thrombosis)	4.5% (5.7% for <50 years)	1.1–3.8
Protein C deficiency	0.145–0.5%	2.7%[c]	?
Protein S deficiency	0.2–0.4%	16%[c]	?
Antithrombin III deficiency	0.02–0.17%	4.4%[c]	?
Hyperhomocysteinemia	5–10% (10–25% with history of DVT; population-dependent, according to folate status)		1.79

APCR/FVL, activated protein C/factor V Leiden; DVT, deep venous thrombosis; RI, recent infection.
[a]From ref. *69*.
[b]From ref. *68*.
[c]Best estimate based on few case controlled studies.

Table 4
Proposed Risk Classification of Patients With Hypercoagulable States

High risk (consider prolonged anticoagulation)
More than one spontaneous thrombotic clinical event
Single spontaneous thrombotic event and a nonmodifiable thrombophilic factor (e.g., antithrombin III, protein C or S deficiency)
Single thrombotic event associated with a nonmodifiable acquired risk factor (e.g., prolonged immobility) and a single hereditary factor
Single thrombotic event associated with more than one allelic hereditary risk factor (e.g., factor V Leiden mutation and prothrombin G20210A mutation)
Single life-threatening thrombosis (PE, cerebral vein thrombosis, mesenteric or portal vein thrombosis) associated with a modifiable acquired risk factor and a nonmodifiable risk factor[a]
Moderate risk (consider temporary warfarin [INR 2–3] followed by antiplatelet therapy)
Single thrombotic event in the presence of a modifiable risk factor
Single thrombotic event associated with a modifiable acquired risk factor and a hereditary risk factor[a]
Low risk (prophylaxis when acquired risk factors are also present)
Asymptomatic in the presence of one or more nonmodifiable hypercoagulable risk factors

Source: Adapted from ref. *73* and personal communication (Fall 2001) from M. Laposata. Suggested treatment regimens are empiric based on clinical experience and uncontrolled studies. Randomized trials are required for definite recommendations.

[a]The choice between a temporary course of warfarin followed by antiplatelet agents vs long-term warfarin therapy is often based on the severity of the initial thrombotic event as well as the overall clinical judgment about the risk of recurrence on a case-by-case basis.

In cases of recurrent cryptogenic infarction despite antiplatelet therapy, long-term anticoagulation with warfarin should be considered, particularly if a nonmodifiable coagulation abnormality is identified. Table 4 offers a suggested risk stratification scheme that may be helpful in some cases. We emphasize that the suggested management strategies have not been rigorously evaluated in clinical trials and are based on our clinical experience and interpretation of the available literature. We caution that, although prolonged low-intensity anticoagulation (INR 2–3) may be effective in preventing thrombotic recurrences *(73)*, it is not without risk. Schulman et al. *(36)* reported 2–3% bleeding complications per year, and Fihn et al. *(74)* reported that the rate of major bleeding complications of warfarin therapy in elderly patients can reach 7–9% per year. The general recommendations we offer

Table 5
List of Some Acquired Risk Factors for Hypercoagulable State

Surgery
Malignancy (Trousseau syndrome)
Immobilization
Trauma
Pregnancy
Oral contraceptives
Hormone replacement therapy
Nephrotic syndrome
Disseminated intravascular coagulation
Thrombotic thrombocytopenic purpura
HELLP syndrome
Polycythemia vera
Myeloproliferative disorders
APS (acquired form)
Obesity

are tentative, and the risk–benefit equation of prolonged anticoagulation must be carefully considered for the individual patient on a case-by-case basis.

Finally, it is important to identify and treat acquired causes of hypercoagulability (e.g., dehydration, cancer, nephrosis) in patients with cryptogenic brain embolic infarcts. It is beyond the scope of this chapter to discuss the optimal management of each of these syndromes. A partial list of acquired thrombophilic disorders is provided in Table 5.

ANTIPHOSPHOLIPID ANTIBODY SYNDROME

Antiphospholipid Antibodies and Risk of Stroke

Among hypercoagulation syndromes, the antiphospholipid (APL) antibody syndrome (APS) is particularly associated with ischemic stroke *(97)*. Antiphospholipid antibodies are a heterogenous group of antibodies that react with phospholipids of cell membranes. Anticardiolipin (ACL) and Lupus anticoagulant (LA) antibodies are subgroups of APL antibodies. ACL antibodies (IgG, IgM, or IgA) react against cardiolipin, a mitochondrial membrane phospholipid used as specific antigen for solid-phase immunological assays. In contrast to the immunological activity of ACL antibodies, LA is defined on the basis of in vitro functional testing of its ability to inhibit phospholipid-dependent clotting factors.

Table 6
Partial List of Disorders Associated With Antiphospholipid Antibodies

Systemic lupus erythematosus
Sjogren's syndrome
Autoimmune thrombocytopenic purpura or autoimmune hemolytic anemia
Myositis
Scleroderma, mixed connective tissue disease, Behcet's, polymyalgia rheumatica
Rheumatoid arthritis
Infection (syphilis, lyme, tuberculosis, human immunodeficiency virus, hepatitis, endocarditis, septicemia)
Medications (phenothiazines, hydralazine, dilantin, quinidine, procainamide, streptomycin, chlorpromazine)
Malignancy (lymphoproliferative disorders, solid tumors, multiple myeloma, leukemia)
Paraproteinemias
von Willebrand's disease
Polyarteritis nodosa, Giant cell arteritis
Stroke, Sneddon's syndrome
Migraine
Myasthenia gravis
Multiple sclerosis

Although frequently found together, they are not always concordant (Table 6). Also, the presence of positive ACL antibodies or LA activity is not specific for thrombotic events, as their production is frequently induced by other factors (Table 6). Definite APS is defined as the occurrence of a clinical episode of thrombosis in any organ together with two laboratory determinations positive for anticardiolipin antibodies or the lupus anticoagulant antibody, at least 6 weeks apart from each other (Table 5). The prevalence of serum anticardiolipin antibodies and LA activity ranges from 1 to 5% in young, healthy adults and from 12 to 30% in older adults.

Among hypercoagulation syndromes, the APS is particularly strongly associated with ischemic stroke *(75)*. Definite APS is defined as the occurrence of a clinical episode of thrombosis in any organ together with two laboratory determinations positive for antiphospholipid (APL) antibodies, at least 6 weeks apart from each other.

APS in its most malignant state causes thrombosis in multiple organs, both venous and arterial. It is a known cause of multiple miscarriages caused by placental infarction. Sneddon's syndrome is a combination of arterial occlusive disease and livedo reticularis skin lesions and is related to APL antibodies. APL antibodies are common in patients with systemic lupus erythematosus (SLE; see Table 6 for a partial list of other disorders associated with APL antibodies). Although it is clear that APL antibodies can be causally related to ischemic stroke, it is not clear that the presence of an elevated antibody titer in a stroke patient indicates that the stroke was caused by an APS. This is especially the case in older individuals, for whom APL titers increase and other stroke risk factors abound.

Cervera *(76)* analyzed the data from 1000 patients with APS and reported a predominance in women (82% of cases). Primary APS occurred in 53% of patients. Secondary APS was associated with SLE in 36% and with other diseases in 11%. Most cases began in the third, fourth, and fifth decades. The age of onset was younger than 15 years in 3% and older than 50 years in 13%. Most patients with later onset (>50 years) were men, and this group suffered from higher incidence of stroke and angina.

APL antibody prevalence in subjects without thrombosis ranges from 1 to 6.5%, rising considerably in the elderly and in patients with SLE *(77,78)*. The association of APL antibodies with stroke is strongest for young adults (<50 years). The reported incidence of APL antibodies ranges from 2 to 46% in this age group *(77,79,80)*. Studies of APL antibody titers among unselected patients with stroke showed a weaker or not significant association. The original Antiphospholipid Antibodies in Stroke Study (APASS) *(81)* reported that 9.7% of patients with a first ischemic stroke are anticardiolipin positive, compared with 4.3% of controls. In the WARSS/APASS *(82)*, APL antibodies were detected in a large proportion (40.7%) of stroke patients, although the presence of these antibodies had no significant effect on stroke recurrence *(83,84)*.

Antiphospholipid Antibodies As Predictors of Recurrent Stroke

The risk of stroke recurrence after APL-associated brain infarction can be high. Levine and coworkers followed 81 patients with focal cerebral ischemia and APL antibodies for 7 years and reported a greater than 50% rate of recurrence of thromboembolic events during this period *(85)*. Patients with the highest anticardiolipin immunoglobulin G (IgG) titers had the shortest time to recurrence. Other groups have also reported an association of stroke risk with APL antibody titers, especially in young patients *(86)* or patients with SLE *(87)*. Khamashta et al. followed retrospectively for a median of 6 years, 147 patients with APL antibodies and a history of thrombosis and reported a 69% rate of recurrent thrombosis (cumulative estimates from all treatment groups) *(88)*. Factors that are thought to increase the rate of recurrence include high IgG anticardiolipin antibody titers *(85,89)*, IgG vs IgM isotype, presence of lupus anticoagulant, and anti-b2GP1 positivity *(90)*.

Conflicting data exist on the association between APL antibodies and stroke recurrence in elderly patients. Heinzlef et al. followed for an average of

2.3 years a prospective cohort of patients older than 60 years with brain infarction and reported on the risk of recurrent ischemic events *(91)*. Although the incidence of prior infarction was significantly higher in patients with positive (>10 IU) anticardiolipin antibodies (26 vs 12%), the incidence of recurrent vascular events was not, even among the subgroup with cryptogenic stroke. The authors concluded that there was no benefit in testing for anticardiolipin antibodies in older patients with brain infarction. Most patients in this study had anticardiolipin rather than other APL antibody profiles, so these results may not be generalizable to other APL antibodies. The original study from the APASS Group reported similar results *(92)*. Other studies have reported conflicting results on the association of APL antibodies with stroke recurrence *(85,89,93,94)*. Further research is needed to define the risk of recurrent stroke in older stroke patients with elevated APL antibodies.

β2 Glycoprotein-1 and Risk of Stroke

β2 Glycoprotein-1 (β2GP-1) is a 50kD plasma protein with high binding affinity for phospholipids (cardiolipin, phosphatidylserine, phosphatidylethanolamine). It is required by many ACL antibodies ("cofactor dependent") associated with SLE and the APL syndrome for cardiolipin binding. ACL antibodies associated with infection or other factors do not display this property. In practice, it may prove useful for selection of patients with positive ACL titers who may be at risk of thrombosis. Consistent with this idea, β2GP-1-dependent ACL IgG was associated with increased risk of first ischemic stroke (15-year adjusted OR 2.2) and myocardial infarction (15-year adjusted OR 1.8) in a sample from the Honolulu Heart Study.

Management of Patients With Elevated Antiphospholipid Antibodies and Stroke

Optimal primary prevention strategies have not been defined in asymptomatic patients with elevated APL antibody titers *(95)*. It is important to identify and address other prothrombotic modifiable risk factors in this group. The prevalence of APL is highest in patients with SLE and increases their risk of thrombosis by a factor of 4.5 *(96)*, suggesting that primary prevention with antithrombotic therapy might be beneficial in this subgroup. Patients with APL antibodies and other identified nonmodifiable thrombophilic disorders (e.g., factor V Leiden mutation) might also benefit from primary prevention with antiplatelet agents or low-intensity anticoagulation. Randomized trials to test these hypotheses are required.

Conflicting data exist regarding the benefit of anticoagulation for secondary stroke prevention in patients with elevated APL antibodies. A nonrandomized retrospective comparison of different treatment strategies in the cohort described by Khamashta et al. *(88)* found that high-intensity anticoagulation (INR > 3) was associated with a significant reduction of stroke recurrence and was superior to aspirin or low-intensity warfarin anticoagulation. Rosove and Brewer reported similar findings in a series of 70 patients *(97)*. Khamashta et al. reported a very high recurrence rate of 1.3 thrombotic events per patient-year following discontinuation of anticoagulation *(88)*. Another group followed 66 patients with APS and prior cryptogenic stroke who were treated with anticoagulation (goal INR 3.5) and found that there was a significant rate of recurrent thrombosis (9 per 100 patient-years) despite anticoagulation *(98)*. Other studies suggest that lower intensity anticoagulation (goal INR 2–3) may be effective *(97,99–101)*. Standard obstetric practice includes anticoagulation with low molecular weight heparin during pregnancy to prevent spontaneous abortion. Despite these findings, the benefits of anticoagulation in patients with APL antibodies and stroke are unclear, potentially because the APL antibody is not causally related to the infarct in all patients in the stroke cohort.

In the WARSS/APASS trial *(83,84,102)*, approx 1800 first-time ischemic stroke patients from the WARSS population *(82)* were enrolled to APASS and followed for approx 2 years for any recurrent arterial or venous thrombo-occlusive event. Of those enrolled, about 40% turned out to be APL antibody positive (28% for anticardiolipin, 19% for lupus anticoagulant, and 7% for both). After risk factor adjustment, there was no observed increase in the risk of recurrent thromboembolism associated with APL antibodies in either the warfarin or the aspirin arm. This suggests that APL antibody status was not an independent predictor of stroke recurrence in the older or treated patient cohort of WARSS/APASS, raising further questions about optimal management in this set of patients. Interestingly, warfarin patients that were both anticardiolipin antibody and lupus anticoagulant positive appeared at greater risk of thromboembolism than warfarin patients who were APL antibody negative (36 vs 26%, $p = 0.11$), although this result did not reach significance.

Overall, data from randomized trials are insufficient at present for firm recommendations to be made. In view of the conflicting data above, it is reasonable to consider either antiplatelet therapy or warfarin anticoagulation for young patients with cryptogenic stroke who have high APL antibody titers on repeated testing. Many experienced stroke physicians will treat with warfarin, for a goal INR of at least 2–3. Some patients with very aggressive disease suffer recurrent stroke whenever their INR drops to a subtherapeutic level, and others may require higher levels of anticoagulation (INR > 3) for stroke prevention *(88)*. For patients older than 60 years, for whom the association between APL antibodies and stroke is weaker *(90)*, or for patients with borderline titers that are not consistently elevated, either low-intensity anticoagulation or antiplatelet therapy may be considered *(103)*. Factors that may influence the decision toward anticoagulation include a history of recurrent stroke, SLE, the presence of lupus anticoagulant, anti-β2GPI antibodies, high APL antibody titers, IgG vs IgM isotype, or the existence of an additional coagulation abnormality.

REFERENCES

1. Bogousslavsky J, Caplan L, eds. Stroke Syndromes, 2nd ed. Cambridge, UK: Cambridge University Press, 2001.
2. Pullicino P. Lenticulostriate arteries. In: Bogousslavsky J, Caplan L, eds. Stroke Syndromes. Cambridge, UK: Cambridge University Press, 2001:428–438.
3. Caplan L, Tettenborn B. Vertebrobasilar occlusive disease: review of selected aspects. 2. Posterior circulation embolism. Cerebrovasc Dis 1992;2:320–326.
4. Gan R, Sacco R, Kargman J, Roberts J, Boden-Albala B, Gu Q. Testing the validity of the lacunar hypothesis: the Northern Manhattan Stroke Study experience. Neurology 1997;48:1204–1211.
5. Ay H, Oliveira-Filho J, Buonanno F, et al. An identifiable subset of lacunar infarctions caused by embolism. Stroke 1999;30:2644–2650.
6. Sacco R, Ellenberg J, Mohr J, et al. Infarcts of undetermined cause: the NINCDS Stroke Data Bank. Ann Neurol 1989;25:382–390.
7. Sacco R, Shi T, Zamanillo M, Kargman D. Predictors of mortality and recurrence after hospitalized cerebral infarction in an urban population: the Northern Manhattan Stroke Study. Neurology 1994;44:626–634.
8. Lechat P, Mas J, Lascault G, et al. Prevalence of patent foramen ovale in patients with stroke. N Eng J Med 1988;318:1148–1152.
9. Kerut EK, Norfleet WT, Plotnick GD, Giles TD. Patent foramen ovale: a review of associated conditions and the impact of physiological size. J Am Coll Cardiol 2001;38:613–623.
10. Hagen P, Scholz D, Edwards W. Incidence and size of patent foramen ovale during the first 10 decades of life: an autopsy study of 965 normal hearts. Mayo Clin Proc 1984;59:17–20.
11. Lamy C, Giannesini C, Zuber M, et al. Clinical and imaging findings in cryptogenic stroke patients with and without patent foramen ovale: the PFO-ASA Study. Atrial Septal Aneurysm. Stroke 2002;33:706–711.
12. Bogousslavsky J, Garazi S, Jeanrenaud X, Aebischer N, Van Melle G. Stroke recurrence in patients with patent foramen ovale. Neurology 1996;46:1301–1306.
13. Di Tullio M, Sacco RL, Gopal A, Mohr JP, Homma S. Patent foramen ovale as a risk factor for cryptogenic stroke. Ann Intern Med 1992;117:461–465.
14. Webster M, Chancellor A, Smith H, et al. Patent foramen ovale in young stroke patients. Lancet 1988;2:11–12.
15. De Belder M, Tourikis L, Leech G, Camm A. Risk of patent foramen ovale for thromboembolic events in all age groups. Am J Cardiol 1992;69:1316–1320.
16. Homma S, Sacco RL, Di Tullio MR, Sciacca RR, Mohr JP. Effect of medical treatment in stroke patients with patent foramen ovale: patent foramen ovale in Cryptogenic Stroke Study. Circulation 2002;105:2625–2631.

17. Cujec B, Mainra R, Johnson DH. Prevention of recurrent cerebral ischemic events in patients with patent foramen ovale and cryptogenic strokes or transient ischemic attacks. Can J Cardiol 1999;15:57–64.
18. Mas JL, Zuber M. Recurrent cerebrovascular events in patients with patent foramen ovale, atrial septal aneurysm, or both and cryptogenic stroke or transient ischemic attack. French Study Group on Patent Foramen Ovale and Atrial Septal Aneurysm. Am Heart J 1995;130:1083–1088.
19. Mas J, Arquizan C, Lamy C, et al. Recurrent cerebrovascular events associated with patent foramen ovale, atrial septal aneurysm, or both. N Engl J Med 2001;345: 1740–1746.
20. De Castro S, Cartoni D, Fiorelli M, et al. Morphological and functional characteristics of patent foramen ovale and their embolic implications. Stroke 2000;31: 2407–2413.
21. Cabanes L, Mas JL, Cohen A, et al. Atrial septal aneurysm and patent foramen ovale as risk factors for cryptogenic stroke in patients less than 55 years of age. A study using transesophageal echocardiography. Stroke 1993;24:1865–1873.
22. Homma S, Di Tullio MR, Sacco RL, Mihalatos D, Li Mandri G, Mohr JP. Characteristics of patent foramen ovale associated with cryptogenic stroke. A biplane transesophageal echocardiographic study. Stroke 1994;25:582–586.
23. Steiner MM, Di Tullio MR, Rundek T, et al. Patent foramen ovale size and embolic brain imaging findings among patients with ischemic stroke. Stroke 1998;29: 944–948.
24. Hausmann D, Mugge A, Daniel W. Identification of patent foramen ovale permitting paradoxic embolism. J Am Coll Cardiol 1995;26:1030–1038.
25. Van Camp G, Schulze D, Cosyns B, Vandenbossche J. Relation between patent foramen ovale and unexplained stroke. Am J Cardiol 1993;71:596–598.
26. Serena J, Segura T, Perez Ayuso MJ, Bassaganyas J, Molins A, Davalos A. The need to quantify right-to-left shunt in acute ischemic stroke: a case-control study. Stroke 1998;29:1322–1328.
27. Nedeltchev K, Arnold M, Wahl A, et al. Outcome of patients with cryptogenic stroke and patent foramen ovale. J Neurol Neurosurg Psychiatry 2002;72:347–350.
28. Stollberger C, Slany J, Schuster I, et al. The prevalence of deep venous thrombosis in patients with suspected paradoxical embolism. Ann Intern Med 1993;119: 461–465.
29. Ruchat P, Bogousslavsky J, Hurni M, Fischer AP, Jeanrenaud X, von Segesser LK. Systematic surgical closure of patent foramen ovale in selected patients with cerebrovascular events due to paradoxical embolism. Early results of a preliminary study. Eur J Cardiothorac Surg 1997;11:824–827.
30. Nighoghossian N, Perinetti M, Barthelet M, Adeleine P, Trouillas P. Potential cardioembolic sources of stroke in patients less than 60 years of age. Eur Heart J 1996;17:590–594.
31. Berkompas D, Sagar K. Accuracy of color Doppler transesophageal echocardiography for the diagnosis of patent foramen ovale. J Am Soc Echocardiogr 1994;7: 253–256.
32. Devuyst G, Bogousslavsky J, Ruchat P, et al. Prognosis after stroke followed by surgical closure of patent foramen ovale: a prospective follow-up study with brain MRI and simultaneous transesophageal and transcranial Doppler ultrasound. Neurology 1996;47:1162–1166.

33. Dearani J, Ugurlu B, Danielson G, et al. Surgical patent foramen ovale closure for prevention of paradoxical embolism-related cerebrovascular ischemic event. Circulation 1999;100(19 Suppl):II171–II175.
34. Homma S, Di Tullio MR, Sacco RL, Sciacca RR, Smith C, Mohr JP. Surgical closure of patent foramen ovale in cryptogenic stroke patients. Stroke 1997;28:2376–2381.
35. Konstantinides S, Geibel A, Olschewski M, et al. A comparison of surgical and medical therapy for atrial septal defect in adults. N Engl J Med 1995:469–473.
36. Schulman S, Granqvist S, Holmstrom M, et al. The duration of oral anticoagulant therapy after a second episode of venous thromboembolism. The Duration of Anticoagulation Trial Study Group. N Engl J Med 1997;336:393–398.
37. Hung J, Landzberg M, Jenkins K, et al. Closure of patent foramen ovale for paradoxical emboli: intermediate-term risk of recurrent neurological events following transcatheter device placement. J Am Coll Cardiol 2000;35:1311–1316.
38. Bridges ND, Hellenbrand W, Latson L, Filiano J, Newburger JW, Lock JE. Transcatheter closure of patent foramen ovale after presumed paradoxical embolism. Circulation 1992;86:1902–1908.
39. Windecker S, Wahl A, Chatterjee T, et al. Percutaneous closure of patent foramen ovale in patients with paradoxical embolism: long-term risk of recurrent thromboembolic events. Circulation 2000;101:893–909.
40. Lethen H, Flachskampf F, Schneider R, et al. Frequency of deep vein thrombosis in patients with patent foramen ovale and ischemic stroke or transient ischemic attack. Am J Cardiol 1997;80:1066–1069.
41. Atherosclerotic disease of the aortic arch as a risk factor for recurrent ischemic stroke. The French Study of Aortic Plaques in Stroke Group. N Engl J Med 1996; 334:1216–1221.
42. Amarenco P, Duyckaerts C, Tzourio C, Henin D, Bousser M, Hauw J. The prevalence of ulcerated plaques in the aortic arch in patients with stroke. N Engl J Med 1992;326:221–225.
43. Mitusch R, Doherty C, Wucherpfennig H, et al. Vascular events during follow-up in patients with aortic arch atherosclerosis. Stroke 1997;28:36–39.
44. Kessler C, Mitusch R, Guo Y, Rosengart A, Sheikhzadeh A. Embolism from the aortic arch in patients with cerebral ischemia. Thromb Res 1996;84:145–155.
45. Kronzon I, Tunick PA. Atheromatous disease of the thoracic aorta: pathologic and clinical implications. Ann Intern Med 1997;126:629–637.
46. Toyoda K, Yasaka M, Nagata S, Yamaguchi T. Aortogenic embolic stroke: a transesophageal echocardiographic approach. Stroke 1992;23:1056–1061.
47. Karalis D, Chandrasekaran K, Victor M, Ross J, Mintz G. Recognition and embolic potential of intraaortic atherosclerotic debris. J Am Coll Cardiol 1991;17:73–78.
48. Amarenco P, Cohen A, Tzourio C, et al. Atherosclerotic disease of the aortic arch and the risk of ischemic stroke. N Engl J Med 1994;1994:1474–1479.
49. Tunick P, Rosenzweig B, Katz E, Freedberg R, Perez J, Kronzon I. High risk for vascular events in patients with protruding aortic atheromas: a prospective study. J Am Coll Cardiol 1994;23:1085–1090.
50. Tunick PA, Kronzon I. Atheromas of the thoracic aorta: clinical and therapeutic update. J Am Coll Cardiol 2000;35:545–554.
51. Stone DA, Hawke MW, LaMonte M, et al. Ulcerated atherosclerotic plaques in the thoracic aorta are associated with cryptogenic stroke: a multiplane transesophageal echocardiographic study. Am Heart J 1995;130:105–108.

52. Agmon Y, Khandheria BK, Meissner I, et al. Independent association of high blood pressure and aortic atherosclerosis: a population-based study. Circulation 2000; 102:2087–2093.
53. Tribouilloy CM, Peltier M, Iannetta Peltier MC, Trojette F, Andrejak M, Lesbre JP. Plasma homocysteine and severity of thoracic aortic atherosclerosis. Chest 2000; 118:1685–1689.
54. Sen S, Oppenheimer SM, Lima J, Cohen B. Risk factors for progression of aortic atheroma in stroke and transient ischemic attack patients. Stroke 2002;33:930–935.
55. Guo Y, Jiang X, Zhang S, Chen S, Li G. Application of transesophageal echocardiography to aortic embolic stroke. Chin Med J (Engl) 2002;115:525–528.
56. Collaboration AT. Collaborative overview of randomised trials of antiplatelet therapy. I. Prevention of death, myocardial infarction, and stroke by prolonged antiplatelet therapy in various categories of patients. BMJ 1994;308:81–106.
57. Hacke W. From CURE to MATCH: ADP receptor antagonists as the treatment of choice for high-risk atherothrombotic patients. Cerebrovasc Dis 2002;13(Suppl 1): 22–26.
58. Ferrari E, Vidal R, Chevallier T, Baudouy M. Atherosclerosis of the thoracic aorta and aortic debris as a marker of poor prognosis: benefit of oral anticoagulants. J Am Coll Cardiol 1999;33:1317–1322.
59. Tunick P, Lackner H, Katz E, Culliford A, Giangola G, Kronzon I. Multiple emboli from a large aortic arch thrombus in a patient with thrombotic diathesis. Am Heart J 1992;124:239–241.
60. Tunick P, Culliford A, Lamparello P, Kronzon I. Atheromatosis of the aortic arch as an occult source of multiple systemic emboli. Ann Intern Med 1991;114:391–392.
61. Nihoyannopoulos P, Joshi J, Athanasopoulos G, Oakley C. Detection of atherosclerotic lesions in the aorta by transesophageal echocardiography. Am J Cardiol 1993;71:1208–1212.
62. Freedberg R, Tunick P, Culliford A, Tatelbaum R, Kronzon I. Disappearance of a large intraaortic mass in a patient with prior systemic embolization. Am Heart J 1993;125:1445–1447.
63. Bansal R, Pauls G, Shankel S. Blue digit syndrome: transesophageal echocardiographic identification of thoracic aortic plaque-related thrombi and successful outcome with warfarin. J Am Soc Echocardiogr 1993;6:319–323.
64. Bruns F, Segel D, Adler S. Control of cholesterol embolization by discontinuation of anticoagulant therapy. Am J Med Sci 1978;275:105–108.
65. Hyman B, Landas S, Ashman R, Schelper R, Robinson R. Warfarin-related purple toes syndrome and cholesterol microembolization. Am J Med 1987;82:1233–1237.
66. Culliford A, Tunick P, Katz E, et al. Initial experience with removal of protruding atheroma from the aortic arch: diagnosis by transesophageal echo, operative technique, and follow-up. J Am Coll Cardiol 1993;21:342A.
67. Hogue CW, Sundt TM, Goldberg M, Barner H, Davila Roman VG. Neurological complications of cardiac surgery: the need for new paradigms in prevention and treatment. Sem Thorac Cardiovasc Surg 1999;11:105–115.
68. Bushnell C, Goldstein L. Diagnostic testing for coagulopathies in patients with ischemic stroke. Stroke 2000;31:3067–3078.
69. Goldstein L, Adams R, Becker K, et al. AHA scientific statement: primary prevention of ischemic stroke. A statement for healthcare professionals from the Stroke Council of the American Heart Association. Stroke 2001;32:280–299.

70. Barinagarrementeria F, Cantu-Brito C, De La Pena A, Izaguirre R. Prothrombotic states in young people with idiopathic stroke. A prospective study. Stroke 1994;25: 287–290.
71. Barinagarrementeria F, Gonzalez-Duarte A, Cantu-Brito C. Prothrombotic states and cerebral ischemia [in Spanish]. Rev Neurol 1998;26:85–91.
72. Chan AK, deVeber G. Prothrombotic disorders and ischemic stroke in children. Sem Pediatr Neurol 2000;7:301–308.
73. Bauer K. The thrombophilias: well-defined risk factors with uncertain therapeutic implications. Ann Intern Med 2001;135:367–373.
74. Fihn S, Callahan C, Martin D, McDonnel M, Henikoff J, White R. The risk for and severity of bleeding complications in elderly patients treated with warfarin. The National Consortium of Anticoagulation Clinics. Ann Intern Med 1996;124: 970–979.
75. Hughes G. Thrombosis, abortion, cerebral disease and lupus anticoagulant. BMJ 1983;187:1088–1091.
76. Cervera R, Piette JC, Font J, et al. Antiphospholipid syndrome: clinical and immunologic manifestations and patterns of disease expression in a cohort of 1000 patients. Arthritis Rheum 2002;46:1019–1027.
77. Petri M. Epidemiology of the antiphospholipid antibody syndrome. J Autoimmun 2000;15:145–151.
78. Vila P, Hernandez M, Lopez-Fernandez M, Battle J. Prevalence, follow-up and clinical significance of the anticardiolipin antibodies in normal subjects. Thromb Haemost 1994;72:209–213.
79. Blohorn A, Guegan Massardier E, Triquenot A, et al. Antiphospholipid antibodies in the acute phase of cerebral ischaemia in young adults: a descriptive study of 139 patients. Cerebrovasc Dis 2002;13:156–162.
80. Nencini P, Baruffi MC, Abbate R, Massai G, Amaducci L, Inzitari D. Lupus anticoagulant and anticardiolipin antibodies in young adults with cerebral ischemia. Stroke 1992;23:189–193.
81. Group A. Anticardiolipin antibodies are an independent risk factor for first ischemic stroke. The Antiphospholipid Antibodies in Stroke Study (APASS) Group. Neurology 1993;43:2069–2073.
82. Mohr J, Thompson J, Lazar R, et al. A comparison of warfarin and aspirin for the prevention of recurrent ischemic stroke. N Engl J Med 2001;345:1444–1451.
83. Mohr JP. Prevention of recurrent ischemic stroke: recent clinical trial results [in Spanish]. Neurologia 2002;17:378–382.
84. Levine S, Brey R, Tilley B, et al. APL and stroke study (APASS). Presented at: 10th International Congress on Antiphospholipid Antibodies, Sept. 29–Oct. 3, 2002, Giardini Naxos, Taormina, Sicily, Italy. Abstract 258.
85. Levine SR, Brey RL, Sawaya KL, et al. Recurrent stroke and thrombo-occlusive events in the antiphospholipid syndrome. Ann Neurol 1995;38:119–124.
86. Kittner SJ, Gorelick PB. Antiphospholipid antibodies and stroke: an epidemiological perspective. Stroke 1992;23:I19–I22.
87. Futrell N, Millikan C. Frequency, etiology and prevention of stroke in patients with systemic lupus erythematosus. Stroke 1989;20:583–591.
88. Khamashta M, Guadrado M, Mujic F, Taub N, Hunt B, Hughes G. The management of thrombosis in the antiphospholipid-antibody syndrome. N Engl J Med 1995; 332:993–1027.

89. Levine S, Salowich-Palm L, Sawaya K, et al. IgG anticardiolipin antibody titer > 40 GPL and the risk of subsequent thrombo-occlusive events and death. A prospective cohort study. Stroke 1997;28:1660–1665.
90. Tanne D, D'Olhaberriague L, Schultz LR, Salowich-Palm L, Sawaya KL, Levine SR. Anticardiolipin antibodies and their associations with cerebrovascular risk factors. Neurology 1999;52:1368–1373.
91. Heinzlef O, Abuaf N, Cohen A, Amarenco P. Recurrent stroke and vascular events in elderly patients with anticardiolipin antibodies: a prospective study. J Neurol 2001;248:373–379.
92. The Antiphospholipid Antibodies in Stroke Study (APASS) Group. Anticardiolipin antibodies and the risk of recurrent thrombo-occlusive events and death. Neurology 1997;48:91–94.
93. Toghi H, Takahashi H, Kashiwaya M, Watanabe K, Hayama K. The anticardiolipin antibody in elderly stroke patients: its effects on stroke types, recurrence, and the coagulation-fibrinolysis system. Acta Neurol Scand 1994;90:86–90.
94. Levine SR, Brey RL, Joseph CL, Havstad S. Risk of recurrent thromboembolic events in patients with focal cerebral ischemia and antiphospholipid antibodies. The Antiphospholipid Antibodies in Stroke Study Group. Stroke 1992;23:I29–I32.
95. Khamashta MA. Primary prevention of thrombosis in subjects with positive antiphospholipid antibodies. J Autoimmun 2000;15:249–253.
96. Love P, Santoro S. Antiphospholipid antibodies: anticardiolipin and the lupus anticoagulant in systemic lupus erythematosus (SLE) and in non-SLE disorders. Ann Intern Med 1990;112:682–698.
97. Rosove M, Brewer P. Antiphospholipid thrombosis: clinical course after the first thrombotic event in 70 patients. Ann Intern Med 1992;117:303–308.
98. Ruiz-Irastorza G, Khamashta MA, Hunt BJ, Escudero A, Cuadrado MJ, Hughes GR. Bleeding and recurrent thrombosis in definite antiphospholipid syndrome: analysis of a series of 66 patients treated with oral anticoagulation to a target international normalized ratio of 3.5. Arch Intern Med 2002;162:1164–1169.
99. Prandoni P, Simioni P, Girolami A. Antiphospholipid antibodies, recurrent thromboembolism and intensity of warfarin anticoagulation. Thromb Haemost 1996;75: 859.
100. Schulman S, Svenungsson E, Granqvist S. Anticardiolipin antibodies predict early recurrence of thromboembolism and death among patients with venous thromboembolism following anticoagulant therapy. Duration of Anticoagulation Study Group. Am J Med 1998;104:332–338.
101. Derksen RH, de Groot PG. Do we know which patients with the antiphospholipid syndrome should receive long-term high dose anti-coagulation? J Autoimmun 2000; 15:255–259.
102. Brey R, Levine S, Thompson J, et al. Baseline frequencies, isotypes, and titers of antiphospholipid antibodies in the Warfarin–Aspirin Recurrent Stroke Study/Antiphospholipid Antibody Stroke Study (WARSS/APASS) collaboration; preliminary results. Stroke 2000;31:280.
103. Knic-Barrie S, Reister O, Connor C, Looney S, Pieriangeli S, Harris E. A retrospective review of 61 patients with antiphospholipid syndrome. Arch Intern Med 1997; 157:2101–2108.
104. Kalashnikova L, Nasonov E, Kushekbaeva A, Gracheva L. Anticardiolipin antibodies in Sneddon's syndrome. Neurology 1990;40:464–467.

14

Less Common Causes of Ischemic Stroke

Raul G. Nogueira and Aneesh B. Singhal

INTRODUCTION

The annual incidence of stroke increases with age. Large-artery atherosclerosis, cardiac embolism, and lacunar disease, which collectively account for 60–70% of all ischemic stroke, primarily affect individuals older than 50 years. The less common causes of stroke (Table 1) predominantly affect young individuals and probably contribute to the number of cryptogenic strokes in all age groups. Stroke-preventive strategies have been studied extensively and preventive guidelines established in conditions like atherosclerosis and embolism. However, few data exist about primary and secondary prevention of stroke from infrequent causes. Here, the diagnosis itself is difficult and often requires a high index of clinical suspicion, and patients are often referred to a tertiary center for treatment. Prevention of a first stroke is an option only in a few conditions, such as sickle cell disease and hypercoagulable states. Prevention after an initial ischemic event involves treatment of the underlying disease whenever possible. In this chapter, we highlight diagnostic features and outline prevention strategies for selected less common stroke etiologies.

CAROTID AND VERTEBRAL ARTERY DISSECTION

Carotid and vertebral artery dissection (CVAD) accounts for approx 2% of all ischemic stroke and 10–25% of stroke in young individuals. There is no gender predilection. The peak incidence is in the fifth decade, although all age groups can be affected. CVAD has been associated with heritable connective tissue disorders (Ehlers–Danlos type IV and Marfan's syndromes), polycystic kidney disease, osteogenesis imperfecta, and fibromuscular dysplasia. An association with migraine and α-1-antitrypsin deficiency has also been proposed. A history of head trauma or brisk neck movements (e.g., after

From: *Current Clinical Neurology: Handbook of Stroke Prevention in Clinical Practice*
Edited by: K. L. Furie and P. J. Kelly © Humana Press Inc., Totowa, NJ

Table 1
Less Common Causes of Stroke

- Arterial dissection
- Cerebral venous sinus thrombosis
- Cerebral vasculitis
- Moyamoya disease
- Migraine
- Cerebral vasoconstriction syndromes
- Hematological and coagulation disorders
  - Sickle cell disease
  - Polycythemia rubra vera
  - Essential thrombocytosis
  - Thrombotic thrombocytopenic purpura
  - Paroxysmal nocturnal hemoglobinuria
  - Leukemias
  - Intravascular lymphoma
  - Disseminated intravascular coagulation
  - Dysfibrinogenemias
  - Waldenstrom's macroglobulinemia
  - Hyperviscosity syndrome
  - Nephrotic syndrome
  - Hyperhomocysteinemia[a]
  - Protein C, protein S, antithrombin III deficiency[a]
  - Factor V Leiden, prothrombin G 20210A mutation[a]
  - Antiphospholipid antibody syndrome[a]
- Inherited
  - Mitochondrial (MELAS)
  - CADASIL
  - Fabry's disease
  - Hereditary endotheliopathy, retinopathy, nephropathy, and stroke
  - Osler–Weber–Rendu syndrome
  - Osteogenesis imperfecta
  - Polycystic kidney disease (arterial dissection)
  - Marfan's syndrome
  - Ehlers–Danlos syndrome
- Vascular anomalies (usually hemorrhagic stroke)
  - Arteriovenous malformations
  - Cavernous malformation
  - Venous anomaly
- Cardiogenic
  - Patent foramen ovale, atrial septal aneurysm[a]
  - Mitral annular calcification
  - Mitral valve prolapse
  - Atrial myxoma and other cardiac tumors
  - Dilated cardiomyopathy
  - Bacterial and fungal endocarditis
  - Marantic (nonbacterial) endocarditis
  - Libman–Sachs endocarditis
- Noncardiogenic embolism
  - Pulmonary arteriovenous malformations
  - Fat embolism
  - Air embolism

[a]Discussed in detail in other chapters.

chiropractic manipulation) can be elicited in many patients, and up to 5% have a family history of spontaneous arterial dissections.

Dissections may be subintimal, which causes lumen stenosis, or subadventitial, which causes aneurysmal dilatation. The classic features of carotid artery dissection include pain (involving the head, face, or neck), Horner's syndrome, and cerebral or retinal ischemia. Cranial neuropathies, usually involving the lower cranial nerves, can be seen in as many as 12% of patients. Vertebral artery dissection typically manifests as posterior head or neck pain followed by ischemia in the vertebrobasilar territory. Occasionally, dissections may extend intracranially and cause subarachnoid hemorrhage. The outcome of CVAD varies according to the location of the dissection, severity of initial ischemia, and extent of collateral flow *(1,2)*. The risk of recurrent dissection is about 2% per month during the first month and 1% per year for at least one decade after the initial dissection. Recurrence of dissection in a previously affected artery is extremely rare. Younger patients and patients with a family history of spontaneous dissections have a greater risk of recurrence *(3)*.

Cerebral angiography, once the gold standard for evaluation of CVAD, has been progressively replaced by computed tomographic angiography (CTA) and magnetic resonance angiography (MRA). Magnetic resonance imaging (MRI) with axial T1 fat-suppressed sequences has the advantage of showing the intramural hematoma in cases which lack luminal changes. Multivessel dissections may be seen in up to 28% of cases *(4)*.

CVAD is not a contraindication for thrombolysis, and tissue plasminogen activator should be considered in the acute stage. The subsequent management of CVAD is largely based on uncontrolled clinical studies and has not been validated by randomized clinical trials *(5)*. Approximately 90% of the stenoses resolve completely, and two of three complete occlusions recanalize within 3 months; additional improvement may be seen until 6 months *(4)*. Although not proven efficacious by a randomized controlled trial, our approach is to initiate anticoagulation with intravenous heparin and then transition to warfarin to achieve an international normalized ratio (INR) goal of 2–3 to prevent propagation and embolization of thrombus. CTA or MRA is performed after 3 months to guide further management. If the stenosis or occlusion has resolved, warfarin is discontinued, and antiplatelet therapy is instituted. If not, oral anticoagulation is maintained for an additional 3 months. Endovascular therapy might be an option in patients with severe stenotic lesions, in patients who fail optimal medical management, and in those with pseudoaneurysms or intracranial dissections (for which there is a risk for subarachnoid hemorrhage). Surgical ligation or arterial bypass procedures are rarely indicated and have been largely replaced by endovascular therapy.

Table 2
International Headache Society Classification of Migraine (1988)

1.1 Migraine without aura (common migraine)
1.2 Migraine with aura
1.21 Migraine with typical aura
1.22 Migraine with prolonged aura (complicated migraine)
1.23 Familial hemiplegic migraine
1.24 Basilar migraine
1.25 Migraine aura without headache (migraine equivalent)
1.26 Migraine with acute onset aura
1.3 Ophthalmoplegic migraine
1.4 Retinal migraine
1.5 Childhood syndromes that may be precursors to or associated with migraine
1.51 Benign paroxysmal vertigo of childhood
1.52 Alternating hemiplegia of childhood
1.6 Complications of migraine
1.61 Status migrainosus
1.62 Migrainous infarction (complicated migraine)
1.7 Migrainous disorder not fulfilling the above criteria

MIGRAINE

Migraine is a primary headache disorder characterized by recurrent attacks of pulsating unilateral or bilateral head pain, often accompanied by nausea, vomiting, photophobia, and phonophobia. Migraine affects 12–15% of the general population, with a threefold higher prevalence in women *(6)*. Migraine can be generally classified according to the presence or absence and duration of accompanying transient neurological manifestations like visual scintillations, scotomas, and motor weakness. The International Headache Society classification of migraine (1988) is outlined in Table 2.

Migraine is considered an independent risk factor for ischemic stroke *(7)*. In individuals younger than 50 years, migraine-associated stroke accounts for roughly 25% of all stroke. The overall incidence of migrainous infarction is 3.36 per 100,000 per year; however, in individuals without other stroke risk factors, the incidence decreases to 1.44 per 100,000 per year *(8)*. Certain migraine subtypes (migraine with typical or prolonged aura; familial hemiplegic migraine; and basilar, retinal, and ophthalmoplegic migraine) have a higher stroke risk. Several case–control studies have demonstrated an approximately fourfold higher stroke risk in women with migraine under age 45 years *(9)*. Within this population, the risk increases to 10-fold in smokers and 14-fold in those taking oral contraceptive pills (OCPs). The risk is high-

Table 3
Differential Diagnosis of Headache in Stroke Patients

Elevated intracranial pressure from large strokes
Embolism to posterior cerebral, middle cerebral, and basilar arteries
Arterial dissection
Cerebral venous sinus thrombosis
Temporal arteritis, inflammatory cerebral vasculitis, infectious arteritis
Antiphospholipid antibody syndrome
Mitochondrial disease (e.g., MELAS)
CADASIL
Cerebral vasoconstriction syndromes (migraine, postpartum angiopathy, drugs)
Reversible posterior leukoencephalopathy (hypertensive encephalopathy, eclampsia)
Cerebral hyperperfusion syndrome

est (odds ratio 34) in young women with migraine who smoke and take OCPs. The association between migraine and stroke is less estblished in older women and men.

Given the high prevalence (20–30%) of headache in patients with cerebrovascular disease (Table 3), it is important to distinguish between (1) stroke of other cause coexisting with migraine, (2) stroke of other cause (e.g., carotid artery dissection) presenting with clinical features of migraine with aura, and (3) stroke occurring during the course of a typical attack of migraine with aura *(10)*.

The mechanism of migrainous infarction is not clear; transient vasoconstriction and migraine-induced arteriopathy with secondary thromboembolism are leading theories. Migrainous infarction is a diagnosis of exclusion and should only be considered after established stroke etiologies have been ruled out. There are no data to suggest that migraine prophylaxis decreases the risk for stroke. Traditionally, calcium channel blockers have been preferred for migraine prophylaxis because of their vasodilatory properties. Contrast cerebral angiography can worsen headache and precipitate stroke in patients with migraine and should be undertaken with caution. Vasoconstrictive drugs like sumatriptan and the ergot derivatives should be avoided in patients with unexplained severe headache, complicated migraine, and stroke.

Recurrence of migrainous stroke is rare. The mainstay of stroke prevention in migraineurs remains aggressive treatment of modifiable risk factors like hypertension, coronary heart disease, obesity, and diabetes. Stroke prophylaxis with aspirin or other antiplatelet agents is reasonable; aspirin is preferred because of its antimigraine effects. Smoking cessation is especially important in young women migraineurs and in individuals who develop new auras or stroke. Women should be encouraged to discontinue smoking before starting oral contraceptives, and women with migraine with aura should be counseled to avoid the use of OCPs *(11)*. If OCPs are to be used, low-dose estrogen or progesterone-only OCPs should be considered.

CADASIL (*see* Chapter 17)

Cerebral autosomal dominant arteriopathy with subcortical infarcts and leukoencephalopathy (CADASIL) is an inherited autosomal dominant disorder that results from mutations in the Notch3 gene (chromosome 19p13.2–13.1) *(12)*. Notch3 encodes for a transmembrane protein component of an intracellular signaling pathway essential for controlling cell fate during development in a wide range of organisms. Stroke (usually lacunar infarction) is the most frequent manifestation. It occurs in 80–85% of patients with usual onset in the fourth-to-fifth decade. Migraine with aura occurs in 40–70%, is usually the first symptom, and develops in the third-to-fourth decade. Other features include mood disturbances (20–30%) and dementia (30%).

Brain MRI shows confluent T2 hyperintensities (leukoaraiosis), with discrete regions of lacunar infarction. Involvement of the anterior temporal pole and the external capsule has high sensitivity and specificity for diagnosis *(13)*. Cardiac ultrasound, cerebrospinal fluid examination, and vascular studies are usually unremarkable. Skin biopsy findings of granular osmophilic material adjacent to the basement membrane of smooth muscle cells of arterioles on electron microscopy has a sensitivity of 45% and specificity of 100% for diagnosis; the sensitivity can be increased to 100% by immunostaining with Notch3 monoclonal antibody. Diagnosis can also be made by mutation detection.

Accurate diagnosis is important for assessing prognosis and for genetic counseling. There is no specific treatment for CADASIL, and stroke prevention involves optimization of stroke risk factor profiles. Acetazolamide has been shown to increase cerebral perfusion and might help improve symptoms of migraine with aura *(14)*.

CEREBRAL VASOCONSTRICTION SYNDROMES (INCLUDING MIGRAINE-ASSOCIATED VASOCONSTRICTION, POSTPARTUM ANGIOPATHY, AND DRUG-INDUCED STROKE)

Reversible cerebral arterial vasoconstriction (RCV) is gaining recognition as an important cause of stroke in young individuals. Typical symptoms include severe “thunderclap” headaches, focal deficits, and seizures *(15)*. RCV can be idiopathic (e.g., postpartum angiopathy, migraine, thunderclap headache) or precipitated by factors like vascular neurosurgery or use of vasoconstrictive drugs like cocaine, amphetamines, ergot derivatives, phenylpropanolamine, and sumatriptan *(16)*. Brain imaging usually shows ischemic strokes in arterial watershed or border zone territories.

Patients with RCV are often misdiagnosed as having primary (inflammatory) cerebral vasculitis and treated with long-term immunosuppressive therapy because features like headache, stroke, and angiographic vasoconstriction are common to both conditions. However, RCV is a noninflammatory and usually self-limited condition. The diagnosis is confirmed by documenting spontaneously reversible cerebral vasoconstriction; serial transfemoral angiography, CTA, or MRA and transcranial Doppler (TCD) ultrasound have been used for this purpose.

Although reversible, the vasoconstriction can persist from days to as long as 6 months, and thunderclap headaches can recur for weeks to months. There is a high risk for stroke (probably resulting from severe large-artery vasoconstriction) at the onset or in the few days after presentation. Worsening arterial spasm has resulted in progressive infarction and death in some patients. Oral and intravenous calcium channel blockers, steroids, magnesium, and even transluminal angioplasty have been used to treat vasospasm and prevent stroke. Recurrence of vasoconstriction after complete symptomatic and angiographic resolution is virtually unknown; therefore, long-term treatment or prophylaxis is not indicated. It is important to counsel patients regarding use of illicit drugs and to avoid further use of vasoconstrictive drugs.

SICKLE CELL DISEASE

A single point mutation with substitution of valine for glutamic acid in the hemoglobin chain results in the formation of hemoglobin S (HbS), an abnormal hemoglobin with lower solubility than normal hemoglobin, and leads to sickle cell anemia. Under hypoxic or acidic conditions, HbS undergoes polymerization, and red blood cells become deformed or sickled, resulting in hemolysis, sludging, and vaso-occlusive phenomena (sickle cell crisis). A relative deficiency of nitric oxide further reduces compensatory vasodilation.

Even without crisis, sickle cell anemia causes a progressive systemic vasculopathy characterized by intimal proliferation, increased fibroblasts, and smooth muscle cells within arterial walls. In the brain, this vasculopathy causes segmental narrowing of the internal carotid and major circle of Willis arteries (present in 80% of patients with sickle cell disease and stroke). A moyamoya pattern is seen in 30% of patients with sickle cell vasculopathy, indicating that the vasculopathy is progressive *(17)*.

Stroke manifests in 10% of individuals with HbSS and 2–5% with HbC. An additional 13% have asymptomatic stroke on MRI. Males and females are equally affected. Ischemic stroke is approximately three times more common than hemorrhagic stroke and can result from large-vessel vasculopathy as well as microvascular occlusion. Infarcts are typically wedge shaped, deep as well as cortical, and usually located in the middle cerebral artery territory. Parenchymal hemorrhage can result from medial necrosis or from venous thrombosis. Subarachnoid hemorrhage can also occur because of increased propensity for aneurysm formation and rupture *(17,18)*.

Sickle cell disease is unique among the several uncommon causes of stroke (Table 1) in that there is real opportunity for primary stroke prevention. In the Stroke Prevention Trial in Sickle Cell Anemia (STOP), 130 children aged 2–16 years with sickle cell disease and without previous stroke were studied with TCD ultrasound to identify those at higher risk for stroke and were randomly assigned to standard care or repeat blood transfusions *(19)*. Time-averaged maximum mean velocities at or above 200 cm/second in the MCA or intracranial internal carotid artery was associated with a stroke risk of 10% per year in untreated subjects, which is 10- to 20-fold higher than in children with sickle cell disease not selected by TCDs. Eleven events occurred in the untreated group, compared to one event in the group treated with transfusions ($p < 0.001$). Based on these results, screening TCDs and transfusions are now an established primary stroke prevention strategy. In children who cannot undergo transfusions, long-term warfarin or antiplatelet agents are alternatives with unproven benefit. Surgical procedures like encephaloduroarteriosynangiosis could be attempted in those who fail medical therapy.

The initial management of stroke in sickle cell disease involves adequate hydration, supplemental oxygen therapy, maintenance of cerebral perfusion, and control of precipitating factors like infection. Thrombolytic treatments like tissue plasminogen activator should be considered and are not contraindicated in this setting. Whether blood transfusion in the acute stage after stroke is beneficial is not known. Stroke recurrence rates are high, approaching 67% in untreated individuals. Secondary prevention with repeated blood transfusions is effective in reducing recurrence rates to 10%, and current guidelines recommend repeat exchange transfusions to reduce total sickle cell hemoglobin values to less than 30% for at least 5 years after stroke or until age 18 years. Hydroxyurea therapy has proven efficacy in reducing sickle cell crisis; however, its role in stroke prevention has not been established. Bone marrow transplantation is potentially curative and might be an option for stroke prevention in individuals with asymptomatic stroke or high risk for stroke. However, questions regarding the timing and efficacy of this therapy remain unanswered *(18)*.

MOYAMOYA DISEASE

Moyamoya disease (MMD) is an idiopathic, nonatherosclerotic, noninflammatory vasculopathy characterized by chronic progressive stenosis of the terminal internal carotid artery and proximal anterior and middle cerebral arteries with formation of a fine network of collateral blood vessels at the base of the brain that angiographically resembles a puff of smoke (*moyamoya* in Japanese) *(20)*. The posterior circulation is rarely involved. MMD should be distinguished from moyamoya syndrome or *angiographic moyamoya*, a term used to describe intracranial vascular stenosis in conditions like sickle cell anemia, cranial irradiation, use of vasoactive drugs, neonatal anoxia, and head trauma. MMD is the most common vascular etiology of childhood stroke and predominantly affects Asians. A family history of MMD is found in 10% of the cases. Histologic examination shows intimal proliferation and degeneration of the internal elastic membrane of large intracranial arteries.

Symptoms include headaches, progressive cognitive decline, seizures, transient ischemic attacks, and ischemic and hemorrhagic strokes. Children tend to present with ischemia because of steno-occlusive changes of the circle of Willis, and adults usually present with bleeding caused by rupture of collaterals formed at a younger age. Aneurysms and arteriovenous malformations may occur in up to 11% of patients.

Conventional angiography remains the gold standard for the diagnosis. MRI and MRA are important for longitudinal follow-up and may be adequate for diagnosis. Positron emission tomography and single-photon emission computed tomography are useful in the assessment of perfusion reserve and help guide therapy.

Medical treatment includes the use of antiplatelet agents such as aspirin and ticlopidine and calcium channel antagonists (nimodipine and nicardipine). Early surgical intervention with encephaloduroarteriosynangiosis might be beneficial in delaying cognitive decline and in improving performance in activities of daily living *(21)*.

CEREBRAL VENOUS SINUS THROMBOSIS

Cerebral venous sinus thrombosis (CVST) is an infrequent condition that affects individuals of all ages, including neonates. It has numerous etiologies, including local infections (mastoiditis, sinusitis), sepsis, dehydration, congenital heart disease, head trauma, prothrombotic states, pregnancy, use of oral contraceptives, Behçet's disease, malignancy, and connective tissue diseases. The lateral and superior sagittal sinuses are most frequently involved.

Symptom onset may be acute, subacute, or chronic, and patients can present with multiple neurological symptoms *(22)*. Patients often manifest headaches or visual symptoms before presenting with focal neurological or encephalopathic features. Clinical characteristics that may help in early recognition of CVST include (1) new onset of headache, particularly in patients at increased thrombotic risk because of cancer, dehydration, pregnancy, hormone therapy, and active or chronic infection; (2) headaches associated with weakness, sensory deficits, visual impairment, or nausea; or (3) a personal or family history of venous thromboembolism

Acutely, the presence of headache, seizures, and symptoms and signs of raised intracranial pressure should raise suspicion for CVST. Head CT can be normal (in up to 30% of cases) or show direct signs of thrombosis within the sinuses (e.g., dense triangle sign and cord sign, which reflect thrombosed sinuses, and the empty delta sign, resulting from nonopacification of the thrombosed superior sagittal sinus after contrast injection). Parenchymal hemorrhages, edema, and hemorrhagic infarctions are indirect signs that help raise suspicion for CVST. Similar changes can be seen on brain MRI, particularly on Fluid-attenuated Inversion Recovery sequences. Newer imaging techniques like MR and CT venography have largely replaced direct angiography for diagnosis and follow-up.

Treatment with antithrombotic agents like heparin has been the subject of debate *(23–25)*. However, a meta-analysis of two randomized controlled trials (the first comparing unfractionated heparin to placebo, the second comparing low-molecular-weight heparin to placebo) showed a dramatic benefit with heparin treatment, with an absolute risk reduction of 14 and 15% in mortality and relative risk reduction of 56 and 70% in death or disability, respectively. Most authorities now concur that early initiation of heparin is beneficial and safe, even in the presence of intracerebral hemorrhage, and heparin remains the first-line agent for treatment of CVST. Thrombolysis with local tissue plasminogen activator infusion or mechanical clot removal has not been tested in clinical trials, but seems a reasonable option for patients with progressive thrombosis and clinical deterioration *(26)*.

Anticoagulation is usually continued with oral warfarin for at least 3–6 months with a target international normalized ratio of 2.0–3.0. Serial MR or CT venography helps assess the response to therapy and guide the duration of treatment. If serial imaging suggests active recanalization, warfarin could be continued for an additional 3 months, or it should be changed to antiplatelet therapy if recanalization is either complete or absent *(27)*. The definitive

Table 4
Diagnostic Evaluation in Cerebral Sinus Thrombosis

Erythrocyte sedimentation rate
Complete blood count
Fasting homocysteine
Vitamin B_{12}
Activated protein C resistance
Functional protein C
Functional protein S
Antithrombin III
Anticardiolipin antibody
Lupus anticoagulant
B_2 glycoprotein
Plasminogen
Prothrombin G20210A polymorphism
Antinuclear antibody
Antineutrophilic cytoplasmic antibodies (ANCAs)
Ophthalmological examination for uveitis
Pathergy test (for Behçet's)

therapy, if possible, is treatment of the predisposing condition resulting in CVST (e.g., antibiotics for mastoiditis or sepsis, rehydration, immunosuppressives for rheumatological diseases, discontinuation of oral contraceptives, vitamin supplementation for homocysteinemia, warfarin for hypercoagulable states). Identification of these conditions requires a full diagnostic examination as outlined in Table 4.

Other treatment and preventive measures include symptomatic treatment (e.g., seizure prophylaxis and treatment, analgesics for headache, measures to reduce raised intracranial pressure, prevention of complications like deep vein thrombosis and aspiration pneumonia). The prognosis of CVST is generally favorable, and more than 80% of patients have a good outcome.

VASCULITIS

Isolated (Granulomatous) Angiitis of the Central Nervous System

Isolated (granulomatous) angiitis of the central nervous system involves small and medium arteries and veins of the brain, spinal cord, and leptomeninges and is, by definition, characterized by neurological involvement out of proportion to systemic symptoms. Typical features include headache, encephalopathy, and multifocal neurological deficits. The clinical course is usually progressive, with a potentially fatal outcome in untreated patients.

Cerebrospinal fluid examination typically shows elevated protein (>100 mg/dL) with moderate lymphocytic pleocytosis (usually <150 cells/mm^3). Brain MRI can show multifocal punctate strokes, diffuse bihemispheric gray and white matter hyperintensities, as well as mass lesions mimicking tumors. Cerebral angiography can be normal or show multifocal arterial irregularities. A brain or leptomeningeal biopsy is required for definitive diagnosis, but has a high false-negative rate. Typical pathological findings include lymphocytic and plasma cell infiltration with or without multinucleated giant cells and granuloma formation. The etiology remains unclear; infectious and immunologic mechanisms have been proposed.

Treatment with cyclophosphamide in combination with low-dose prednisone can result in long-term remission or cure in some patients. There is no standard protocol for treatment; however, early treatment is important given the progressive nature of the disease.

Systemic Vasculitis and Connective Tissue Diseases

Giant cell (temporal) arteritis is a chronic systemic vasculitis of large-and medium-size vessels that characteristically involves the cranial branches of the arteries originating from the aortic arch (mostly the superficial temporal, posterior ciliary, ophthalmic, internal maxillary, facial, and occipital arteries). The incidence increases after the age of 50 years and peaks between 70 and 80 years of age. Women are affected twice as often as men. The American College of Rheumatology criteria for giant cell arteritis include age 50 years or older at onset, new localized headache, temporal artery tenderness or decreased pulse, erythrocyte sedimentation rate 50 mm/hour or higher, and biopsy showing necrotizing arteritis or a granulomatous process with multinucleated giant cells (≥3 criteria: sensitivity of 93.5%, specificity of 91.2%).

Typical clinical features include polymyalgia rheumatica (40–60%), scalp tenderness, and jaw claudication (~50%). Stroke is an uncommon complication (~7%); however, sudden visual loss can occur in up to 20% and is a feared complication. Initial pulsed intravenous methylprednisolone (1000 mg daily for 3 days) must be given to patients with recent or impending visual loss *(28)*.

All suspected cases must be subjected to a temporal artery biopsy, and treatment should not be delayed for purposes of biopsy because pathological abnormalities persist for at least 2 weeks after initiation of therapy. A long-segment biopsy, directed to sites of visible or palpable abnormalities of the temporal artery, should be obtained. If the clinical suspicion is high, the contralateral artery should be biopsied. Color duplex ultrasonography of the temporal artery can show the "dark halo" sign and appears to be a promising noninvasive diagnostic test; however, it has not been validated.

Treatment generally involves the use of oral high-dose corticosteroids, which can be tapered gradually over 1–2 years. Relapses can occur in 30–50% of the patients.

Polyarteritis nodosa (PAN) is a systemic necrotizing angiitis that affects small and medium arteries. The disease can affect any organs, with the usual exception of the lungs and the follicular arteries of the spleen. Stroke can result from the vasculitis itself or be related to long-standing hypertension or to cardioembolism secondary to cardiac involvement. PAN can be associated with hepatitis B or C (20–30% of all cases) and human immunodeficiency virus infections as well as hairy cell leukemia.

Diagnosis is based on visceral angiography (celiac, mesenteric, and renal) and tissue biopsy (usually from muscle, sural, or superficial peroneal nerves, rectum, testes, kidney, or skin). Treatment consists of corticosteroids and cyclophosphamide. Antiviral therapy with interferon γ-2b plus ribavirin and plasma exchange should be considered for PAN associated with viral hepatitis. *Microscopic polyangiitis* is a recently defined subtype of PAN that tends to affect smaller vessels and is characterized by glomerulonephritis, pulmonary hemorrhage, and the presence of peripheral antineutrophilic cytoplasmic antibody (P-ANCA) (80% of the patients).

Wegener's granulomatosis is characterized by the triad of granulomatous vasculitis of the upper and lower respiratory tract, focal and segmental glomerulonephritis, and small-vessel vasculitis. Cerebrovascular disease (including ischemic infarct, subarachnoid and parenchymal hemorrhages, and venous thrombosis) can result from necrotizing vasculitis, hypertensive small-vessel disease, or contiguous extension of granulomas. C-ANCA has a specificity of 98% and a sensitivity of 96% in active disease and 65% in initial or inactive disease. Angiogram is usually normal. Tissue diagnosis (lung, renal, sural nerve) is often required. Treatment includes corticosteroids and cyclophosphamide. Cotreatment with trimethoprin–sulfamethoxazole significantly reduces the relapse rate. Methotrexate may be used for the less-aggressive forms of the disease.

Central nervous system vasculitis or vasculopathy and stroke may also occur with other systemic diseases (such as systemic lupus erythematous, rheumatoid arthritis, scleroderma, Sjögren's syndrome, Churg–Strauss disease, cryoglobulinemia, lymphomatoid granulomatosis, Sneddon syndrome, sarcoidosis, Behçet's disease, Susac syndrome, Degos's disease, Cogan's syndrome, ulcerative colitis, Kawasaki disease, and Henoch–Schonlein purpura), infections (e.g., meningovascular syphilis, tuberculous meningitis, some bacterial and fungal meningoencephalitidies, and varicella zoster virus), malignancies (leukemias, lymphomas, and carcinomas), and drugs (e.g., cocaine, amphetamines, phenylpropanolamine, and LSD [lysergic acid diethylamide). Drug-induced stroke can result from vasoconstriction (*see* pages 236–237) as well as from inflammatory vasculitis; counseling is essential for primary and secondary stroke prevention *(28,29)*.

FABRY'S DISEASE

Fabry's disease is an X-linked recessive lysosomal storage disorder caused by α-galactosidase A deficiency. Intracellular accumulation of the glycolipid substrate of this enzyme leads to severe painful neuropathy with progressive renal, cardiovascular, and cerebrovascular dysfunction, and early death. Ischemic stroke, mostly involving the vertebrobasilar territory, is the most common cerebrovascular manifestation. Intracerebral and subarachnoid hemorrhages can also occur. The diagnosis is confirmed by documenting markedly decreased α-galactosidase A activity in plasma, isolated leukocytes, or cultured fibroblasts or lymphoblasts. Treatment includes enzyme replacement with intravenous infusions of α-galactosidase A. Gene therapy and substrate deprivation are promising future therapeutic options.

MITOCHONDRIAL ENCEPHALOMYOPATHY, LACTIC ACIDOSIS, AND STROKELIKE EPISODES (*see* Chapter 17)

Mitochondrial encephalomyopathy, lactic acidosis, and strokelike episodes (MELAS) is a maternally inherited disorder caused by mitochondrial deoxyribonucleic acid (DNA) mutations encoding for transfer RNA. It affects males and females equally. Clinical features of MELAS include recurrent strokelike episodes, encephalopathy, seizures, migraines, episodic vomiting, dementia, visual defects, ataxia, short stature, proximal muscle weakness, hearing loss, and diabetes. Neuroimaging reveals areas of infarction in a nonvascular distribution. Muscle biopsy may show ragged red fibers.

The diagnosis of MELAS is confirmed by enzyme activity measurements or molecular analysis. Treatment is mostly palliative and empiric. Ubiquinone (Coenzyme Q_{10}), idebenone, thiamine, riboflavin, menadione, nicotinamide, ascorbic acid, vitamin E, and creatine monohydrate have been used. Seizures usually respond to conventional antiepileptic medications. However, valproic acid should be used with caution and always coadministered with L-carnitine because of its well-documented inhibition of carnitine uptake.

REFERENCES

1. Schievink WI. Spontaneous dissection of the carotid and vertebral arteries. N Engl J Med 2001;344:898–906.
2. Stapf C, Elkind MS, Mohr JP. Carotid artery dissection. Annu Rev Med 2000;51: 329–347.

3. Schievink WI, Mokri B, Piepgras DG, Kuiper JD. Recurrent spontaneous arterial dissections: risk in familial vs nonfamilial disease Stroke 1996;27:622–624.
4. Mas JL, Bousser MG, Hasboun D, Laplane D. Extracranial vertebral artery dissections: a review of 13 cases. Stroke 1987;18:1037–1047.
5. Lyrer P, Engelter S. Antithrombotic drugs for carotid artery dissection. Cochrane Database Syst Rev 2000;4:CD000255.
6. MacGregor EA, Brandes J, Eikermann A. Migraine prevalence and treatment patterns: the global Migraine and Zolmitriptan Evaluation survey. Headache 2003;43: 19–26.
7. Buring JE, Hebert P, Romero J, et al. Migraine and subsequent risk of stroke in the Physicians' Health Study. Arch Neurol 1995;52:129–134.
8. Henrich JB, Sandercock PA, Warlow CP, Jones LN. Stroke and migraine in the Oxfordshire Community Stroke Project. J Neurol 1986;233:257–262.
9. Tzourio C, Tehindrazanarivelo A, Iglesias S, et al. Case–control study of migraine and risk of ischaemic stroke in young women. BMJ 1995;310:830–833.
10. Welch KM. Relationship of stroke and migraine. Neurology 1994;44:S33–S36.
11. Bousser MG, Conard J, Kittner S, et al. Recommendations on the risk of ischaemic stroke associated with use of combined oral contraceptives and hormone replacement therapy in women with migraine. Cephalalgia 2000;20:155–156.
12. Joutel A, Corpechot C, Ducros A, et al. Notch3 mutations in CADASIL, a hereditary adult-onset condition causing stroke and dementia. Nature 1996;383:707–710.
13. Markus HS, Martin RJ, Simpson MA, et al. Diagnostic strategies in CADASIL. Neurology 2002;59:1134–1138.
14. Chabriat H, Pappata S, Ostergaard L, et al. Cerebral hemodynamics in CADASIL before and after acetazolamide challenge assessed with MRI bolus tracking. Stroke 2000;31:1904–1912.
15. Call GK, Fleming MC, Sealfon S, Levine H, Kistler JP, Fisher CM. Reversible cerebral segmental vasoconstriction. Stroke 1988;19:1159–1170.
16. Singhal AB, Koroshetz W, Caplan LR. Cerebral vasoconstriction syndromes. In: Bogousslavsky J, Caplan LR, eds. Uncommon Causes of Stroke. Cambridge, UK: Cambridge University Press, 2001:114–123.
17. Ohene-Frempong K, Weiner SJ, Sleeper LA, et al. Cerebrovascular accidents in sickle cell disease: rates and risk factors. Blood 1998;91:288–294.
18. Adams RJ. Stroke prevention and treatment in sickle cell disease. Arch Neurol 2001; 58:565–568.
19. Adams RJ, McKie VC, Hsu L, et al. Prevention of a first stroke by transfusions in children with sickle cell anemia and abnormal results on transcranial Doppler ultrasonography. N Engl J Med 1998;339:5–11.
20. Natori Y, Ikezaki K, Matsushima T, Fukui M. "Angiographic moyamoya": its definition, classification, and therapy. Clin Neurol Neurosurg 1997;99(Suppl 2): S168–S172.
21. Fukui M. Guidelines for the diagnosis and treatment of spontaneous occlusion of the circle of Willis ("moyamoya" disease). Clin Neurol Neurosurg 1997;99:S238–S240.
22. Bousser MG. Cerebral venous thrombosis: diagnosis and management. J Neurol 2000; 247:252–258.
23. de Bruijn SF, de Haan RJ, Stam J. Clinical features and prognostic factors of cerebral venous sinus thrombosis in a prospective series of 59 patients. J Neurol Neurosurg Psychiatry 2001;70:105–108.

24. Einhaupl KM, Villringer A, Meister W, et al. Heparin treatment in sinus venous thrombosis. Lancet 1991;338:597–600.
25. de Bruijn SF, Stam J. Randomized, placebo-controlled trial of anticoagulant treatment with low-molecular-weight heparin for cerebral sinus thrombosis. Stroke 1999;30:484–488.
26. Wasay MR, Bakshi S, Kojan G, et al. Nonrandomized comparison of local urokinase thrombolysis vs systemic heparin anticoagulation for superior sagittal sinus thrombosis. Stroke 2001;32:2310–2317.
27. Buonanno FS. Cerebral sinovenous thrombosis. Curr Treat Options Cardiovasc Med 2001;3:417–427.
28. Moore PM, Richardson B. Neurology of the vasculitides and connective tissue diseases. J Neurol Neurosurg Psychiatry 1998;65:10–22.
29. Nadeau SE. Neurologic manifestations of systemic vasculitis. Neurol Clin 2002;20: 123–150.

15

Perioperative Stroke Risk Assessment and Management

David M. Greer and Ferdinando S. Buonanno

To prevent stroke in patients undergoing surgical procedures, it is critical first to understand the potential mechanisms. Specific procedures, particularly cardiac surgery, have a high risk of ischemic injury related to reduced cerebral perfusion, disruption of atheromatous material, and formation of intracatheter or intracardiac thrombi. The patients undergoing these types of procedures are also high risk; they generally have multiple vascular risk factors and underlying cardiac disease. Noncardiac surgical procedures also present a risk for recurrent ischemic injury in patients with a prior stroke history.

This chapter presents the methods of stratifying stroke risk in patients undergoing cardiac surgery, outlines preoperative testing and management, and suggests intraoperative strategies to reduce stroke risk. We also discuss the management of stroke patients who require noncardiac, elective surgical procedures.

PREDICTORS OF STROKE RISK DURING CORONARY ARTERY BYPASS GRAFT

The incidence of stroke following coronary artery bypass graft (CABG) surgery has remained stable over the past two decades and is reported to occur in 0.8 to 6% of patients who undergo isolated CABG *(1)*. Stroke following CABG is an important predictor of increased length of hospital and intensive care unit stay, morbidity, and mortality. Hogue and colleagues prospectively collected data on 5113 patients undergoing CABG at Washington University St. Louis, MO, and found that postoperative stroke correlated strongly with mortality for both men and women *(2)*. Roach and colleagues evaluated 2108 patients from 24 US institutions and found that patients with an adverse neurological outcome had higher in-hospital mortality rates, longer hospitalizations, and higher rates of discharge to facilities for intermediate or long-

From: *Current Clinical Neurology: Handbook of Stroke Prevention in Clinical Practice*
Edited by: K. L. Furie and P. J. Kelly © Humana Press Inc., Totowa, NJ

Table 1
Predictors of Major Adverse Outcomes (Including Stroke)

Correlate	Odds ratio	Confidence intervals	Points
Pre-CABG creatinine ≥ 3.0 mg/dL	4.4	2.8–7.0	12
Age ≥ 80 years	4.0	2.6–6.1	11
Cardiogenic shock	3.2	1.9–5.4	10
Emergent operation	2.8	2.0–4.0	9
Age 70–79 years	2.5	1.8–3.4	8
Prior CABG	2.3	1.7–3.1	7
Ejection fraction < 30%	2.1	1.5–3.1	6
Liver disease (history)	2.1	1.1–4.1	6
Age 60–69 years	1.9	1.4–2.6	5
Pre-CABG creatinine 1.5–3.0 mg/dL	1.9	1.4–2.4	5
Stroke or TIA (history)	1.6	1.2–2.1	4
Ejection fraction 30–49%	1.4	1.1–2.0	3
Chronic obstructive pulmonary disease (history)	1.5	1.1–1.8	3
Female gender	1.4	1.1–1.8	3
Hypertension (history)	1.3	1.0–1.6	2
Urgent operation	1.3	1.0–1.6	2

Source: Adapted from ref. *5*.

term care *(3)*. Postoperative events that correlate with stroke occurrence include the need for ventilatory assistance for longer than 24 hours and an intensive care unit stay for longer than 2 days *(4)*.

Numerous preoperative risk factors have been examined, mostly retrospectively, in an attempt to predict which patients are at greatest risk of stroke during CABG. For predictors of perioperative adverse effects, Fortescue et al. assessed 9498 patients undergoing isolated CABG at 12 academic medical centers (Table 1). They developed a scoring system based on the weight of impact of each independent risk factor. The risk factors that correlated with increased rates of stroke and other adverse outcomes included higher age, preoperative renal insufficiency, urgent or emergent operation, cardiogenic shock, prior stroke or transient ischemic attack (TIA), low ejection fraction, prior CABG, female gender, and a history of liver disease, chronic obstructive pulmonary disease, or hypertension *(5)*. Scores greater than 16 carry a 40–50% higher risk of adverse outcomes. Scores greater than 26 carry a sevenfold increase in risk. Others have found additional preoperative risk factors that may be associated with stroke, including diabetes *(6,7)* and alcohol consumption *(3)*.

As cardiac procedures are increasingly performed in older patients, the rates of adverse outcomes in this population, including stroke, have increased. Craver and colleagues compared 152 patients aged 70 years or older undergoing aortic valve replacement (AVR), with or without concomitant CABG, to patients aged 20–69 *(8)*. They found a higher perioperative stroke rate and longer postoperative hospital stay for the older patients, but relatively similar survival curves and morbidity rates. Kohl et al. examined AVR in octogenarians and found an overall mortality rate of 13% (9% for AVR alone, 24% for AVR-CABG combined) *(9)*. Atrial fibrillation is an important postoperative factor predicting stroke risk *(10)*.

There are additional stroke risk factors that may be discovered only intraoperatively, including atherosclerosis of the ascending aorta. In fact, some postulate that the presence of aortic atherosclerosis is the single most important risk factor for neurological injury *(11)*. Unfortunately, this risk factor is often not appreciated or properly quantified preoperatively, and is only detected on intraoperative palpation of the aorta or by transesophageal echocardiography (TEE).

Mizuno et al. used TEE to evaluate the intimal thickness of aortic atherosclerosis in 315 patients, and found that an intimal thickness greater than 5 mm carried a significantly greater risk of perioperative stroke *(12)*. Hartmann et al. examined an additional 189 patients with TEE intraoperatively and found a high degree of correlation of stroke incidence with the severity of aortic atherosclerosis *(13)*. Van der Linden and colleagues looked at 921 patients who underwent TEE at the time of CABG; the investigators further elucidated that disease in the ascending aorta was the most important risk factor for postoperative stroke: 8.7% of patients with aortic atherosclerotic disease had a stroke vs 1.8% in the population without significant disease *(14)*.

The risk factors for the development of aortic atherosclerosis and atheroembolization during cardiac surgery were retrospectively analyzed by Kolh and colleagues *(15)*. Of 5486 patients who underwent cardiac surgical procedures, 107 (1.9%) developed atheroembolic syndromes. These patients were older and had a higher incidence of hypertension, cerebrovascular disease, and aortoiliac disease. Autopsies were performed in 27 of these patients, and showed diffusely diseased aortas with calcification, mural thrombus, and ulceration.

Knowing the high rate of stroke incurred in patients with severe aortic atherosclerosis, many have postulated that the key to stroke prevention is the development of techniques to limit the embolization of particulate debris *(16)*. To that end, surgical techniques have been developed in an attempt to minimize damage when the ascending aorta is known to have severe atherosclerotic disease. Trehan et al. reported on 104 patients who were found to have mobile arch atheromas by intraoperative TEE *(17)*. These patients subsequently underwent modifications of surgical technique, including aortic arch atherectomy, CABG combined with transmyocardial laser revascularization, off-pump CABG, and minimally invasive direct coronary artery bypass. The perioperative stroke rate for these patients was 0.96%, and there were no embolic events in the 88 patients who underwent off-pump CABG.

Postoperative encephalopathy that occurs following cardiac procedures must be carefully distinguished from ischemic stroke because the causes and outcomes may differ between the two groups. Encephalopathy and subsequent cognitive impairment are felt to be secondary to the microembolization of particulate and gaseous matter (primarily at the time of cardiotomy suction), as well as from intraoperative hypotension *(18)*. McKhann and coworkers prospectively applied five preoperative variables for risk of stroke or encephalopathy to 2711 CABG patients *(19)*. Older age, prior stroke, the presence of a carotid bruit, hypertension, diabetes, and cardiac bypass (CPB) time were all significantly associated with the development of postoperative encephalopathy, but only prior stroke, hypertension, and diabetes predicted stroke risk. Both stroke and postoperative encephalopathy were associated with increased length of stay and mortality.

The presence of cerebrovascular disease has been shown to correlate with an increased risk of stroke during cardiac procedures. Hirotani and colleagues collected data on 472 patients undergoing CABG *(20)*. They found a correlation between the severity of extracranial carotid artery stenosis and postoperative stroke. Seven patients in this study with symptomatic carotid stenosis underwent carotid endarterectomy (CEA) prior to CABG, and none had strokes. Whether this technique should be applied to the asymptomatic population is more controversial and is the subject of the next section.

SCREENING FOR CEREBROVASCULAR DISEASE

In many centers, patients undergoing cardiac surgery have preoperative screening for cerebrovascular disease. Notable exceptions are younger patients, for whom the presence of atherosclerotic disease of the cerebrovasculature is much less common, and in cases of emergency operations. The method of screening is primarily carotid duplex imaging, which optimally includes evaluation of the extracranial vertebral arteries and of the ophthalmic arteries.

Archbold and colleagues evaluated 529 patients undergoing urgent cardiac surgery, 8% of whom were screened with carotid duplex because of prior stroke or TIA, or because of the presence of an anterior cervical bruit *(21)*. Of these patients, 25% had an internal carotid artery (ICA) stenosis of greater than 60%. The investigators concluded that screening should be performed for all patients with a history of stroke or TIA, all patients with a carotid bruit, and all patients older than 65 years.

Salasidis et al. analyzed 387 patients who underwent preoperative duplex scanning *(22)*. They found in this population that 8.5% had severe carotid disease (≥80% stenosis). The factors associated with stenosis included older age, previous CEA, preoperative neurological symptoms, and peripheral vascular disease. Those who had postoperative events were older and more likely to have peripheral vascular disease and prior CEA. This study suggested that the presence of peripheral vascular disease may be a helpful screening trigger.

Additional methods of assessing the cerebrovascular system preoperatively include transcranial Doppler, computed tomographic angiography (CTA), and magnetic resonance angiography (MRA). Transcranial Doppler can give information regarding the hemodynamic significance of an asymptomatic internal carotid artery lesion, perhaps indicating patients at higher risk of stroke secondary to hypoperfusion (watershed-type injury) *(23)*. CTA can give additional information regarding the existence of prior strokes, as well as useful anatomical information regarding the degree of vascular stenosis or occlusion. Its sensitivity for detection of complete occlusion of the internal carotid artery is not quite 100%, and for cases in question, conventional transfemoral cerebral angiography should be performed. CTA must be used with caution in patients with renal insufficiency or with known contrast hypersensitivity. Magnetic resonance imaging (MRI) with MRA may provide insight into the presence of both acute and chronic strokes *(24)*, but MRA may overestimate the degree of vascular stenosis. Its accuracy may be improved using gadolinium as a contrast agent *(25)*.

MANAGEMENT OF PATIENTS WITH CAROTID ARTERY DISEASE

There have been no randomized studies regarding the performance of a combined CEA and CABG vs staged the procedures. Furlan and Craciun retrospectively analyzed 144 patients with angiographically documented ICA stenosis of 50% or more in asymptomatic patients *(26)*. Patients either underwent combined CEA-CABG or CABG alone. There were no differences in outcomes between the two groups, and the authors concluded that asymptomatic ICA stenosis (>90%) or occlusion does not increase stroke risk during CABG.

The data to support combined CEA-CABG for patients with symptomatic carotid disease is stronger. Multiple studies, albeit not controlled or randomized, randomized, have suggested a benefit from performing the combined operation to limit neurological events perioperatively. Zacharias and colleagues evaluated 189 patients who received combined CEA-CABG and had 5 years of follow-up *(27)*. Operative death occurred in 5 of the 189 patients, and there were a total of five strokes as well. CEA was always performed first, with concomitant vein harvesting. The mean arterial pressure (MAP) was kept above 60 mmHg to prevent stroke caused by hypoperfusion. This study argued against performing a staged procedure (CEA followed by CABG at a later date) in patients with active coronary artery disease because of the high postoperative rate of myocardial infarction (MI) (up to 7% in some studies) *(28,29)*. This study also argued the cost-effectiveness of doing the combined procedure vs the staged procedure.

Others, however, propose performing staged CEA followed by CABG. Antunes and colleagues reported on 77 patients (83 CEAs) who had staged CEA then CABG, 74% of whom were asymptomatic *(32)*. There were two strokes (2.4%) and three MIs (3.6%). They concluded that staged CEA, then CABG was a reasonable option.

Some smaller studies, however, have suggested that CABG should be performed prior to CEA because of a potentially higher rate of MI. Giangola et al. examined 57 patients with symptomatic carotid disease, 28 of whom had a combined procedure *(30)*. There were five MIs in the combined procedure group, and two of these patients died. In 12 patients who underwent CABG followed by CEA, there were no strokes, MIs, or deaths. In a study by Horst and colleagues, 63 patients underwent combined CEA-CABG, and the perioperative mortality rate was 7.9%, all attributed to cardiac complications *(31)*.

Still other studies have proposed a lower rate of complications for the combined procedure. Kaul et al. reported on 408 patients who underwent combined CEA-CABG, 63% of whom were asymptomatic from their carotid disease *(33)*. In 60% of these patients, the disease was bilateral, and 12 patients had bilateral CEAs performed at the time of surgery. Their reported combined mortality rate from stroke and MI was 2.45%.

Estes and colleagues argued that the same benefit and cost-effectiveness can be applied to patients with asymptomatic disease *(34)*. They compared the stroke, MI, and mortality rate between symptomatic patients and asymptomatic patients who underwent combined CEA-CABG and found that there were in fact more strokes in the patients with symptomatic disease. They proposed low morbidity associated with the combined procedure, as well as patient convenience and cost savings for the group with asymptomatic disease.

There appears to be no difference in outcome between men and women who undergo combined CEA-CABG *(35)*.

The timing of CPB during the combined procedure is particularly important. Bonacchi and colleagues compared two groups of patients who underwent combined CEA-CABG *(36)*. The first group underwent CPB during both procedures; the second had CEA performed prior to the initiation of CPB. The second group had less morbidity associated with the procedure, as well as better overall outcomes. There was significantly more renal dysfunction in the first group.

A review by Borger and Fremes *(37)* concluded that a combined CEA-CABG should be performed in patients with symptomatic carotid stenosis, but that patients with asymptomatic disease should only undergo CEA if considered in a high-risk population (e.g., those with severe bilateral disease). In the absence of data from randomized trials, we recommend that at institutions in which there is a low operative morbidity and mortality rate for both CEA and CABG, the procedure may be safely combined and applied to both symptomatic and asymptomatic patients with little if any additional risk to the patient and with the added benefit of cost-effectiveness and patient convenience.

MANAGEMENT OF CAROTID OCCLUSION AND INTRACRANIAL STENOSIS

Patients with a completely occluded carotid artery present another intriguing challenge. Suematsu and colleagues studied 11 patients with total occlusion prior to CABG *(38)*. Four of these patients underwent elective CABG, and five underwent emergency CABG. One patient underwent surgical anastamosis of the extracranial-to-intracranial circulation (bypass from superficial temporal artery to middle cerebral artery), and one underwent combined CEA-CABG. Only one patient who had a transient neurological episode. At most institutions, the common management of total carotid occlusion is to maintain adequate MAPs during the CABG (>70 mmHg) and without attempted revascularization of the carotid circulation. Although the aforementioned bypass procedure continues to undergo further investigation (currently in a multicenter study supported by the National Institutes of Health), its use in this setting is unsubstantiated.

Similarly, for patients with intracranial cerebrovascular stenoses and those with vertebral or basilar artery stenoses, the most prudent management is maintenance of adequate mean arterial pressures intraoperatively to prevent stroke secondary to hypoperfusion. Hirotani et al. determined a stroke rate of 3.1% in patients with no significant vertebral artery disease, but the rate was 16.7% for patients with vertebral artery stenosis greater than 50% (although the number of patients studied was small and the difference did not meet statistical significance *[39]*). In fact, eight patients in this study with vertebral artery occlusion prior to CABG did not have strokes.

There have been limited reports in the literature regarding the use of prophylactic angioplasty of intracranial vascular stenoses prior to CABG to prevent stroke secondary to hypoperfusion *(40)*. Perhaps more promising are intraoperative techniques designed to maintain adequate perfusion pressure, including off-pump CABG, intraaortic balloon pump use during CABG, and the Super Pulse dynamic pulsatile cardiopulmonary bypass devices *(41)*.

POSTOPERATIVE STROKE

Patients who have undergone cardiac surgery remain at risk for delayed ischemic stroke in the postoperative period. Several studies have correlated postoperative atrial fibrillation and low cardiac output with delayed stroke onset, and these conditions must be assiduously monitored and treated *(6,7)*. Another related factor is moderate-to-severe left ventricular dysfunction *(42)*. Clearly, if a patient has known extracranial or intracranial vascular stenoses, their risk of stroke from hypoperfusion is ongoing in the postoperative period, and MAPs should be maintained at a level similar to that maintained during the procedure.

Multiple imaging modalities may be useful in evaluating postoperative stroke. Computed tomographic imaging is a useful early screening tool to differentiate between hemorrhagic and ischemic damage, but may be insensitive to acute changes and cannot readily distinguish subacute from chronic infarcts *(43)*. MRI may be a more useful tool, especially with the use of diffusion-weighted imaging, which can easily detect acute infarction in the postoperative setting *(44)*. Further MRI techniques include perfusion-weighted imaging, which can help determine additional territory at risk for ischemic injury that may be amenable to treatment with blood pressure manipulation *(45)*. In addition, magnetic resonance spectroscopy has been implemented in detecting areas of frontal lobe hypometabolism in postoperative cardiac patients, correlating with neuropsychological dysfunction *(46)*.

MANAGEMENT OF ANTICOAGULATION DURING ELECTIVE SURGICAL PROCEDURES

Patients with atrial fibrillation and mechanical heart valves are at strong risk for thromboembolic complications and are frequently maintained on warfarin anticoagulation *(47)* (Table 2). The proper management of their anticoagulation in the perioperative setting of elective procedures is of paramount

Table 2
Estimated Rates of Thromboembolism Associated With Various Indications for Oral Anticoagulation and Reduction in Risk Caused by Anticoagulant Therapy

Indication	Rate without therapy (%)	Risk reduction with therapy (%)
Acute venous thromboembolism[a]		
Month 1	40	80
Months 2 and 3	10	80
Recurrent venous thromboembolism[a,b]	15[c]	80
Nonvalvular atrial fibrillation	4.5[c]	66
Nonvalvular atrial fibrillation and previous embolism	12[c]	66
Mechanical heart valve	8[c]	75
Acute arterial embolism, month 1	15	66

Source: Adapted from ref. *47*.

[a]The increase in the risk of venous thromboembolism associated with surgery (estimated to be 100-fold) is not included in these rates.

[b]The term refers to patients whose last episode of venous thromboembolism occurred more than 3 months before evaluation, but who require long-term anticoagulation because of high risk of recurrence.

[c]The rate shown is per year.

importance because additional factors increase the risk of thrombosis in this setting. The risks of perioperative bleeding must be weighed against the risk of thromboembolic complications. Some procedures, such as colonoscopy or minor surgeries, may be performed while warfarin is continued, provided that the international normalized ratio (INR) in the perioperative period is in the 1.5–2.0 range. However, this level of anticoagulation is unacceptable for many other procedures, including regional (spinal or epidural) anesthesia as well as some neurosurgical and plastic surgical procedures *(48)*.

Abrupt cessation of warfarin therapy creates "a gap between the rapidly rising levels of factors VII and IX and a slow normalization of protein C and S levels, mirrored by a hypercoagulable state associated with some thromboembolic events and increased levels of fibrinopeptide A" *(49)*. In one study of patients on warfarin for MI, 9 of 47 patients who had abrupt withdrawal of warfarin had thromboembolic complications within 4 weeks *(50)*. Palareti et al. performed a prospective study in 32 patients with abrupt vs gradual withdrawal of warfarin and found higher levels of prothrombin fragments F1+2, as well as thrombin–antithrombin III levels, in the abrupt cessation

Table 3
Bridging With Low Molecular Weight Heparin Perioperatively for Patients With Normal Renal Function

Pre-op day 6	Last day of warfarin
Pre-op day 5	Start dalteparin100 U/kg sq every 12 hours (usually 7–9 AM and 7–9 PM)
Pre-op day 4	Same
Pre-op day 3	Same
Pre-op day 2	Same
Pre-op day 1	Same, last dalteparin dose is in morning; no evening dose (this will ensure 24 hours off the drug; may need longer if renal insufficiency present)
Procedure Day	May resume dalteparin 100 U/kg sq every 12 hours once surgeons are confident of adequate hemostasis; usually 8–12 hours postoperatively; if taking oral medications, may take daily warfarin dose (no loading dose) after dalteparin resumed
Postop day 1	Dalteparin 100 U/kg sq every 12 hours; usual daily warfarin dose; check prothrombin time and INR
Postop days 2–5	As above; adjust warfarin as needed

Note that a 5-day overlap of dalteparin and warfarin is needed, and it is recommended that the prothrombin and INR are in range for the last 2 of those days.

group *(51)*. Other studies have shown elevated thrombin–antithrombin and fibrinopeptide A levels during the acute warfarin withdrawal period *(52)*. Of note, it has been recommended that, for dental surgery, warfarin anticoagulation should be continued because of the risk of a thromboembolic event far outweighing the risk of local bleeding that cannot be controlled *(53)*.

Johnson and Turpie performed a prospective study using low-molecular-weight heparin (dalteparin) in 112 patients undergoing invasive surgical procedures, necessitating the temporary cessation of warfarin anticoagulation. There were no thromboembolic events in any patient, and only 1 patient had a major episode of bleeding in the rectus muscle injection site *(54)*. Tinmouth et al. performed a similar prospective study in 27 patients, and reported two episodes of minor bleeding and one transient ischemic attack *(55)*. Formal recommendations were put forth in 2001 regarding the management of oral anticoagulation during invasive procedures by bridging therapy with low-molecular-weight heparin perioperatively to reduce the risk of stroke *(56)*.

We recommend the following algorithm for patients on full anticoagulation who require procedures and yet minimal time off full anticoagulation (Table 3). (Note, this assumes normal renal function; dose adjustments are necessary for patients with renal insufficiency.) The last dose of Coumadin should be given 6 days prior to surgery. Starting the following day, dalteparin 100 U/kg sq should be given every 12 hours (usually 7–9 AM and 7–9 PM). This is continued until the day prior to the procedure, when only the morning dose is given. This ensures 24 hours off the drug; again, longer withholding may be necessary with renal impairment. On the day of the procedure, dalteparin may be resumed at 100 U/kg sq every 12 hours once surgeons are confident of adequate hemostasis, usually 8–12 hours postoperatively. If the patients are able to take oral medications, they may resume their usual daily warfarin dose (no loading dose) that night after dalteparin is resumed. Dalteparin is overlapped with warfarin for at least 5 days, with a recommended overlap of a therapeutic INR range for the last 2 days.

REFERENCES

1. Gardner TJ, Horneffer PJ, Manolio TA, et al. Stroke following coronary artery bypass grafting: a 10-year study. Ann Thorac Surg 1985:40:574–581.
2. Hogue Jr. CW, Sundt III T, Barzilai B, et al. Cardiac and neurologic complications identify risks for mortality for both men and women undergoing coronary artery bypass graft surgery. Anesthesiology 2001;95:1074–1078.
3. Roach GW, Kanchuger M, Mangano CM, et al. Adverse cerebral outcomes after coronary bypass surgery: Multicenter study of postoperation ischemia reseach group and the Ischemia Research and Education Foundation Investigators. N Engl J Med 1996;335:1857–1863.
4. Herlitz J, Wognsen GB, Haglid M, et al. Risk indicators for cerebrovascular complications after coronary artery bypass grafting. Thorac Cardiovasc Surg 1998;46: 20–24.
5. Fortescue EB, Kahn K, Bates DW. Development and validation of a clinical prediction rule for major adverse outcomes in coronary bypass grafting. Am J Cardiol 2001;88:1251–1258.
6. Hogue CW Jr, Murphy SF, Schechtman KB, et al. Risk factors for early or delayed stroke after cardiac surgery. Circulation 1999;100:642–647.
7. Engelman DT, Cohn LH, Rizzo RJ. Incidence and predictors of TIAs and strokes following coronary artery bypass grafting: report and collective review. Heart Surg Forum 1999;2:242–245.
8. Craver JM, Goldstein J, Jones EL, et al. Clinical, hemodynamic, and operative descriptors affecting outcome of aortic valve replacement in elderly vs young patients. Ann Surg 1984;199:733–741.
9. Kolh P, Lahaye L, Gerard P, Limet R. Aortic valve replacement in the octogenarians: perioperative outcome and clinical follow-up. Eur J Cardiothorac Surg 1999; 16:68–73.
10. Shah SI, Movsowitz HD, Meyerowitz C, et al. Cardiac surgery in patients at or above 75 years old: analysis of perioperative and long-term outcome. Am J Geriatr Cardiol 1994;3:44–50.
11. Vaage J, Jensen U, Ericsson A. Neurologic injury in cardiac surgery: aortic atherosclerosis emerges as the single most important risk factor. Scand Cardiovasc J 2000: 34:550–557.

12. Mizuno T, Toyama M, Tabuchi N, et al. Thickened intima of the aortic arch is a risk factor for stroke with coronary artery bypass grafting. Ann Thorac Surg 2000;70: 1565–1570.
13. Hartmann GS, Yao, FS, Bruefach III M, et al. Severity of aortic atheromatous disease diagnosed by trans-esophageal echocardiography predicts stroke and other outcomes associated with coronary artery surgery: a prospective study. Anesth Analg 1996;83:701–708.
14. Van der Linden J, Hadjinikolaou L, Bergman P, Lindblom D. Postoperative stroke in cardiac surgery is related to the location and extent of atherosclerotic disease in the ascending aorta. J Am Coll Cardiol 2001;38:131–135.
15. Kolh PHH, Torchiana DF, Buckley MJ. Atheroembolization in cardiac surgery: the need for preoperative diagnosis. J Cardiovasc Surg 1999;40:77–81.
16. Vaage J, Jensen U, Ericsson A. Neurologic injury in cardiac surgery: aortic atherosclerosis emerges as the single most important risk factor. Scand Cardiovasc J 2000: 34:550–557.
17. Trehan N, Mishra M, Kasliwal R, Mishra A. Reduced neurological injury during CABG in patients with mobile aortic atheromas: a 5 year follow up study. Ann Thorac Surg 2000;70:1558–1564.
18. Taggart DP, Westaby S. Neurological and cognitive disorders after coronary artery bypass grafting. Curr Opin Cardiol 20001;16:271–276.
19. McKhann GM, Grega MA, Borowicz LM Jr, et al. Encephalopathy and stroke after coronary artery bypass grafting; incidence, consequences, and prediction. Arch Neurol 2002;59:1422–1428.
20. Hirotani T, Kameda T, Kumamato T, et al. Stroke after coronary artery bypass grafting in patients with cerebrovascular disease. Ann Thorac Surg 2000;70:1571–1576.
21. Archbold RA, Barakat K, Magee P, Curzen N. Screening for carotid artery disease before cardiac surgery: is current clinical practice evidence based? Clin Cardiol 2001;24:26–32.
22. Salasidis GC, Latter DA, Steinmetz OK, et al. Carotid artery duplex scanning in preoperative assessment for coronary artery revascularization: the association between peripheral vascular disease, carotid stenosis, and stroke. J Vasc Surg 1995;21:154–160.
23. Kistler JP, Furie KL. Carotid endarterectomy revisited. N Engl J Med 2000;342: 1743–1745.
24. Schaefer PW. Applications of DWI in clinical neurology. J Neurol Sci 2001;186: S25–S35.
25. Okumura A, Araki Y, Nishimura Y, et al. The clinical utility of contrast-enhanced 3D MR angiography for cerebrovascular disease. Neurol Res 2001;23:767–771.
26. Furlan AJ, Craciun AR. Risk of stroke during coronary artery bypass graft surgery in patients with internal carotid artery disease documented by angiography. Stroke 1985;16:797–799.
27. Zacharias A, Schwann TA, Riordan CJ, et al. Operative and 5-year outcomes of combined carotid and coronary revascularization: review of a large contemporary experience. Ann Thorac Surg 2002;73:491–498.
28. Ennix CI Jr, Lawrie GM Jr, Morris GC, et al. Improved results of carotid endarterectomy in patients with symptomatic coronary disease: an analysis of 1546 consecutive carotid operations. Stroke 1979;10:122–125.
29. Peric M, Huskic R, Nezic D, et al. Cardiac events after combined surgery for coronary and carotid artery disease. Eur J Cardiothorac Surg 1997;11:1074–1080.

30. Giangola G, Migaly J, Riles TS, et al. Perioperative morbidity and mortality in combined vs staged approaches to carotid and coronary revascularization. Ann Vasc Surg 1996;10:138–142.
31. Horst M, Geissler HJ, Mehlhorn U, et al. Simultaneous carotid and coronary artery surgery: indications and perioperative outcome. Thorac Cardiovasc Surg 1999;47: 328–332.
32. Antunes PE, Anacleto G, de Oliveira JM, et al. Staged carotid and coronary surgery for concomitant carotid and coronary artery disease. Eur J Cardiothorac Surg 2002; 21:181–186.
33. Kaul TK, Fields BL, Riggins LS, et al. Coexistent coronary and cerebrovascular disease: results of simultaneous surgical management in specific patient groups. Cardiovasc Surg 2000;8:355–365.
34. Estes JM, Khabbaz KR, Barnatan M, et al. Outcome after combined carotid endarterectomy and coronary artery bypass is related to patient selection. J Vasc Surg 2001;33:1179–1184.
35. Roddy SP, Darling RC 3rd, Abrishamchian AR, et al. Combined coronary artery bypass with carotid endarterectomy: Do women have worse outcomes? J Vasc Surg 2002;36:555–558.
36. Bonacchi M, Prifti E, Frati G, et al. Concomitant carotid endarterectomy and coronary bypass surgery: should cardiopulmonary bypass be used for the carotid procedure? J Card Surg 2002;17:51–59.
37. Borger MA, Fremes SE. Management of patients with concomitant coronary and carotid vascular disease. Sem Thorac Cardiovasc Surg 2001;13:192–198.
38. Suematsu Y, Nakano K, Sasako Y, et al. Conventional coronary artery bypass grafting in patients with total occlusion of the internal carotid artery. Heart Vessels 2000;15:256–262.
39. Hirotani T, Kameda T, Kumamoto T, et al. Stroke after coronary artery bypass grafting in patients with cerebrovascular disease. Ann Thorac Surg 2000;70:1571–1576.
40. Kihara S, Shimakura T, Tanaka SA, et al. Staged coronary artery bypass grafting after percutaneous angioplasty for intracranial vascular stenosis. J Thorac Cardiovasc Surg 2001;122:608–610.
41. Higami T, Kozawa S, Asada T, et al. Coronary artery bypass grafting using the "Super Pulse" dynamic pulsatile cardiopulmonary bypass device in patients with cerebrovascular occlusive disease. Ann Thorac Cardiovasc Surg 2000;6:173–178.
42. Stamou SC, Hill PC, Dangas G, et al. Stroke after coronary artery bypass: incidence, predictors and clinical outcome. Stroke 2001;32:1508–1513.
43. Wijdicks EF, Jack CR. Coronary artery bypass grafting-associated ischemic stroke. A clinical and neuroradiological study. J Neuroimaging 1996;6:20–22.
44. Wityk RJ, Restrepo L. Cardiac surgery and magnetic resonance imaging of the brain. Arch Neurol 2002;59:1074–1076.
45. Wityk RJ, Goldsborough MA, Hillis A, et al. Diffusion- and perfusion-weighted brain magnetic resonance imaging in patients with neurologic complications after cardiac surgery. Arch Neurol 2001;58:571–576.
46. Bendszus M, Reents W, Franke D, et al. Brain damage after coronary artery bypass grafting. Arch Neurol 2002;59:1090–1095.
47. Kearon C, Hirsh J. Management of anticoagulation before and after elective surgery. N Engl J Med 1997;336:1506–1511.

48. Gallus AS, Baker RI, Chong BH. Consensus guidelines for warfarin therapy. Recommendations from the Australasian Society of Thrombosis and Haemostasis. Med J Aust 2000;172:600–605.
49. Hemostasis and Thrombosis, chapter 132 Also, Schofield KP, Thompson JM, Poller L. Protein C response to induction and withdrawal of oral anticoagulation treatment. Clin Lab Haematol 1987;9:255–262.
50. Grip L, Blomback M, Schulman S. Hypercoagulable state and thromboembolisin following warfarin withdrawal in post-myocardial-infarction patients. Eur Heart J 1991;12:1225–1233.
51. Palareti G, Legnani C, Guazzaloca G, et al. Activation of blood coagulation after abrupt or stepwise withdrawal of oral anticoagulant—a prospective study. Thromb Haemost 1994;72:222–226.
52. Genewein U, Haeberli A, Straub PW, et al. Rebound after cessation of oral anticoagulant therapy: the biochemical evidence. Brit J Haemat 1996;92:479–485.
53. Wahl MJ. Dental surgery in anticoagulated patients. Arch Intern Med 1998;158; 1610–1616.
54. Johnson J, Turpie AGG. Temporary discontinuation of oral anticoagulants: role of low molecular weight heparin. Thromb Haemost 1999;82(Suppl):62–63.
55. Tinmouth AH, Morrow BH, Cruickshank MK, et al. Dalteparin as periprocedure anticoagulation for patients on warfarin and at high risk of thrombosis. Ann Pharmacother 2001;35:669–674.
56. Ansell J, Hirsh J, Dalen J, et al. Managing oral anticoagulant therapy. Chest 2001; 19:22S–38S.

16

Serum Biomarkers in Prediction of Stroke Risk and Outcome

Rachel Farrell and Peter J. Kelly

INTRODUCTION

Only half of the risk of clinical atherosclerotic disease can be predicted by established risk factors of age, gender, hypertension, hyperlipidemia, smoking, and diabetes. The remainder is likely to be accounted for by genetic and other factors. Measurement of serological markers of processes known to be important in the pathogenesis of atherosclerosis and thrombosis may contribute to the ability to predict risk of incident and recurrent stroke and outcome following stroke.

An ideal biomarker for prediction of vascular risk and outcome should have several properties. The marker assay should be inexpensive and standardized with acceptable variability. It should predict clinically relevant events in a manner independent of, and additive to, established vascular risk factors. Population-specific normal values should be available to guide interpretation of results *(1)*. To date, most work has been directed toward markers of inflammation (including matrix metalloproteinases [MMPs] and fibrinogen) and nutrition, particularly total plasma homocysteine (tHcy).

MARKERS OF INFLAMMATION

Inflammation is an important contributor to the development of atherosclerosis and unstable plaque. In prospective studies, markers of inflammation are associated with the risk of a first coronary event, outcome after unstable coronary ischemia, first ischemic stroke, and outcome following stroke. Several molecules involved in inflammatory processes have been studied as predictors of vascular risk. These include cell adhesion molecules (e.g., soluble intercellular adhesion molecule 1 [sICAM-1], p-selectin), cytokines (particularly interleukin-6 [IL-6]), and circulating proteins with concentrations that

From: *Current Clinical Neurology: Handbook of Stroke Prevention in Clinical Practice*
Edited by: K. L. Furie and P. J. Kelly © Humana Press Inc., Totowa, NJ

are affected by inflammatory processes (C-reactive protein [CRP], serum amyloid A [SAA], albumin, fibrinogen) *(2–4)*. Most attention has focused on CRP as a potential primary and secondary risk predictor.

High-Sensitivity CRP in Primary Prediction of Stroke Risk

Several prospective studies have demonstrated that high-sensitivity CRP is a strong independent predictor of stroke in populations free of clinical vascular disease. In a nested case–control analysis from the Physicians' Health Study, CRP measured years previously was higher in individuals who subsequently developed stroke compared to controls (median CRP 1.38 vs 1.13 mg/dL, $p = 0.02$). Individuals in the third and fourth quartiles of the CRP distribution had twice the risk of ischemic stroke (95% confidence interval [CI] 1.1–3.3) than those in the lowest quartile. Although the risk of ischemic stroke adjusted for other vascular risk factors was not reported, CRP independently predicted the risk of myocardial infarction in this sample *(5)*.

In an analysis from the prospective community-based Leiden 85-plus study, baseline CRP was twofold higher in individuals who died from stroke and other noncardiovascular causes compared to controls who survived. There was no difference in CRP between subjects who died from stroke compared to those who died from noncardiovascular causes. The authors concluded that CRP was a strong, but nonspecific, risk factor of fatal stroke in their elderly study sample *(6)*.

In a population-based cross-sectional analysis of 8850 individuals from the Third National Health and Nutrition Examination Study (NHANES), CRP was strongly associated with past history of self-reported stroke. The odds ratio (OR) of stroke when the highest tertile was compared to the lowest tertile was 1.71 (95% CI 1.11–2.64) after adjustment for established vascular risk factors. For each 1 mg per deciliter increase in CRP, the adjusted odds ratio of stroke increased by 19% (95% CI 5–34%) *(7)*.

In an analysis of 1462 subjects from the Framingham cohort, the risk of first stroke or transient ischemic attack (TIA) increased in a dose-dependent manner across increasing quartiles of the baseline (prestroke) CRP distribution. In this study, CRP was a strong independent predictor of first stroke or TIA. After adjustment for other risk factors, the relative risk of stroke or TIA in the highest compared to the lowest CRP quartile was 2.1 (95% CI 1.19–3.83) in women, but ceased to be statistically significant in men *(8)*.

CRP has also been associated with the development of asymptomatic atherosclerosis in prospective studies. In 3173 subjects without clinical vascular disease from the Framingham offspring cohort, CRP was associated with internal carotid artery stenosis (narrowing >25% of lumen diameter) measured by Doppler ultrasound. After adjusting for age, the odds ratio of carotid stenosis in the highest compared to the lowest CRP quartile was 1.62 for men and 3.9 for women. These values fell after accounting for established vascular risk factors. CRP remained a significant independent predictor of carotid stenosis in women (OR 2.97, 95% CI 1.72–5.25), but not men *(9)*.

CRP has also been shown by Van Der Meer et al. *(10)* to be a good predictor of atherosclerosis throughout the vascular tree. They studied a group of patients participating in the Rotterdam study. Baseline CRP levels were measured, and the patients were assessed prospectively over a mean of 6.5 years for progression of atherosclerosis. Atherosclerosis was assessed at the onset of the trial and at the third review by ultrasonographic measurement of carotid plaque, aortic and iliac calcification, and ankle–arm indices. The adjusted odds ratio for progression of generalized atherosclerosis was 4.6 (95% CI 2.2–9.5). The odds ratio for progression of carotid plaque was 1.7 (95% CI 1.0–3.1). High CRP levels correlated strongly with disease progression, and the odds ratios for progression were as high as those associated with the traditional cardiovascular risk factors.

Direct Comparisons of CRP to Other Markers of Vascular Risk

To compare the predictive value of CRP directly with other established and potential markers (inflammatory, lipid related, and homocysteine [Hcy]) of vascular risk, Ridker and colleagues measured 12 different serum markers in a nested case–control study of apparently healthy postmenopausal women from the Women's Health Study *(11)* (Fig. 1). Included were 366 women, 122 who developed subsequent cardiovascular events (coronary death, nonfatal myocardial infarction, stroke, coronary revascularization) and 244 controls. The measured markers were high sensitivity CRP, SAA, sICAM-1, IL-6, total cholesterol (TC), low-density lipoprotein cholesterol (LDLc), high-density lipoprotein cholesterol (HDLc), TC:HDLc ratio, lipoprotein(a), apolipoprotein A-I, apolipoprotein B-100, and tHcy.

The relative risk of cardiovascular events was significantly increased for women in the highest quartile of the distributions of tHcy and several inflammatory (CRP, SAA, sICAM-1, IL-6) and lipid (TC, LDLc, TC:HDLc) markers. In this sample, CRP was a better predictor of subsequent events than tHcy, IL-6, LDLc, or HDLc; the relative risk in individuals in the highest CRP quartile was almost twice that in the highest quartiles of tHcy, IL-6, or LDLc.

After adjustment for other markers and established vascular risk factors, only CRP (relative risk 1.5, 95% CI 1.1–2.1) and the TC:HDLc ratio (relative risk 1.4, 95% CI 1.1–1.9) remained as independent predictors of vascular risk. For each lipid and inflammatory variable studied, an additive effect was

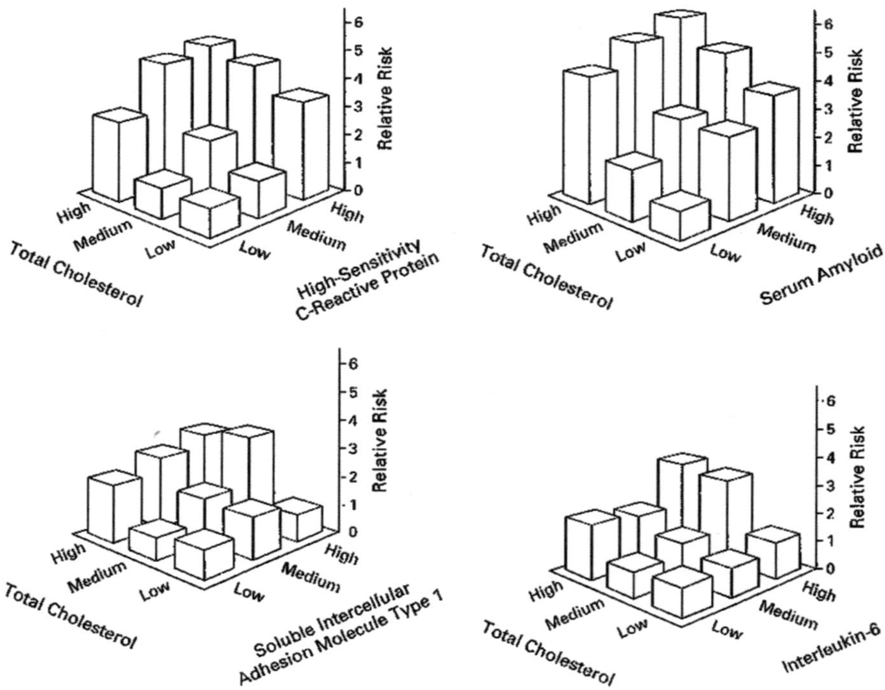

Fig. 1. Relative risk of cardiovascular events among apparently healthy postmenopausal women according to baseline levels of total cholesterol and markers of inflammation. (Reproduced with permission from ref. *11*.)

present, such that risk was higher in the highest quartile and lowest in the lowest quartile of both measures combined.

Furthermore, CRP accurately predicted events in those for whom LDLc levels were considered safe (i.e., <130 mg/dL) under National Cholesterol Education Program guidelines. Finally, these data and other data from the Physicians' Health Study *(5)* indicate that the predictive power of CRP and lipid markers (TC:HDLc) combined is greater than the product of each marker alone *(12)* (Fig. 2).

Ridker and coworkers *(13)* again directly compared the ability of CRP and LDL-C to predict future cardiovascular events, including stroke, in almost 28,000 apparently healthy women. They confirmed their previous findings that women in the highest quintiles of the CRP distribution had an increased risk of events independent of age, plasma cholesterol, and other vascular risk factors. The adjusted relative risks of first cardiovascular event were 2.0 and 2.3 in the fourth and highest quintiles, respectively. CRP predicted subsequent vas-

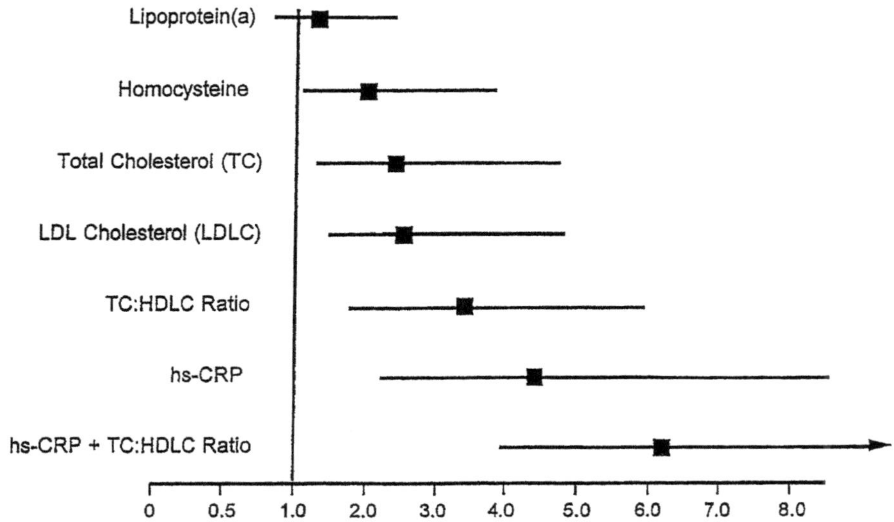

Fig. 2. Relative risk of future cardiovascular events according to different serum biomarker concentrations. (Reproduced with permission from ref. *12*.)

cular events better than LDLc in this study, and the combination of CRP and LDLc provided better prognostic information than each marker alone *(13)*.

CRP and Prediction of Stroke Outcome

Several studies have investigated the relationship between HSCRP and outcome following stroke. Muir et al. *(14)* prospectively studied a cohort of patients admitted with stroke who had CRP measured within 72 hours of onset. Survival in those with CRP values greater than the geometric mean (>10.1 mg/L) was significantly worse than in those with levels below this value. Older age, stroke severity, and higher CRP levels were strong independent predictors of mortality, particularly in the first 3 months (hazard ratio [HR] 1.23). In this study, an increase in CRP by 1 log-unit carried the same predictive ability for adverse outcome as an increase of 4 points on the National Institutes of Health Stroke Scale (NIHSS).

Di Napoli and colleagues *(15)* investigated the correlation between CRP (measured at admission, 48–72 hours, and discharge) and outcome. The discharge CRP threshold of 1.5 mg/dL had optimal sensitivity and specificity for prediction of adverse outcome based on likelihood ratio testing of receiver operating curves. Discharge CRP (HR 7.42) and stroke severity were strong independent predictors of death or further cardiovascular events at 1 year (Fig. 3).

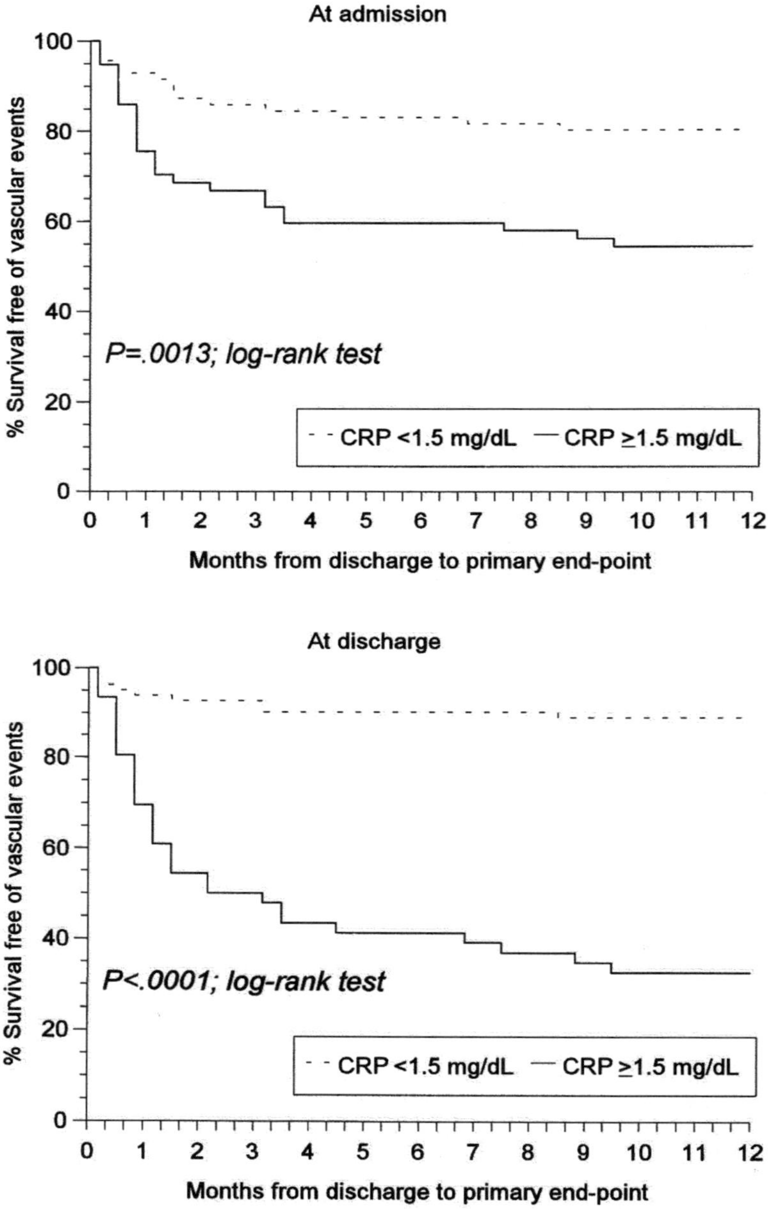

Fig. 3. Kaplan–Meier curves showing cumulative freedom from risk of death or any new vascular event within 1 year in acute stroke patients with CRP levels at admission and at discharge above or below 1.5 mg/dL. (Reproduced with permission from ref. *15*.)

Discharge CRP above 1.5 mg/dL was also associated with disability at 1 year. Only 6.5% of patients with high CRP were independent at 1 year compared to 37% with CRP less than 1.5 mg/dL. There was no association between CRP level on admission and death, but admission CRP predicted new vascular events (HR 3.71) *(15)*. The same group directly compared the ability of early (<24 hours) CRP and fibrinogen to predict outcome at 1 year after stroke. As both are acute phase response proteins, they were significantly correlated, and each was predictive of death and recurrent vascular events. However, only CRP and stroke severity were independent predictors of outcome on multivariable analysis *(16)*.

Winbeck and coworkers *(17)* studied the relationship of outcome with the timing of acute CRP measured after stroke (<12 hours of onset, 12–24 hours, 48 hours). CRP values rose consistently during the first 48 hours after symptom onset. Stroke severity (measured by the Barthel Index) and CRP measured between 12 and 24 hours were the most reliable independent predictors of unfavorable outcome (Barthel Index < 85) and death or recurrent vascular events at 1 year. High levels at 24–48 hours also predicted poor outcome, but the level prior to 12 hours did not.

The pathophysiological mechanisms underlying these associations remain unclear. At least three stimuli for inflammation and increased hepatic CRP synthesis exist in patients with stroke. These include the burden of preexisting atherosclerosis, the extent of cerebral tissue infarcted, and the presence of systemic infection, which commonly complicates stroke. Although several of these studies attempted to control for the confounding influence of infection and stroke severity, it remains unclear whether the relationship between HSCRP and poor outcome simply relates to larger stroke volumes or more frequent infectious complications.

Measurement of CRP in Clinical Practice

A combined American Heart Association and Centers for Disease Control and Prevention guideline made recommendations for measurement of inflammatory markers in clinical practice *(18)*. For primary prevention, they recommended CRP screening for individuals judged at intermediate risk (10–20% over 10 years) of vascular disease by global risk assessment. Although initial studies suggested that high sensitivity CRP measurement may have some utility in identification of individuals at high risk of recurrent stroke and other vascular events, the data are insufficient to recommend routine screening of patients following stroke in clinical practice. In our practice, we empirically measure CRP in selected patients who have made a moderate-to-good functional recovery following their initial stroke and in whom evidence of infection is absent. In this selected group, we wait until 6 months following onset, a time when the inflammatory response following stroke is likely to have resolved. We emphasize that the benefits of this strategy remain unproven.

Although there is no specific therapy to reduce CRP, individuals with higher levels may be targeted for more intensive measures for vascular risk reduction, such as diet, exercise, blood pressure control, and weight loss. Data from the Cholesterol and Recurrent Events (CARE) study *(19)* and Air Force/Texas Coronary Atherosclerosis Prevention Study *(20)* indicate that 3-hydroxy-3-methyl-glutaryl reductase inhibitors (statins) lower CRP independent of their effects on LDLc. Furthermore, the attributable risk reduction from aspirin and statins in these and other trials was greater in individuals with elevated CRP, suggesting that statins may benefit this group regardless of lipid levels *(21)*. The potential benefit of statin therapy in reducing vascular events in individuals with average lipid values and high CRP is currently being assessed in clinical trials.

HOMOCYSTEINE AND RISK OF STROKE

The Homocysteine Hypothesis of Atherosclerosis

Homocystinuria was originally described in 1962 as a metabolic disorder associated with mental retardation in children from Northern Ireland. Vascular complications leading to death in childhood or adolescence were common, usually peripheral venous thrombosis, pulmonary embolism, and ischemic stroke. Neuropathological studies showed occlusion of cortical veins and the dural sinuses, with infarction in the underlying parenchyma. Intraarterial thrombosis of leptomeningeal and small deep cortical arteries with adjacent cerebral infarction also was described. In large-and medium-size arteries, abnormalities included intimal and medial thickening, proliferation of fibrous connective tissue, and degeneration of the internal elastic lamina, which caused focal fibrous plaques. Increased lipid deposition or inflammatory cell infiltration was not a feature.

In 1969, McCully *(22)* proposed that modest elevations in plasma tHcy, which are common in the general population, might act as an initiating factor promoting intimal injury, leading to fibrosis, secondary lipid deposition, and the development of complex atherosclerotic plaque. Thus began the "homocysteine hypothesis" of atherosclerosis.

Biochemistry of Homocysteine Metabolism

Hcy is a sulfur-containing amino acid (thiol) formed in vivo from the essential amino acid methionine (Fig. 4). Once formed, Hcy is metabolized via one of two major degradation reactions, remethylation or transsulfura-

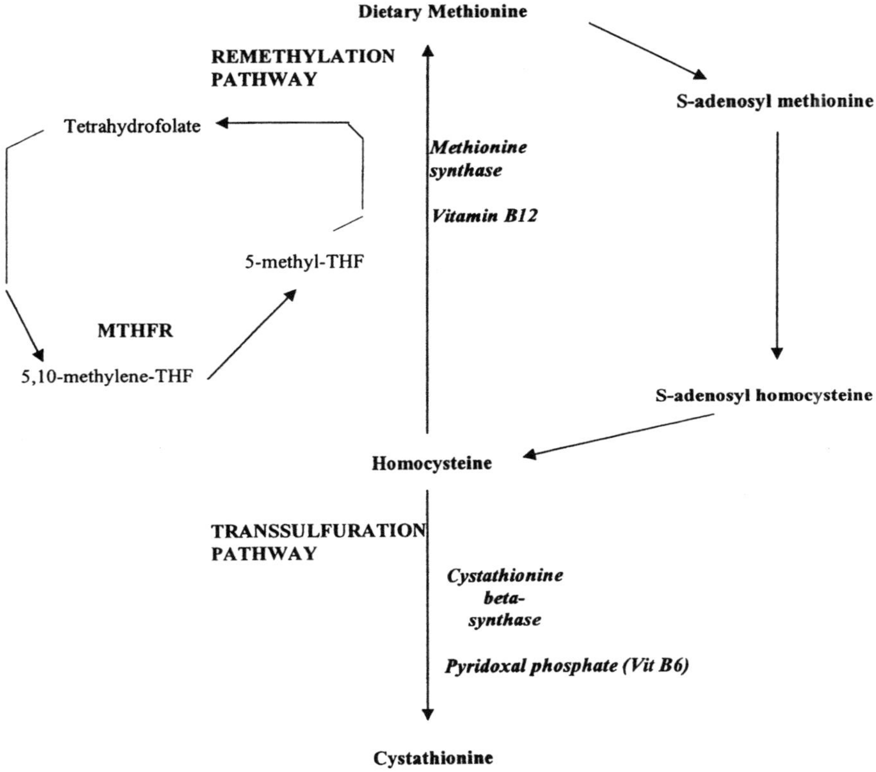

Fig. 4. Metabolism of homocysteine in vivo (THF, tetrahydrofolate).

tion. In the remethylation reaction, a methyl group is added to a single Hcy molecule, forming methionine. One of two methyl group donors is usually utilized in vivo: betaine derived from dietary choline or 5-methyl tetrahydrofolate (THF), a derivative of dietary folic acid (catalyzed by methionine synthase). Cobalamin (vitamin B_{12}) acts as an essential cofactor in this reaction. In the transsulfuration reaction, cystathionine β-synthase (CBS) catalyzes the removal of a sulfhydryl group to form cysteine. Pyridoxal 5'-phosphate, the major circulating form of vitamin B_6, is an important cofactor for this reaction.

Once formed, 5–10% of reduced tissue Hcy is exported to the plasma, where most of it rapidly undergoes oxidation to form a pool of disulfide moieties. Approximately 70–80% of circulating Hcy exists as protein-bound disulfide, primarily to cysteine residues of circulating albumin. About 2–3% exists as free reduced Hcy, and the remaining unbound portion exists as mixed Hcy–cysteine or Hcy–Hcy disulfides. tHcy refers to the circulating pool of free and protein-bound Hcy-derived moieties measured in most assays *(23)*.

Determinants of Plasma tHcy in the General Population

Plasma tHcy rises with age and is higher in age-matched men compared to women. The gender difference is greatest among premenopausal women and age-matched men. tHcy levels are also higher in those with impaired renal function because of impaired renal elimination. As vitamins B_6, B_{12}, and folic acid are essential cofactors for enzymes involved in Hcy degradation, plasma concentrations of these vitamins are negatively correlated with plasma tHcy. A common polymorphism (677C→T) in the gene for methylenetetrahydrofolate reductase (MTHFR) is associated with elevated tHcy in the general population. Medications that interfere with folate metabolism (phenytoin, carbamazepine, methotrexate) are also associated with elevated tHcy.

Although no clear consensus has been established regarding the tHcy level above which an increased risk of vascular disease may exist, elevated tHcy is generally classified as mild (15–30 μmol/L), moderate (31–100 μmol/L), and severe (>100 μmol/L) *(24–26)*.

The prevalence of mild-to-moderately elevated tHcy varies from 10 to 20% according to the nutritional status of the specific population. National cereal grain folic acid supplementation programs have been introduced in the United States and Canada with the aim of reducing the incidence of neural tube defects secondary to maternal folate deficiency. Data from the Framingham study indicate that the resulting improvement in folate status in the general population has resulted in a reduction in mean plasma tHcy of approx 9% and a reduction in the prevalence of elevated tHcy (>13 μmol/L) from approx 20 to 10%, a relative reduction of 48% *(27)* (Fig. 5).

Mechanisms of Ischemic Stroke Associated With Elevated Homocysteine

Accelerated Atherosclerosis

Relatively few precise data exist on the exact pathophysiological mechanisms of ischemic stroke associated with elevated tHcy. In patients with homocystinuria caused by CBS deficiency, pathological studies have confirmed McCully's observations of patchy arterial lesions involving arterioles and small and large arteries. However, to our knowledge, these changes have been associated with intraarterial luminal thrombosis and cerebral embolism in only two cases.

Studies have reported associations between mild-to-moderate hyper-tHcy and markers of early atherosclerosis, such as abnormal endothelial-dependent vasodilation, carotid intimal-media thickening, and early carotid stenosis. However, the precise role of mild-to-moderately elevated tHcy in the pathogenesis of cerebrovascular atherosclerosis remains unresolved.

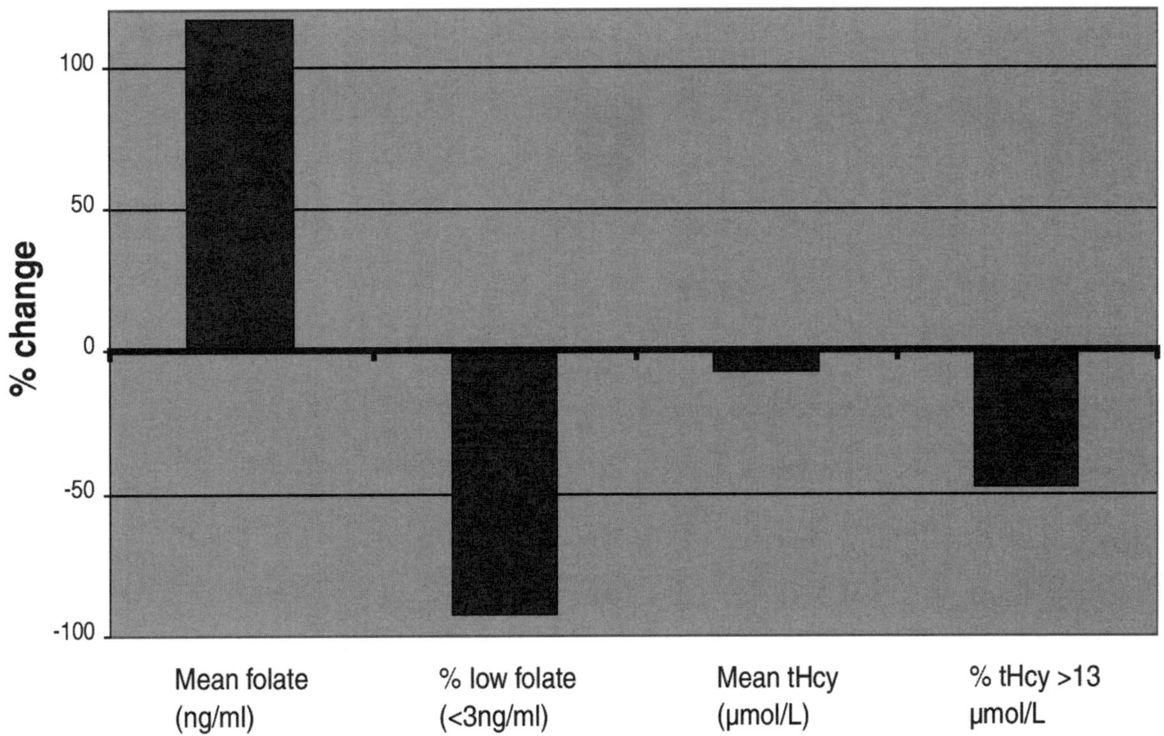

Fig. 5. Change in folate and tHcy in Framingham offspring cohort since folic acid fortification in the United States. (From data presented in ref. *27*.)

Several studies have investigated whether tHcy is associated with greater stroke risk among subtypes primarily related to atherosclerosis compared to others. One recent study found that mean tHcy was significantly greater in stroke because of large-artery and small-artery (lacunar) disease compared to cardioembolic stroke and controls, with a graded increase in odds ratio that was greatest in the large-artery subgroup *(28)*. Several other studies found no evidence of subtype-specific increased risk, but these studies may have been limited by small sample sizes and failure to control for important confounders such as vitamin status and MTHFR genotype. Given these conflicting data, it is unclear whether elevated tHcy is associated with a differential stroke risk between subtypes.

Thrombosis and Embolism

Consistent data indicate that thrombophilia is likely to predispose to stroke in patients with homocystinuria caused by CBS deficiency. Markers of platelet activation and thrombin generation such as urinary thromboxane B2 and plasma F1.2 are elevated, and activated protein C is diminished (consistent with compensatory increased fibrinolytic activity) in these patients. Venous infarction secondary to spontaneous cerebral venous thrombosis is a well-established mechanism of stroke in these patients. Rare reports also exist of spontaneous arterial system thrombosis with secondary embolism in homocystinuric patients *(29,30)*.

In sporadic stroke, tHcy may contribute to the development of arterial thromboembolism in conditions associated with blood stasis. A study that investigated the pathogenesis of left atrial thrombus in patients with stroke caused by atrial fibrillation reported that mean tHcy was higher in patients with thrombus verified by transesophageal echocardiography (20.75 vs 13.34 μmol/L, $p < 0.001$). After controlling for other variables known to predispose to left atrial thrombus (spontaneous echo contrast and atrial dilation), high tHcy (>15 μmol/L) was a strong independent predictor of the risk of left atrial thrombus (adjusted OR 14.25, 95% CI 2.7–75.1) *(31)*.

Craniocervical Arterial Dissection

Two studies implicated mild-to-moderate hyper-tHcy as an independent risk factor for ischemic stroke related to cervical artery dissection, possibly related to weakening of vascular connective tissue protein fibrils because of replacement of cysteine–cysteine cross-bridges by protein-bound Hcy–cysteine disulfides. Consistent with these observations, we have also described a young adult with CBS-deficient homocystinuria with retinal embolism because of dissection of the cervical carotid artery. These preliminary observations require confirmation in larger studies *(32,33)*.

Epidemiological Studies of Homocysteine and Risk of Stroke

Case-Control Studies

In the 1990s, numerous epidemiological studies demonstrated an association between elevated tHcy and ischemic stroke. Early studies reported a significantly higher frequency of elevated tHcy (fasting and after methionine loading) in patients with stroke compared to healthy controls. For example, Clarke and colleagues reported an adjusted odds ratio of 3.2 associated with postmethionine load hyper-tHcy in 123 Irish subjects with premature vascular disease *(34)*. Brattstrom reported that mean fasting tHcy was significantly higher in 70 cases following stroke compared to 66 controls *(35)*. Similar findings were reported by Coull and coworkers *(36)*. Graham and colleagues reported a 1.7-fold adjusted increase in the odds of stroke among 211 cases and 800 controls in the European Concerted Action Project *(37)*. Supporting these results, Eikelboom and coworkers found an adjusted 2.2-fold increase in the odds of ischemic stroke when the highest and lowest quartiles of the tHcy distributions were compared in 229 cases and 205 controls *(28)*.

In the United States, scant data exist on the relationship of stroke with tHcy since the introduction of cereal grain folic acid fortification in 1998. Fortification has increased folate and reduced tHcy concentrations in the US population, with a greater effect in individuals with higher prefortification tHcy, such as those with vascular disease.

In a case-control study, we found identical tHcy distributions in 320 post-fortification, folate-replete US subjects (180 stroke or TIA, 140 matched controls) (geometric mean 10.8 vs 10.31 μmol/L, $p = 0.5$). After adjusting for vascular risk factors, tHcy did not predict stroke or TIA (OR 0.92, 95% CI 0.4–2.1) *(38)*. Although confirmation in prospective studies is required, these data suggest that tHcy may have limited utility for prediction of vascular risk in populations in which folate supplementation has been introduced.

Prospective Studies

Unlike case-control studies, data from prospective studies have reported a less-robust association between tHcy and stroke. In a nested case-control analysis among men aged 40–59 years from the British Regional Heart Study, Perry and coworkers found that tHcy concentrations were significantly higher in 141 cases compared to 118 controls, with a graded increase in risk of stroke in the second, third, and fourth quartiles of tHcy distribution *(39)*. Similar results were reported from the Framingham study, which found a graded increase in risk across increasing quartiles of the tHcy distribution among 1947 subjects *(40)*. Bots and coworkers reported similar findings in a nested case-control analysis from the Rotterdam study *(41)*.

In a population-based cross-sectional study, the relationship among tHcy, vitamin status, and internal carotid artery stenosis (>25%) in 1041 elderly Framingham Heart Study subjects was studied. When the prevalence of carotid stenosis greater than 25% in the fourth and first quartiles of tHcy distribution was compared, an inverse correlation was found ($p < 0.001$ in men, $p = 0.03$ in women) *(42)*. A nested case-control study from the Atherosclerosis Risk in Communities (ARIC) cohort examined intimal-medial thickening (a marker for early atherosclerosis) of the extracranial carotid artery in 257 asymptomatic matched pairs aged 45–64 years. An inverse correlation was present between wall thickness and tHcy (OR 3.15 when subjects in the top quintile were compared to those in the bottom quintile, $p < 0.001$) *(43)*.

In contrast to these findings, no difference in mean tHcy was found between 74 stroke cases and 269 controls in a nested analysis of a Finnish population-based cohort *(44)*. In a nested analysis of a sample from the Physicians' Health Study, 109 patients with stroke were compared to 427 healthy controls. Only a small, nonsignificant increase in risk of stroke was associated with elevated tHcy (ORs for top compared to bottom tHcy quintiles were 1.4 [crude] and 1.2 [adjusted]) *(45)*. Fallon and colleagues reported only a small increase in the risk of stroke (adjusted HR 1.3) among 2254 men in a Welsh community-based study *(46)*.

The reasons for the conflicting results of these studies are not clear. It has been suggested that the findings of the Finnish study may be explained based on the exceptionally low prevalence of hyperhomocyst(e)inemia in the Finnish population. The weak association found in the US study may be related to the likelihood that tHcy levels among US physicians are lower than those of the general US population because of better vitamin intake in this group. Thus, both the US and Finnish studies may have lacked statistical power to detect an association between tHcy and stroke. Alternatively, tHcy may simply act as a marker for low folate and B vitamin status, and population-specific nutritional differences may contribute to the varying results of prospective studies. tHcy also rises in the first and subsequent weeks after stroke. This may have contributed to the frequent positive associations reported in case–control studies, which measured tHcy in the early poststroke period.

Prevention and Treatment of Hyperhomocysteinemia in the General Population

Impact of Vitamin Supplements on tHcy

In a meta-analysis, the Homocysteine Lowering Trialists Collaboration *(47)* reviewed the pooled data from randomized trials that investigated vitamin therapy for elevated tHcy. Supplemental folic acid was most effective

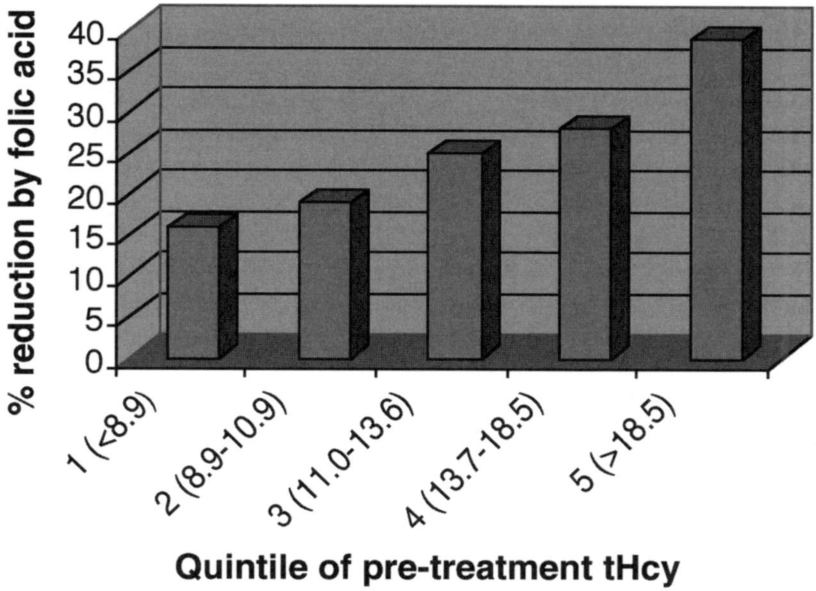

Fig. 6. Impact of folic acid supplementation on plasma tHcy, stratified by quintile of pretreatment tHcy. There is a dose–response relationship between the tHcy-lowering effect of folic acid and pretreatment tHcy, such that individuals with higher initial tHcy experience greatest reductions ($p < 0.001$). (From data presented in ref. *46*.)

at reducing tHcy, with an cross-study pooled reduction of 25%. Supplementation with B_{12} (0.02–1 mg daily, mean dose 0.5 mg) conferred an additional pooled reduction of 7%, but B_6 supplementation (2–50 mg daily, mean dose 16.5 mg) provided no additional effect.

Although the doses of folic acid varied from 0.4 to 10 mg, no difference in tHcy-lowering effect was present between studies that administered less than 1 mg (mean dose 0.5 mg) and higher doses after standardization for pretreatment folate and tHcy levels (Fig. 6).

In contrast, the pooled benefit of folic acid supplementation was markedly influenced by pretreatment tHcy and folate levels (Fig. 6). Individuals in the highest pretreatment tHcy quintile had a 39% Hcy reduction, compared to 16% among those in the lowest pretreatment quintile, with near-identical effects when the results were stratified by pretreatment folate quintile. Other data suggest that the MTHFR 677C→T polymorphism may also modify the tHcy-lowering response to folic acid supplements.

Benefit of Vitamin Supplements for Risk of Stroke and Vascular Disease

The benefit of tHcy reduction for vascular disease risk is less clear. Based on a meta-analysis of observational data, Boushey and coworkers estimated a reduction in vascular disease risk of 30–40% associated with an absolute reduction in tHcy by 3–4 μmol/L *(48)*.

tHcy reduction has been reported to improve surrogate markers of atherosclerosis in patients with stroke and vascular disease, including endothelium-dependent vasodilation, plasma thrombomodulin, carotid plaque area, and abnormal stress electrocardiogram findings. However, the validity of some of these markers as precursors for clinically relevant vascular disease has not been well established. A clinical trial of vitamin supplements after coronary angioplasty reported a significant reduction in restenosis rates of 48% compared to placebo *(49)*. In an extension of this trial, the frequency of major adverse vascular events (death, nonfatal myocardial infarction, revascularization) was reduced by 32% by tHcy-lowering vitamins ($p = 0.03$) *(50)*.

Two large randomized trials investigated tHcy-lowering vitamin supplement therapy for secondary stroke prevention. The VITATOPS (Vitamins to Prevent Stroke) study is comparing supplements (2 mg folic acid, 500 μg B_{12}, 50 mg B_6>) to placebo in 8000 subjects with recent stroke or TIA for prevention of recurrent stroke, myocardial infarction, and vascular death at 2.5 years *(51)*. The Vitamins in Stroke Prevention study is comparing the efficacy of high (2.5 mg folic acid, 400 μg B12, 25 mg B6) and low (200 μg folic acid, 6 μg B12, 0.2 mg B6) for secondary prevention of stroke or myocardial infarction in 3600 subjects with recent stroke. This trial was prematurely terminated and publication of its findings is pending.

Guidelines for tHcy Screening and Management

Routine population screening of tHcy is not recommended because of the cost of testing, inconsistent data from prospective studies regarding the utility of tHcy for prediction of vascular risk, and lack of data from clinical trials indicating a clear benefit of tHcy-lowering treatment. The clinical practice adopted by our group and others is to reserve tHcy measurement for young patients with stroke or TIA or other patients at high risk of vascular disease (those with a strong family history or past history of early-onset vascular disease, impaired renal function, or elevated CRP). The Nutrition Committee of the American Heart Association recommended an upper limit of 10 μmol/L as a reasonable goal for tHcy-lowering strategies; the recommendation was based on a single study reporting the benefit of vitamin therapy for preventing progression of carotid plaque in adults younger than 60 years *(52)*.

For primary prevention, the American Stroke Association recommends an emphasis on meeting recommended daily allowances of folic acid, B_{12}, and B_6 by consumption of vegetables, fruits, legumes, meat, fish, and fortified ready-to-eat breakfast cereals *(53)*.

In patients with elevated tHcy, serum levels of folate, vitamin B_{12}, and B_6 should be measured, and drugs associated with elevated tHcy should be discontinued if possible. If B_{12} is low, appropriate further investigations should be conducted to clarify the underlying cause, and B_{12} should be repleted. If vitamin levels are not low, then patients should be advised to consume the diet recommended by the American Stroke Association, and tHcy should be rechecked 4–6 weeks later. If tHcy remains elevated, a multivitamin containing 400 mg folic acid, 2 mg B_6, and 6 μg B_{12} may be prescribed. If tHcy remains above 10 μmol/L, higher dose vitamins (1 mg folic acid, 25 mg B_6, 0.5 mg B_{12}) may be prescribed. Although the above recommendations are reasonable, inexpensive, and low risk, we emphasize that their efficacy remains to be proven in clinical trials.

PREDICTION OF HEMORRHAGE FOLLOWING STROKE THROMBOLYSIS

Reperfusion following ischemic stroke is associated with injury to the blood–brain barrier, leading to cerebral edema and hemorrhage. These are major causes of stroke-related secondary brain injury, early neurological death, and disability, particularly in patients treated with tissue plasminogen activator (tPA). MMPs are a group of proteolytic, zinc-dependent enzymes involved in many aspects of normal development, such as connective tissue remodeling, angiogenesis, tissue development, and tumor cell invasion. However, they are highly destructive when involved in inflammatory processes of the central nervous system. In animal models, MMP2 and MMP9 act as gelatinases, degrading major proteins in the basal lamina of the cerebral microcirculation (laminin, fibronectin, and type IV collagen). During acute cerebral ischemia in animals, local inflammatory processes result in upregulation of expression of cell adhesion molecules and MMPs, progressive loss of basal lamina structural proteins, and disruption of the integrity of the microvascular blood–brain barrier. This is associated with ischemic edema and hemorrhagic transformation of the infarct, particularly in the presence of higher cerebral perfusion pressures or exogenous tPA *(54–56)*.

Plasma levels of MMP2 and MMP9 are frequently raised after acute stroke in humans. This has raised the prospect that MMPs may have clinical utility to predict hemorrhagic change after tPA-treated ischemic stroke. Clinical studies have examined the time course of MMP elevation after stroke *(57)*.

Montaner et al. *(58)* measured MMP9 and MMP2 levels in tPA-untreated patients at less than 6, 12, 24, and 48 hours after onset of cardioembolic stroke. Plasma MMP9 peaked at admission (<12 hours from onset) and correlated with stroke severity (NIHSS) and infarct volume on computed tomography at 48 hours *(58)*. In a later analysis of the same sample, there was no association between either MMP2 or MMP9 and hemorrhagic transformation, but subgroup analysis revealed a peak of MMP9 at 24 hours in all patients with early symptomatic parenchymal hematoma. MMP9 was also an independent predictor of late hemorrhagic transformation after adjusting for hypertension and lack of recanalization.

In another study of 250 unselected ischemic stroke patients, admission plasma MMP9 was higher in those who had subsequent hemorrhage, including those assessed within the time window for intravenous tPA therapy. Admission MMP9 above 140 ng/mL had a 61% positive and 97% negative predictive value for subsequent hemorrhage. After adjusting for temperature, blood pressure, early computed tomographic changes, and anticoagulant use, high MMP9 independently predicted hemorrhagic transformation (OR 12, 95% CI 3–51) *(59)*.

In the only study examining MMPs in tPA-treated human stroke, plasma MMP9 measured within 3 hours of stroke onset was highest among patients who subsequently developed a parenchymal hematoma compared to those with hemorrhagic infarction or without hemorrhage. A threshold of 191.3 ng/mL had a positive predictive value of 67% and negative predictive value of 100% for subsequent hematoma development. Early (<3 hours) MMP9 was an independent predictor of subsequent parenchymal hematoma on regression analysis (OR 9.62, 95% CI 1.3–70.3) *(60)*.

These data indicate that measurement of MMPs, particularly MMP9, in the acute stage after ischemic stroke may potentially provide useful additional information to predict patients more likely to develop symptomatic intracranial hematomas if treated with tPA. Further research is required to confirm the validity of these initial findings before MMP measurement can be considered for tPA risk stratification in acute stroke.

REFERENCES

1. Pearson TA, Mensah GA, Alexander RW, et al. Markers of inflammation and cardiovascular disease. Application to clinical and public health practice. Circulation 2003;107;499–511.
2. Ridker PM, Hennekens CH, Roitman-Johnson B, Stampfer MS, Allen J. Plasma concentration of soluble intercellular adhesion molecule-1 and risks of future myocardial infarction in apparently healthy men. Lancet 1998;351:88–92.
3. Ridker PM, Buring JE, Rifai N. Soluble P-selectin and the risk of future cardiovascular events. Circulation 2001;103:491–495.

4. Blann AD. Inflammation, cell adhesion molecules and stroke: tools in pathophysiology and epidemiology. Stroke 2002;33:2141–2143.
5. Ridker PM, Cushman M, Stampfer MS, Tracey RP, Hennekens CH. Inflammation, aspirin and the risk of cardiovascular disease in apparently healthy men. N Engl J Med 1997;336:973–979.
6. Gussekloo J, Schaap MC, Frolich M, Blauw G, Westendorp R. C-reactive protein is a strong but non-specific risk factor of fatal stroke in elderly persons. Arterioscl Thromb Vasc Biol 2000;20:1047–1051.
7. Ford E, Giles WH. Serum C-reactive protein and self reported stroke: findings from the Third National Health and Nutrition Examination Survey. Arterioscler Thromb Vasc Biol 2000;20:1052–1056.
8. Rost NS, Wolf PA, Kase CS, et al. Plasma concentration of C-reactive protein and risk of ischemic stroke and transient ischemic attack. Stroke 2001;32:2575–2579.
9. Wang T, Byung-Ho N, Wilson P, et al. Association of C-reactive protein with carotid atherosclerosis in men and women. The Framingham Heart Study. Arterioscler Thromb Vasc Biol 2002;22:1662–1667.
10. Van Der Meer I, de Maat MP, Hak AE, et al. C-reactive protein predicts progression of atherosclerosis measured at various sites in the arterial tree. The Rotterdam Study. Stroke 2002;33:2750–2755.
11. Ridker PM, Hennekens CH, Buring JE, Rifai N. C-reactive protein and other markers of inflammation in the prediction of cardiovascular disease in women. N Engl J Med 2000;342:836–843.
12. Ridker PM. High sensitivity C-reactive protein. Potential adjunct for global risk assessment in the primary prevention of cardiovascular disease. Circulation 2001; 103:1813–1818.
13. Ridker PM, Rafai N, Rose L, Buring J, Cook N. Comparison of C-reactive protein and low density lipoprotein cholesterol levels in the prediction of first cardiovascular events. N Engl J Med 2002;347:1557–1565.
14. Muir KW, Weir CJ, Alwan Wafa, Squire IB, Lees KR. C-reactive protein and outcome after ischemic stroke. Stroke 1999;30:981–985.
15. Di Napoli M, Papa F, Bocola V. C-reactive protein in ischemic stroke. An independent prognostic factor. Stroke 2001;32:917–924.
16. Di Napoli M, Papa F, Bocola V. Prognostic influence of increased C-reactive protein and fibrinogen levels in ischemic stroke. Stroke 2001;32:113–138.
17. Winbeck K, Poppert H, Thornleif E, Conrad B, Sander D. Prognostic relevance of early serial C-reactive protein measurements after first stroke. Stroke 2002;33: 2459–2464.
18. Pearson TA, Mensah GA, Alexander RW, et al. Markers of inflammation and cardiovascular disease. Application to clinical and public health practice. A statement for healthcare professionals from the Centers for Disease Control and Prevention and the American Heart Association. Circulation 2003;107:499–511.
19. Ridker PM, Rifai N, Pfeffer MA, Sacks F, Braunwald E. Longterm effects of pravastatin on concentration of C-reactive protein. The Cholesterol and Recurrent Events Investigators. Circulation 1999;100:230–235.
20. Ridker PM, Rifai N, Clearfield D, Downs JR, Weis SE, Miles JS, Grotto A. Measurement of C-reactive protein for the targeting of statin therapy in primary prevention of acute coronary events. N Engl J Med 2001;334:1959–1965.

21. Di Napoli PM, Papa F. Inflammatory hemostatic markers and antithrombotic agents in relation to long term risk of cardiovascular events in first ischemic stroke patients. Stroke 2002;32:1763–1771.
22. McCully K. Vascular pathology of homocysteinemia: implications for the pathogenesis of atherosclerosis. Am J Pathol 1969;56:111–128.
23. Mudd SH, Levy HL, Kraus JP. Disorders of transsulfuration. In: Valle D, ed. The Metabolic and Molecular Basis of Inherited Disease, 8th ed. New York: McGraw Hill, 2001.
24. Selhub J, Jacques PF, Rosenberg IH, et al. Serum total homocysteine concentrations in the Third National Health and Nutrition Examination Survey (1991–1994): population reference ranges and contribution of vitamin status to high serum concentrations. Ann Intern Med 1999;131:331–339.
25. Selhub J, Jacques P, Wilson PWF, Rush D, Rosenberg IH. Vitamin status and intake as primary determinants of homocysteinemia in an elderly population. JAMA 1993; 270:2693–2698.
26. Rozen R. Genetic modulation of homocysteinemia. Semin Thromb Hemost 2000; 26:255–261.
27. Jacques PF, Selhub J, Bostom AG, Wilson PWF, Rosenberg IH. The effect of folic acid fortification on plasma folate and total homocysteine concentrations. N Engl J Med 1999;340:1449–1454.
28. Eikelboom JW, Hankey GJ, Anand SS, Lofthouse E, Staples N, Baker RI. Association between high homocyst(e)ine and ischemic stroke due to large- and small-artery disease but not other etiologic subtypes of ischemic stroke. Stroke 2000;31:1069–1075.
29. Coppola A, Davi G, De Stefano V, Mancini FP, Cerbone AM, Di Minno G. Homocysteine, coagulation, platelet function, and thrombosis. Semin Thromb Hemost 2000; 26:243–254.
30. D'Angelo A, Selhub J. Homocysteine and thrombotic disease. Blood 997;90:1–11.
31. Ay H, Arsara EM, Tokgozoghi SL, Ozer N, Saribas O. Hyperhomocysteinemia is associated with left atrial thrombus in stroke patients with nonvascular atrial fibrillation. Stroke 2003;34:909–912.
32. Gallai V, Caso V, Paciaroni M, et al. Mild hyperhomocyst(e)inemia: a possible risk factor for cervical artery dissection. Stroke 2001;32:714–718.
33. Pezzini A, Del Zotto E, Archetti S, et al. Plasma homocysteine concentration, C677T MTHFR genotype, and 844ins68bp CBS genotype in young adults with spontaneous cervical artery dissection and atherothrombotic stroke. Stroke 2002;33:664–669.
34. Clarke R, Daly L, Robinson K, et al. Hyperhomocysteinemia: an independent risk factor for vascular disease. N Engl J Med 1991;324:1149–1155.
35. Brattstrom L, Israelsson B, Norrving B, et al. Impaired hemocysteine metabolism in early-onset cerebral and peripheral occlusive arterial disease. Effects of pyridoxine and folic acid treatment. Atherosclerosis 1990;81:51–60.
36. Coull BM, Malinow MR, Beamer N, Sexton G, Nordt F, de Garmo P. Elevated plasma homocysteine concentration as a possible independent risk factor for stroke. Stroke 1990;21:4:572–576.
37. Graham I, Daly LE, Refsum HM, et al. Plasma homocysteine as a risk factor for vascular disease. The European Concerted Action Project. JAMA. 1997;277:1775–1781.

38. Kelly PJ, Shih VE, Kistler JP, et al. Low vitamin B_6 but not homocysteine is associated with increased risk of stroke and transient ischemic attack in the era of folic acid grain fortification. Stroke. 2003;34:e51–e54.
39. Perry IJ, Refsum H, Morris RW, Ebrahim SB, Ueland PM, Shaper AG. Prospective study of serum total homocysteine concentration and risk of stroke in middle-aged British men. Lancet 1995;346:1395–1398.
40. Bostom AG, Rosenberg IH, Silbershatz H, et al. Nonfasting plasma total homocysteine levels and stroke incidence in elderly persons: the Framingham Study. Ann Int Med 1999;131:352–355.
41. Bots ML, Launer LJ, Lindemans J, et al. Homocysteine and short-term risk of myocardial infarction and stroke in the elderly: the Rotterdam Study. Arch Intern Med 1999;159:38–44.
42. Selhub J, Jacques PF, Bostom AG, et al. Association between plasma homocysteine concentrations and extracranial carotid-artery stenosis. N Engl J Med 1995; 332:286–291.
43. Malinow MR, Nieto FJ, Szklo M, Chambless LE, Bond G. Carotid artery intimal-medial wall thickening and plasma homocyst(e)ine in asymptomatic adults. The Atherosclerosis Risk in Communities Study. Circulation 1993;87:1107–1113.
44. Alfthan G, Pekkanen J, Jauhiainen M, et al. Relation of serum homocysteine and lipoprotein(a) concentrations to atherosclerotic disease in a prospective Finnish population based study. Atherosclerosis 1994;106:9–19.
45. Verhoef P, Hennekens CH, Malinow MR, Kok FJ, Willett WC, Stampfer MJ. A prospective study of plasma homocyst(e)ine and risk of ischemic stroke. Stroke 1994;25:1924–1930.
46. Fallon UB, Elwood P, Ben-Shlomo Y, Ubbink JB, Greenwood R, Smith GD. Homocysteine and ischaemic stroke in men: the Caerphilly study. J Epidemiol Community Health 2001;55:91–96.
47. Lowering blood homocysteine with folic acid based supplements: metaanalysis of randomised trials. Homocysteine Lowering Trialists Collaboration. BMJ 1998;316: 894–898.
48. Boushey CJ, Beresford SA, Omenn GS, Mohilsky AG. A quantitative assessment of plasma homocysteine as a risk factor for vascular disease. Probable benefits if increasing folic acid intakes. JAMA 1995;275:1049–1057.
49. Schnyder G, Roffi M, Flammer Y, Pin R, Hess OM. Effect of homocysteine-lowering therapy with folic acid, vitamin B(12), and vitamin B(6) on clinical outcome after percutaneous coronary intervention: the Swiss Heart study: a randomized controlled trial. JAMA 2002;288:973–979.
50. Schnyder G, Roffi M, Pin R, et al. Decreased rate of coronary restenosis after lowering of plasma homocysteine levels. N Engl J Med 2001;345:1593–600.
51. VITATOPS Trial Study Group. Homocysteine VITATOPS (Vitamins to Prevent Stroke) Trial: rationale and design of an international large, simple, randomised trial of homocysteine lowering multivitamin therapy in patients with recent transient ischemic attack or stroke. Cerebrovascular Dis 2002;13:2:120–126.
52. Malinow MR, Bostom AG, Krauss RM. Homocyst(e)ine, diet, and cardiovascular diseases. A statement for healthcare professionals from the Nutrition Committee, American Heart Association. Circulation 1999;99:178–182.

53. Goldstein L, Adams, R, Becker K, et al. Primary prevention of ischemic stroke: a statement for healthcare professionals from the Stroke Council of the American Heart Association. Stroke 2001;32:280–299.
54. Rosenberg GA, Estrada EY, Dencoff JE. Matrix metalloproteinases and TIMPs are associated with blood brain barrier opening after reperfusion in rat brain. Stroke 1998;29:2189–2195.
55. Rosenberg GA. Matrix Metalloproteinases in neuroinflammation. Glia 2002;39: 279–291.
56. Romanic AM, White RF, Arleth AJ, Ohlstein EH, Barone FC. Matrix metalloproteinase expression increases after cerebral focal ischemia in rats: inhibition of MMP9 reduces infarct size. Stroke 1998;29:1020–1030.
57. Montaner J, Alvarez-Sabin J, Molina C, et al. Matrix metalloproteinase expression after human cardioembolic stroke. Temporal profile and relation to neurological impairment. Stroke 2001;32:1759–1766.
58. Montaner J, Alvarez-Sabin J, Molina CA, et al. Matrix metalloproteinase expression is related to hemorrhagic transformation after cardioembolic stroke. Stroke 2001;32:2762–2767.
59. Castellanos M, Leira R, Serona J, et al. Plasma metalloproteinase-9 concentration predicts hemorrhagic transformation in acute ischemic stroke. Stroke 2003;34: 40–46.
60. Montaner J, Molina C, Monasterio J, et al. Matrix metalloproteinase-9 pretreatment level predicts intracranial hemorrhagic complications after thrombolysis in human stroke. Circulation 2003;107:598–603.

17

Genetic Susceptibility and Early Stratification of Stroke Risk

Peter J. Kelly and Karen L. Furie

STROKE AS A GENETICALLY INFLUENCED PHENOTYPE

Traditionally, risk for stroke and cardiovascular disease has been considered to be predominantly mediated by environmental factors such as smoking and dietary determinants of hypertension and hyperlipidemia. In addition to environmental factors, family and twin studies have indicated that genetic factors may be associated with increased stroke risk *(1,2)*. Early data also suggest that, in addition to established determinants of stroke outcome (age; stroke severity, location, or mechanism), genetic factors may influence survival and recurrence following hemorrhagic and ischemic stroke.

Genetic influence on a complex phenotype such as stroke is likely to be mediated by the interaction of environmental factors with polymorphisms in several genes, each of which may have a relatively modest influence on important intermediate phenotypic traits (e.g., susceptibility to thrombosis) *(1,2)*.

Although methodological and statistical problems in the field are still being addressed, research examining genetic susceptibility to complex disease phenotypes such as stroke is progressing at a rapid pace *(3,4)*. This research has several goals. First, it may uncover evidence of previously unrecognized biological mechanisms contributing to the pathogenesis of stroke (e.g., apolipoprotein E [apo E] in sporadic lobar hemorrhage, Notch3 in cerebral small-vessel disease). Second, pharmacogenomic strategies may identify the genetic and molecular mechanisms underlying the variation in response to stroke therapies (e.g., unresponsiveness to aspirin therapy). In clinical practice, this may allow selection of patients for such therapies based on genetic determinants of their likelihood of response.

Eventually, low-cost, high-throughput technology may be used to screen panels of genomic markers rapidly to identify inherited susceptibility to conditions such as hypertension, atherosclerosis, and thrombosis, thus allowing targeted prevention strategies for high-risk individuals at a preclinical stage

From: *Current Clinical Neurology: Handbook of Stroke Prevention in Clinical Practice*
Edited by: K. L. Furie and P. J. Kelly © Humana Press Inc., Totowa, NJ

Table 1
Comparison of Linkage and Association Strategies for Investigation of Genetic Susceptibility to Stroke

	Linkage	Association
Affected family members	Index case + 1 (minimum)	Index case only
Multiplex families	Desirable	Not needed
Genetic resolution	Limited (megabases)	Higher (disease-causative allele or within kilobases of same)
Statistical power	Limited if several small gene influences	Higher for a given case sample size

of the disease. Although this scenario may seem futuristic, similar preclinical screening for the *BRCA1* and *BRCA2* genes is already available in some US centers for women with a positive family history of breast cancer. The ethical and counseling implications of this approach are considerable. Strong regulatory protections will also be required to safeguard against discrimination in insurance and employment.

LINKAGE AND ASSOCIATION STRATEGIES FOR GENETIC STUDIES OF STROKE

Unlike highly penetrant, early-onset disorders, linkage analysis has disadvantages for the study of complex late-onset phenotypes such as stroke *(3)* (Table 1). Reasons include incomplete penetrance of the stroke phenotype, genetic heterogeneity, frequent lack of availability of multiplex family data, and relatively low genetic resolution of linkage strategies. Association studies circumvent the requirement for multiplex family data, provide better statistical power to detect gene–disease relationships, and offer higher genetic resolution to detect disease-causing alleles when dense marker maps are used.

However, to date, many association (case-control) studies of candidate genetic variants (mainly single-nucleotide polymorphisms [SNPs]) have yielded nonreproducible results *(3,4)*. Reasons include failure to control for bias caused by population stratification, poor selection of controls, inadequate sample size (type 2 error), lack of replication in an independent data set, multiple hypothesis testing without appropriate statistical corrections (type 1 error), and publication bias. A consensus is now emerging for the design, analysis, and publication of association studies for complex disorders; this should greatly reduce problems associated with earlier studies.

Because of the relative limitations of linkage approaches, association-based strategies are more likely to reveal susceptibility genes for common stroke in most populations *(2,3)*. An exception is the Icelandic population, for whom excellent genealogical data, access to centralized health information, and relative ethnic homogeneity have made a linkage-based investigation of common disease phenotypes feasible *(5)*. For other populations, the improved power of an association design will enhance the ability to detect modest relationships between gene markers and disease. The inclusion of unaffected family members (e.g., siblings) as the primary control group will circumvent the problem of false-positive findings caused by population stratification bias. Large studies have already successfully employed association-based strategies to discover susceptibility genes for complex stroke-related phenotypes (Table 2). Examples include the apo E2, E3, E4 polymorphism that predisposes to lobar hemorrhage, and an angiotensin-converting enzyme (ACE) insertion–deletion polymorphism that predisposes to hypertension.

The discovery of genetic variants predisposing to disease susceptibility by association methods is based on mapping of linkage disequilibrium (allelic association) between genetic markers and disease-associated polymorphisms. Important methodological issues regarding the use of high-density SNP marker maps in association studies have been clarified in a "proof-of-concept" study of the apo E4 susceptibility gene for Alzheimer's disease *(6)*. These include the optimal SNP density, importance of SNP allele frequency, use of exonic vs intronic SNP markers, and appropriate statistical approaches.

By studying 60 SNPs at 28-kb intervals (on average) in a 1.7-Mb region around the apo E gene in patients with Alzheimer's disease, Martin and coworkers *(6)* demonstrated significant associations between seven SNPs close (<32 kb) to the functional apo E polymorphism. The associations were consistently significant in both case-control and family-based tests and showed a strong trend across adjacent loci. After Bonferroni correction for multiple comparisons, the findings remained highly significant for three marker SNPs (p values 10^{-5} to 10^{-20}). Intronic and exonic SNPs with moderate (>0.3) allele frequencies were most informative. This study also indicated that typing "haplotype-tagging" SNPs may greatly increase the efficiency of genomic screening in complex diseases. An international collaborative project to define genomewide haplotype associations ("hap-map") is currently under way.

CHARACTERIZATION OF HOMOGENOUS STROKE PHENOTYPES

For genetic stroke studies, it is important to consider the problem of heterogeneity among ischemic stroke syndromes *(7)*. In general, it is crucial to define

Table 2
Recent Advances in Stroke Genetics

Stroke syndrome	Phenotype	Genes	Inheritance	Strategy
Cerebral amyloid angiopathy	Lobar ICH	APP, BRI, CST3	Monogenic	Linkage
Cavernous angioma	Lobar/deep ICH	KRIT1	Monogenic	Linkage
CADASIL	Ischemic stroke, migraine, dementia	NOTCH3	Monogenic	Linkage
Homocystinuria	Ischemic stroke	CBS	Monogenic	Linkage
Arterial dissection	Ischaemic stroke	COL3A1, COL1A1, lysine hydroxylase, PKD1, Fibrillin, α1-antitrypsin	Monogenic	Linkage
Sporadic ICH	Lobar ICH	ApoE	Polygenic	Association
Sporadic ischemic stroke?	_ LDL cholesterol and total cholesterol, OR 1.68 (1.4, 2.1)	ApoE	Polygenic	Association, meta-analysis
Sporadic stroke	Ischemic and hemorrhagic stroke (95% ischemic)	STRK1 (5q12) PDE4 Gene?	Polygenic	Linkage
Sporadic stroke	Ischemic stroke	MTHFR	Polygenic	Association, meta-analysis

carefully the phenotype of interest before attempting either family-based or population-based studies. Genes predisposing to thromboembolic stroke are unlikely to be of major importance in patients with stroke caused by other causes (e.g., hemorrhage, lacunar disease, or endocarditis). Inclusion of such cases is likely to cause misclassification bias and loss of statistical power. Therefore, restriction of cases to carefully selected subtypes or defined pathophysiological mechanisms within those subtypes (e.g., arterial dissection) is highly desirable.

INHERITED STROKE SUSCEPTIBILITY: EVIDENCE FROM FAMILY AND TWIN STUDIES

Epidemiological studies have reported that a family history of stroke is associated with incident and prevalent stroke *(1,2)*. The Framingham Offspring Study found that an increased risk of stroke was associated with parental history of coronary artery disease (CAD) (odds ratio [OR] 3.3), paternal stroke, or transient ischemic attack (TIA) (OR 2.4) or maternal stroke or TIA (OR 1.4). A Canadian study reported a strong association between incident cerebral infarction or TIA and family history of stroke (OR 2.33) or CAD (OR 2.14) in a first-degree relative. These studies did not find that a family history of stroke increased the risk of incident stroke after controlling for other stroke risk factors, suggesting that the effect may have been mediated through genetic influences on common risk factors. However, a Finnish study reported that a parental history of stroke was an independent predictor of stroke risk in both men (OR 1.9) and women (OR 1.8). The Family Heart Study demonstrated a strong association between a family history of stroke and incident stroke independent of other stroke risk factors. This study found an adjusted odds ratio of 2.00 (confidence interval [CI] 1.13–3.54) for prevalent stroke for cases with a positive paternal history and an odds ratio of 1.4 (CI 0.8–2.5) for those with a positive maternal history of stroke. Woo and colleagues reported that having a first-degree relative with a history of intracerebral hemorrhage (ICH) was associated with increased risk of hemorrhagic stroke independent of other risk factors (OR 6.3, 95%CI 1.8–22) *(8)*.

When interpreting the results of family studies of common disease phenotypes, it is important to consider that clustering within families is likely because of the combined influences of shared environmental exposures and genetic susceptibility. Thus, the phenotypic variance may be considered the sum of environmental and genetic influences, the latter because of dominant and background genetic effects. The heritability h^2 of a common phenotype is an estimate of the proportion of phenotypic variance caused by the influence of multiple background genes. A twin study estimated heritability rates of 0.17

for the phenotype of stroke-related death and 0.32 for stroke-related hospital admission *(9)*.

Other data from twin studies also suggest a genetic influence on atherosclerosis and stroke. Twin studies on CAD have reported lower concordance rates (0.25–0.28) among dizygotic compared to monozygotic twins (0.48–0.9). Brass found a concordance rate for stroke of 3.6% in dizygotic twins compared to 17.7% in monozygotic twin pairs *(10)*. A Danish study reported higher concordance (10%) for stroke-related death in monozygotic compared to dizygotic twins (5%) *(9)*.

STROKE AS A PHENOTYPE OF MONOGENIC DISORDERS

Cerebral Autosomal Dominant Arteriopathy With Subcortical Infarcts and Leukoencephalopathy

Cerebral autosomal dominant arteriopathy with subcortical infarcts and leukoencephalopathy (CADASIL) is an autosomal dominant syndrome characterized by cerebral microvasculopathy, diffuse white matter change on magnetic resonance imaging (MRI) (leukoaraiosis), midlife onset of lacunar and subcortical ischemic stroke, migraine, mood disorders, seizures, and dementia (Fig. 1) *(11)*. Although uncommon, it is becoming increasingly recognized as an important and underdiagnosed cause of familial stroke and migraine in the general population. CADASIL shows linkage with a gene locus on chromosome 19 for Notch3, a member of a protein family involved in intercellular signaling and cell fate determination during embryogenesis *(11,12)*.

The Notch3 gene product is a large transmembrane protein, with an intracellular portion involved in signal transduction and an extracellular ligand-binding domain containing 34 epidermal growth factor (EGF)-like repeats, encoded by the first 23 exons of the gene. An analysis of the Notch3 gene in 60 unrelated patients from CADASIL kindreds found that the cohort exhibited marked clustering of highly stereotyped mutations; approx 65% had missense mutations in the first 5 gene exons, all of which resulted in loss or gain of a cysteine residue in an EGF repeat. These data were subsequently confirmed by a Dutch study, which also described three new mutations of similar type. A British study found mutations in Notch3 in 48 of 83 index cases with suspected CADASIL, 73% of which were in exon 4, and 94% were clustered in exons 3–6 *(13)*. The mechanism by which these mutations lead to the CADASIL phenotype is unclear at this time, but may be mediated by abnormal folding of the extracellular Notch3 domain or abnormal ligand binding caused by an unpaired cysteine residue within the EGF-like repeats.

The diagnosis of CADASIL is usually suggested by an appropriate clinical history and a family history of stroke, migraine, or dementia, often with evi-

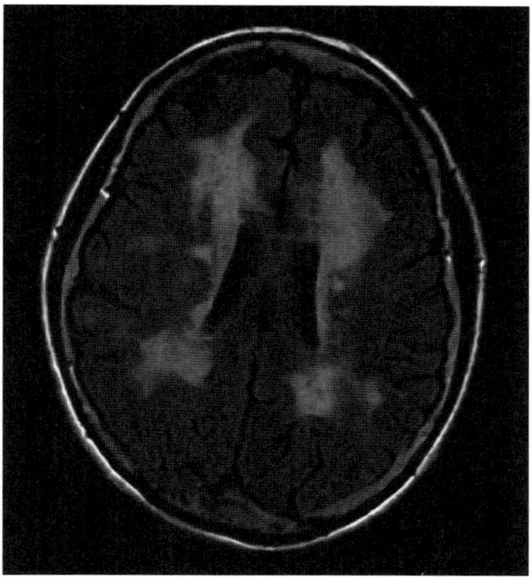

Fig. 1. Axial flair MRI showing subcortical white matter abnormality in CADASIL.

dence of subcortical stroke and diffuse white matter change on fluid-attenuated inversion recovery or T2-weighted MRI. Recent data suggest that the presence of moderate-to-severe white matter involvement of the anterior temporal lobe or external capsule on MRI has high sensitivity as a marker for genetically proven CADASIL *(13)*. Although confidence intervals were not provided, anterior temporal involvement had greater specificity than external capsule change (86 vs 44%). Early reports described the presence of granular osmiophilic material in the smooth muscle basement membrane of small arteries or arterioles on full-thickness skin biopsy as a highly sensitive and specific pregenetic screening technique for CADASIL. However, later studies reported lower sensitivity data. In the most systematic assessment of the utility of skin biopsy to date, Markus and colleagues reported 45% sensitivity and 100% specificity of skin arteriolar granular osmiophilic material as a marker for subsequent proven CADASIL *(13)*. Joutel and colleagues *(14)* reported that the sensitivity of skin biopsy could be enhanced to 100% by immunostaining with a monoclonal antibody against Notch3. However, these findings have not yet been replicated.

Although much has been learned in recent years about the genetics and clinical manifestations of CADASIL, the range of phenotypic expression and correlation of genotype to phenotype remains to be defined fully. The disorder is likely to remain underdiagnosed in the United States because most kindreds reported in the literature have been from Europe. Survival with minimal clinical manifestations in the seventh and eighth decades has been reported in several individuals with proven Notch3 mutations. One report of a Notch3 mutation occurring *de novo* in a patient with sporadic lacunar subcortical stroke has been published, and reports have appeared of CADASIL-associated mutations in families with migraine, but without stroke or dementia.

The prevalence of Notch3 mutations in patients with apparently sporadic ischemic stroke, particularly lacunar and migraine-associated stroke, has not been extensively investigated. In the only study to date that systematically screened for CADASIL mutations (in exons 3 and 4) in patients with lacunar stroke, only 1 of 218 British patients had a CADASIL-causing mutation in exon 4 *(15)*. The prevalence of mutations among the entire cohort was less than 0.5%, increasing to 11% among individuals younger than 50 years. Another study reported no exon 3 or 4 mutations among 70 subjects with ischemic stroke of all subtypes *(16)*. In practice, it has been suggested that genetic screening be considered for individuals with early-onset ischemic subcortical stroke, particularly if leukoaraiosis is present on MRI or if migraine, dementia, or a strong family history of stroke is present.

Stroke Associated With Homocystinuria

Homocystinuria was originally described by Carson in 1962, as a previously unrecognized metabolic disorder resembling Marfan's syndrome in children from Northern Ireland *(17)*. Onset usually occurs in infancy, with failure to thrive and motor and behavioral developmental delay. In some cases, onset occurs in early childhood, with intellectual impairment, focal or generalized seizures, and venous or arterial thrombosis. Milder phenotypes have been described, with onset in the second, third, or fourth decades. These are usually related to specific mutations in the cystathionine β-synthase gene. Affected children have a characteristic physical appearance, with fine, fair hair and a malar flush. They are usually tall, often with abnormalities of both the axial (pectus carinatum or excavatum, spinal kyphosis or scoliosis) and appendicular (arachnodactyly, tibial bowing, pes cavus) skeleton. In later childhood, progressive myopia and closed-angle glaucoma may occur because of loosening and dislocation of the ocular lens. Vascular complications are common, usually peripheral venous thrombosis, pulmonary embolism, and ischemic stroke. Plasma total and free homocysteine are elevated, usually with elevated methionine and low cysteine levels. Urinary homocysteine is also elevated, and a red-purple color develops on addition of sodium cyanide and nitroprusside to the urine, indicating the presence of sulphydryl-containing reducing substances.

Homocystinuria is inherited in an autosomal recessive fashion. It is usually caused by missense mutations in the gene for cystathionine β-synthase (CBS), a homocysteine-degrading enzyme essential for the conversion of methionine to cysteine *(17)*. To date, 92 such mutations have been reported. A 919G→A substitution (predicting a glycine-to-serine change at position 307 of the protein) is the most common mutation in populations of northwest coastal European (Celtic) descent. An 833T→C substitution (predicting an isoleucine-to-threonine alteration at position 278) is the most common mutation in patients of non-Celtic descent. This mutation is associated with a milder clinical phenotype, later onset, and an excellent therapeutic response to pyridoxine supplements. Rarely, the homocystinuria phenotype also occurs because of mutations in other proteins involved in homocysteine metabolism, such as methylenetetrahydrofolate reductase (MTHFR) and cobalamin-transporter proteins.

Several mechanisms are likely to contribute to the increased frequency of stroke and other vascular complications in children and young adults with homocystinuria. Pathological studies have demonstrated patchy arterial lesions (intimal fibrosis, smooth muscle proliferation, luminal narrowing, and degeneration of the internal elastic lamina) of cerebral arterioles and small and large arteries *(18)*. Clinical studies have described impaired endothelial-dependent vasodilation and increased expression of markers of endothelial activation, suggesting endothelial injury. These and other data suggest that elevated homocysteine may contribute to premature atherosclerosis and thrombosis.

Thrombophilia related to severely elevated homocysteine also directly contributes to the pathogenesis of stroke in patients with homocystinuria *(19,20)*. Spontaneous cerebral venous thrombosis is a well-established mechanism of stroke in these patients. Reports also exist of spontaneous arterial system thrombosis with secondary embolism (Fig. 2). Markers of platelet activation and thrombin generation such as urinary thromboxane B2 and plasma F1.2 are elevated, and activated protein C is diminished (consistent with compensatory increased fibrinolytic activity) in patients with homocystinuria, consistent with a thrombophilic state.

Finally, we have reported carotid artery dissection in a single patient with homocystinuria *(19)*. Other authors have speculated that displacement of the ocular lens may be related to weakening of vascular connective tissue protein fibrils caused by replacement of cysteine–cysteine cross-bridges by protein-bound homocysteine–cysteine disulfides. It is possible that a similar mechanism may contribute to vascular dissection.

A

B

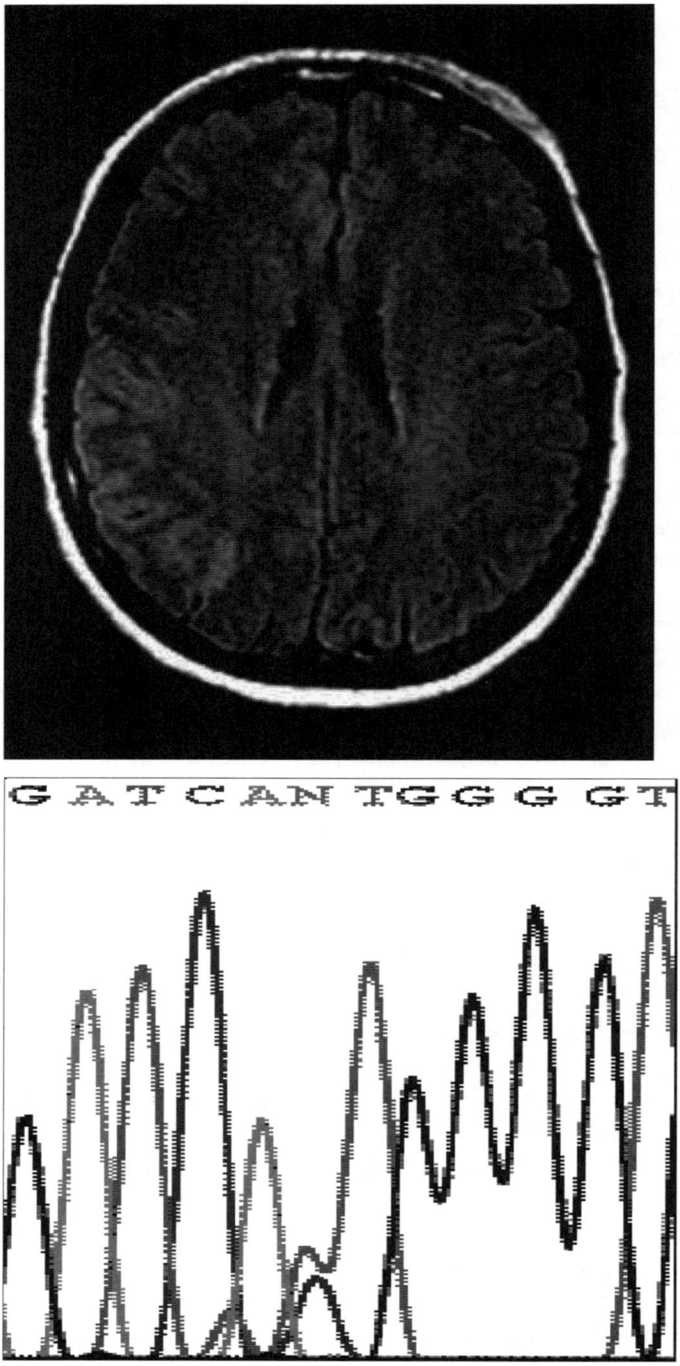

As vitamin B_6 is an essential cofactor for CBS activity, supplementation with pyridoxine (200–600 mg per day) is usually prescribed. Patients generally exhibit either dramatic reduction in plasma homocysteine or minimal response, which permits their classification as responders or nonresponders, respectively. Since characterization of the CBS genetic abnormalities underlying most cases of homocystinuria, it has become clear that the phenotypic response to B_6 correlates with specific CBS mutations, which in turn may determine residual enzyme activity. For patients who exhibit normalization of homocysteine with B_6, usually no other specific measures are required, although supplemental folic acid and B_{12} are sometimes also prescribed.

A methionine-restricted diet with cysteine supplementation is generally prescribed for patients unresponsive to pyridoxine. Several groups have reported that this delays or reduces the incidence of complications, including stroke *(21,22)*. However, compliance can be problematic for patients diagnosed in childhood or early adulthood. Betaine (600–900 mg per day) has been reported to reduce homocysteine levels in pyridoxine-unresponsive patients, particularly those poorly compliant with dietary measures.

Mitochondrial Myopathy, Encephalopathy, Lactic Acidosis, and Stroke-Like Episodes

The majority of proteins comprising the mitochondrial respiratory chain are encoded by nuclear deoxyribonucleic acid (DNA). However, each mitochondrion also contains 2–10 copies of circular double-stranded DNA (mitochondrial DNA, mtDNA) within the matrix, which encodes 13 polypeptides, all subunits of respiratory chain complexes, 22 transfer ribonucleic acids (RNAs), and 2 ribosomal RNAs. As each cell may contain thousands of mitochondria, the cellular copy number of mtDNA is very large.

The mtDNA differs from nucleic DNA in that its genes are tightly packed together with virtual absence of introns. This fact, combined with the vulnerability of mtDNA to damage by oxygen free-radical species produced during oxidative phosphorylation, renders mtDNA particularly susceptible to the development of pathological mutations during replication. Such mutations produce functional deficiencies of one or more elements of the respira-

---

Fig. 2. (*Opposite page*) **(A)** Axial FLAIR MRI showing right parietal embolic infarct secondary to intra-carotid thrombosis (not shown) in a female patient with homocystinuria. **(B)** Sequence analysis of the cystathionine-β synthase gene revealed a T–C substitution at position 833 of the gene, predicting an isoleucine-to-threonine amino acid substitution in the enzyme. This is the commonest mutation associated with B_6-responsive homocystinuria.

tory chain, leading to submaximal adenosine triphosphate synthesis. Any cell thus affected will have a population of normal wild-type mitochondria and one of mutant mitochondria, a phenomenon termed *heteroplasmy*. The vulnerability of a particular tissue type to pathological damage depends on the relative proportion of wild-type to mutant mitochondria and on the energy requirements of that tissue. Therefore, the development of clinical problems most often occurs in tissues that have high energy consumption, such as nervous tissue, skeletal and cardiac muscle, liver, and endocrine glands.

The MELAS syndrome (myopathy, encephalopathy, lactic acidosis, and strokelike episodes) was first described in 1984 by Pavlakis *(23)*. Approximately 80% of patients with this disorder have an A→G mutation at position 3243 of the mitochondrial gene encoding leucine-specific transfer RNA *(24)*. Other point mutations in this gene have also been described. The phenotypic manifestations of MELAS are highly variable. The disorder is usually maternally inherited, although clinical manifestations may be lacking in the mother. Characteristic manifestations include episodic acute strokelike episodes (hemianopsia, hemiparesis, or neglect syndromes), often with headache, vomiting, or stupor. Diffusion MRI frequently shows evidence of cortical hyperintensity in the occipital and parietal lobes in a nonvascular distribution. Serial MRI studies may show resolution of this signal change, which has been attributed to cytotoxic edema. Hydrogen magnetic resonance spectroscopy demonstrates reduced pH with elevated brain lactate signal.

Other clinical manifestations include short stature, seizures, ataxia, sensorineural hearing impairment, pigmentary retinopathy, and progressive opthalmoplegia. A slowly progressive myopathy may develop that is characterized by exercise-induced fatigue or muscle pains and muscle wasting. Vomiting or headache provoked by exercise may occur. Endocrine disturbances, particularly diabetes mellitus and thyroid disorders, are common.

The diagnosis of MELAS is based on a suggestive clinical history, with a family history suggestive of maternally transmitted disease. Light microscopy of skeletal muscle frequently shows subsarcolemmal stippling of muscle fibers (ragged red fibers) with modified Gomori trichrome stain and intense uptake of stains specific for succinate dehydrogenase. Segmental reduction of cytochrome-*c* oxidase staining is also frequently seen. Electron microscopy often reveals increased numbers of morphologically abnormal mitochondria, which may contain abnormal crystalline inclusion bodies. However, muscle histology may be normal in affected patients because of sampling error, cytoprotective effects of wild-type mitochondria, or lack of expression of mtDNA mutations in skeletal muscle of that individual.

Serum biochemistry may reveal elevation of resting lactate concentration, but normal resting serum lactate concentration is frequently observed in affected patients (35 of 50 patients studied in one series). Bicycle or treadmill ergometry may reveal a rapid abnormal rise in serum lactate levels. Cerebrospinal fluid lactate and protein concentrations may be normal or elevated in patients with central nervous system involvement.

Biochemical studies of cultured fibroblasts usually demonstrate reduced cytochrome-*c* oxidase and complex 1 activity of the mitochondrial respiratory chain. The diagnosis is confirmed by genetic analysis of leucocyte mtDNA.

Craniocervical Arterial Dissection in Monogenic Connective Tissue Disorders

Craniocervical arterial dissection accounts for 10–20% of cases of ischemic stroke in patients younger than 30 years. Case reports and small case series have reported associations between stroke because of craniocervical arterial dissection and missense mutations in the following genes coding for connective tissue proteins: (1) the COL3A1 gene, which encodes procollagen 3 and is the underlying genetic abnormality in Ehlers–Danlos syndrome type IV; (2) the lysine hydroxylase gene, which is abnormal in Ehlers–Danlos syndrome type VI; (3) the COL1A1 gene, which encodes the procollagen 1 α-chain and is the genetic basis of osteogenesis imperfecta; (4) the fibrillin gene, which is associated with abnormal elastin microfibril assembly in Marfan syndrome; (5) the α-1 antitrypsin gene, which is associated with reduced inhibition of circulating elastase, a major protease involved in connective tissue degradation; and (6) the PKD1 gene, which is associated with intracranial aneurysm formation and polycystic kidney disease. To date, a systematic evaluation of the prevalence of mutations in these genes in a large consecutive series of patients with sporadic craniocervical arterial dissection has not been performed.

Other Monogenic Stroke Syndromes

Other monogenic disorders associated with hemorrhagic or ischemic stroke include cerebral cavernous angiomas, Fabry's disease, sickle cell disease, and cerebral amyloid angiopathy (Table 2).

GENETIC SUSCEPTIBILITY TO COMMON STROKE: POLYGENIC INFLUENCES

For common stroke, it is highly unlikely that any one genetic defect will prove to predispose to all cases of any particular stroke subtype or stroke-related trait *(1–3)*. Rather, these phenotypes are more likely to result from the interaction of environmental factors, with multiple polymorphisms in several genes encoding key proteins involved in the pathophysiology of the trait or subtype. This genetic heterogeneity increases the difficulty involved in identification of specific genetic determinants of stroke phenotypes. Genetic association studies of candidate genes and polymorphisms have been widely used for the investigation of inherited susceptibility to stroke. These designs treat the candidate polymorphism like a conventional environmental exposure. Compared to similar studies of environmental risk factors, genetic association studies have the major advantage that the exposure (i.e., gene variant) is clearly defined and is not modified as a consequence of the disease.

Linkage Studies of Common Stroke

In an Icelandic population *(5)*, using the pedigrees of 476 patients with stroke, investigators detected significant linkage (Log of Odds [LOD] 4.4, $p = 3.9 \times 10^{-6}$) to a region on chromosome 5q12, which contains a putative stroke-related gene (STRK1). This population-based sample consisted of individuals affected as follows: 95% ischemic stroke (13% large artery, 16% small vessel, 23% cardioembolism, 39% undetermined, and 4% other cause) and 5% hemorrhage. Although the gene appears to contribute more to ischemic stroke, there was no statistically significant difference in the LOD score between ischemic and hemorrhagic stroke. Using a multiplicative model, siblings of individuals with this gene carried almost a twofold higher risk of stroke. When fine mapping of the locus was performed, markers within the gene for phosphodiesterase 4D (PDE4D) were most strongly associated with stroke, particularly subgroups due to carotid disease and cardiac embolism *(25)*. Although PDE4D is a promising candidate gene within this population, these findings remain to be confirmed by other groups at this time.

Association Studies of Common Stroke

Genetic Susceptibility to Thrombosis

Arterial thrombosis is a major intermediate biological process in ischemic stroke, particularly embolism originating from the heart or craniocervical arteries. Prothrombotic proteins (e.g., fibrinogen, von Willebrand factor) and homocysteine are associated with increased risk of stroke in epidemiological studies. Antithrombotic therapies have proven benefit for stroke prevention and treatment. Thus, there is a strong *a priori* rationale for study of genes encoding thrombosis pathway proteins as candidates for inherited susceptibility to stroke *(26)*.

Platelet Proteins

Platelet surface receptor glycoproteins GPIa–GPIIa and GPIIb–GPIIIa mediate platelet binding to collagen and fibrinogen, respectively, promoting thrombus adherence and stability. A common polymorphism (1565T→ C or Pl^{A2}) in the GPIIIa gene is associated with enhanced platelet activation and may affect fibrinogen binding. Several studies have reported strong associations among Pl^{A2} allele, CAD, and stroke, suggesting a role in arterial thrombosis in vivo *(27–29)*. However, a large cohort study found no such effect. Similarly, a common allele in the GPIa gene (807T) has been associated with increased GPIa–GPIIa platelet receptor density, enhanced collagen adhesion, and CAD in younger adults, women, and smokers. In a Japanese population, a polymorphism causing a phenylalanine-to-valine substitution in the enzyme that inactivates platelet-activating factor, platelet-activating factor acetylhydrolase, was independently associated with increased risk of ischemic stroke.

Coagulation Pathway Proteins

Plasma fibrinogen and von Willebrand Factor levels are associated with increased risk of ischemic stroke and CAD. Fibrinogen level shows moderate heritability and has been associated with a common β-fibrinogen promoter polymorphism (455G→A) *(30)*. This SNP is a marker for a common haplotype associated with carotid atherosclerosis and CAD. An α-fibrinogen variant (Thr312Ala) has been associated with embolic stroke and pulmonary embolism, suggesting formation of unstable thrombus caused by ineffective fibrin cross-linking. Supporting this hypothesis, an interaction with this variant was found with a common polymorphism in factor XIII (Val34Leu), which mediates clot stability by promotion of fibrin cross-linking *(31)*. Both factor V Leiden, which confers abnormal in vivo resistance to the endogenous anticoagulant activity of activated protein C, and the 20210A→G prothrombin gene polymorphism, which is associated with increased prothrombin levels in vivo, have been implicated as potent genetic modifiers on the clinical risk of venous thrombosis. However, data are conflicting concerning their potential role in arterial thromboembolism and ischemic stroke, with some studies reporting positive and others no association between these variants and stroke.

In general, it is likely that several common polymorphisms may each confer a small risk of venous and arterial thromboembolism, and that these effects are additive when multiple variants exist in the same individual. Many studies to date have defined stroke very broadly, often including hemorrhages as well as ischemic strokes. The effect of interactions between these genetic factors, cardiac pathology (e.g., atrial fibrillation), and hemostatic activation in embolic stroke has yet to be elucidated.

Genetic Predisposition to Hypertension

Hypertension is a major risk factor for ischemic and hemorrhagic stroke and is an important stroke-related intermediate trait. Genetic influences have been estimated to account for one-third to one-half of the predisposition to hypertension, with constitutional (age, sex, body mass) and environmental (sodium consumption, alcohol intake, and smoking) factors accounting for the remainder. Familial aggregation of hypertension independent of environmental factors has been described in several studies. Adoption studies have found higher correlation of systolic and diastolic hypertension between parents and biological children compared to adopted children and between biological siblings compared to adoptive siblings. Twin studies have reported higher correlation of systolic and diastolic blood pressure among monozygotic compared to dizygotic twins.

Several genes encoding proteins involved in the physiology of blood pressure homeostasis are candidates for the phenotypes of hypertension and, by extension, ischemic and hemorrhagic stroke. One of these is the gene for ACE. The ACE gene has two major alleles, one with insertion (I) and the other with deletion (D) of a 287-nucleotide basepair sequence. This polymorphism has a major influence on plasma ACE concentrations, accounting for up to half the variance in one report. Zee and others found that the D allele was significantly more common in hypertensive patients with familial hypertension compared to normotensive controls *(32)*. Subsequent studies evaluating the potential association between the I–D polymorphism and hypertensive phenotype have yielded conflicting results. Several studies have reported associations between the DD genotype and myocardial infarction. In the largest study to date, the DD genotype was associated with a 10% increase in the risk of myocardial infarction (95% CI 0–21%) in almost 11,000 subjects in the ISIS trial *(33)*.

Several studies have examined the potential association between the D allele and ischemic stroke, with conflicting results. A meta-analysis of published studies found a small, but significant, association (OR 1.3) between the DD genotype and stroke risk, consistent with the range reported for CAD *(34)*. Others have found a positive association between DD genotype and lacunar, but not atherothrombotic or cardioembolic, infarction. A meta-analysis of 23 studies (9833 subjects) found that the D allele was positively associated with common carotid intima-media thickness ($p < 0.01$), with a stronger association among higher-risk populations *(34)*. These conflicting results are likely to be at least partly because of ethnic differences in study populations, small sample size, inclusion bias, and failure to define stroke subtypes.

The angiotensinogen (AGT) gene is also a candidate for hypertension and ischemic stroke *(35)*. Early studies using a GT short tandem repeat marker found significant linkage between the AGT locus and hypertension. Subsequent studies confirmed linkage between the AGT locus and hypertension in

British, African Caribbean, Mexican American, and French Canadian cohorts, although no linkage was demonstrated in a European study and a study in China. Sequence analysis of the AGT gene has revealed a variant causing a methionine-to-threonine (M235T) substitution, which was significantly more frequent in hypertension cases than controls. The presence of the T allele was found to correlate with plasma AGT concentration. A recent meta-analysis of 127 studies *(35)* found an allele-specific dose-dependent increase in plasma AGT (5% [95% CI 2–8%] with MT, 11% [95% CI 7–15%] with TT genotypes). The risk of hypertension was also increased in white (OR 1.08 [95% CI 1.01–1.15] with MT, 1.19 [95%CI 1.19–1.3 with TT) and Asian (OR 1.29 [95% CI 0.96–1.74] with MT, 1.6 [95% CI 1.19–2.15] with TT) subjects. However, no increased risk of CAD was detected in this analysis. Two other meta-analyses also reported significant associations between the AGT 235T allele and hypertension. These data suggest a relative risk of 20–30% associated with the AGT 235T allele, which may translate into a significant attributable risk for certain ethnic populations in which this allele is highly prevalent (allele frequencies are approx 0.9 in African American, 0.7 in Asian, and 0.4 in Caucasian populations).

The pathogenic mechanism of the AGT 235T variant has yet to be elucidated. One possibility is that it is a marker for a functional mutation (a G→A substitution at position (6 in the AGT gene promotor region), which exists in strong linkage disequilibrium with the 235T polymorphism, and causes a significant increase in the basal rate of AGT transcription.

Two relatively small studies investigated for an association between the AGT 235T polymorphism and ischemic stroke and carotid atherosclerosis *(36,37)*. Although no association was found, no definite conclusions can be drawn as these studies were underpowered to detect an association, if present *(36–38)*. In contrast, two studies *(39,40)* have reported that this variant is associated with MRI white matter abnormalities presumed secondary to microangiopathic cerebral disease. A third study found no such association in a smaller sample of patients with essential hypertension *(41)*.

Other candidate genes for human hypertension, and hypertension-associated stroke, include those encoding subunits of the renal epithelial sodium channel and atrial natriuretic peptide (ANP) gene. Both are implicated in the phenotype of hypertension with dietary sensitivity to salt, which is partially genetically determined and is common in African Americans. Single base-pair substitutions in the α- and β-subunits of ENaC are the basis for Liddle's syndrome, a rare autosomal dominant syndrome of hypertension, low plasma renin, and hypoaldosteronism, which is associated with a gain of function of the renal tubular sodium channel. Large epidemiological studies have failed to demonstrate a clear association between individual ENaC polymorphisms and hypertension. ANP counteracts the renin–angiotensin–aldosterone system by promoting urinary sodium and water excretion and causing vasodilation. Polymorphisms in the ANP gene have begun to be scrutinized for possible associations with salt-sensitive hypertension, particularly in African Americans. One study found that an allele at a HpaII restriction enzyme site was significantly more frequent in hypertensive compared to normotensive controls. To our knowledge, no data exist on the role of ENaC and ANP polymorphisms in predisposition to stroke.

Genetic Predisposition to Hyperhomocyst(e)inemia and Stroke

MTHFR is a key enzyme involved in homocysteine degradation. It catalyzes the formation of 5-methyl tetrahydrofolate, an essential cofactor in the detoxification of homocysteine to methionine. In 1988, a thermolabile variant of MTHFR was described that has low specific activity at body temperature and unusually severe reduction in activity after heating. A single 677C→T basepair substitution in the human MTHFR gene predicts expression of the thermolabile variant *(42)*. The T allele dose correlates highly with plasma homocyst(e)ine, and mild-to-moderate elevated homocyst(e)ine is more prevalent in TT homozygotes compared to CT heterozygotes and wild-type CC controls. This relationship is modified by plasma folate status because the greatest elevation in homocyst(e)ine occurs in TT homozygotes with folate concentrations that are in the lower half of the reference range *(43)*.

The MTHFR 677C→T polymorphism has been investigated as a candidate stroke susceptibility allele. To date, however, association studies examining the relationship of the TT genotype with stroke have yielded conflicting results. To address power limitations of previous studies, we performed a meta-analysis of all studies published prior to 2001 *(44)*. Among 19 included studies (2788 strokes, 3962 nonstrokes), the pooled odds ratios associated with TT genotype was 1.23 (95% CI 0.96–1.58, $p = 0.1$). A subsequent association study in a large (more than 3600 subjects) Chinese sample reported an odds ratio that was almost identical to this estimate (OR 1.27, 95% CI 1.04–1.56) *(45)*.

The importance of the 677C→T variant as a risk factor for cerebrovascular disease may differ according to the allele frequencies and folate status in the population studied. Available data suggest that the T allele is relatively common in Asian and most European populations, but less common in African Americans. This concept is supported by another meta-analysis examining the risk of CAD associated with the TT genotype *(43)*. In more than 23,000 subjects, the pooled odds ratio of coronary disease was 1.16 (95% CI 1.05–1.28), increasing to 1.44 (95% CI 1.12–1.83) in subjects with low folate status. Although the magnitude of risk associated with this polymorphism is relatively low for an individual, the population-attributable risk is likely to be substantial because the variant is common in the general population (TT genotype prevalence 10–22%). It may be particularly important in populations outside North America in which low folate status is common.

Apolipoprotein E Genotype and Stroke

Apolipoprotein E (APOE for gene, apo E for protein) is a 299-amino acid protein synthesized in the liver, brain, and other tissues. It is normally found in association with low-density lipoprotein (LDL) and high-density lipoproteins, in which it functions as a ligand-promoting particle binding to cell surface receptors. The APOE gene is polymorphic, with three alleles (E2, E3, E4) coding for three isoforms, differing from each other by possession of a cysteine or arginine residue at positions 112 and 158. The substitution at residue 158 affects the LDL receptor binding site, which impairs clearance of LDL cholesterol. A spectrum of total and LDL cholesterol exists, depending on apo E isoform (lowest with E2, intermediate with E3, highest with E4). Conversely, E2/E2 homozygotes are predisposed to type III hyperlipidemia, characterized by low cholesterol and hypertriglyceridemia. APOE genotype is estimated to account for 7% of interindividual variability of total and LDL cholesterol.

The APOE4 allele has been reported to be an independent risk factor for CAD and atherosclerosis. Surprisingly, this effect remains after inclusion of LDL cholesterol on multivariate analysis. Some authors have hypothesized that this may be because of an isoform-specific antioxidant effect of apo E, which is most potent with E2 and least strong with E4. This effect may modulate the progression and clinical manifestation of atherosclerosis. Several studies have examined the potential association between APOE genotype and stroke. Many of these were limited by small sample size, combination of ischemic and hemorrhagic stroke, inclusion bias, and failure to define ischemic stroke subtypes. A meta-analysis of these reported a significant excess of the E4 allele in cases with stroke, with a summary odds ratio for stroke of 1.68 (CI 1.36–2.09, $p < 0.001$) *(46)*. No significant difference was found in E2 allele frequency, but E3 was significantly more common in control subjects, suggesting a protective effect.

In addition to predisposing to atherosclerosis and incident stroke, experimental and clinical studies suggest that apo E may modulate the neuronal injury response to various central nervous system lesions. In vitro and animal studies have shown that apo E has isoform-specific antioxidant, immunomodulatory, and neurotrophic effects that may underlie this effect. Initial clinical studies indicated that APOE genotype may influence outcome after stroke and traumatic brain injury *(47–50)*. Possession of the E4 allele has been associated with reduced survival after sporadic hemorrhagic stroke *(49)*, although no correlation between specific alleles and hemorrhage volume or perilesional edema has been found *(51)*. In contrast to these findings, one study reported an unexpected positive association between E4 allele and survival after ischemic stroke *(52)*. No influence of the E4 allele was reported on functional outcome following rehabilitation for stroke, but this may have been related to insufficient statistical power *(53)*.

Cerebral amyloid angiopathy is a cerebral microangiopathy characterized by amyloid deposition and degenerative changes (fibrinoid necrosis and cracking) in the media of arterioles and small arteries, frequently leading to multiple lobar hemorrhagic strokes *(54)*. It has become recognized as the most common underlying cause of lobar brain hemorrhage in the elderly *(55)*. APOE genotype is an important modifier of the pathological progression and clinical manifestation of cerebral amyloid angiography. Possession of the E4 allele is pathologically associated with greater deposition of β-amyloid in the vessel wall. In contrast, the E2 allele is associated with vessel degeneration, development of hemorrhages, and earlier age of hemorrhage onset. Both alleles are associated with higher risk of recurrent hemorrhage; possession of the uncommon E2/E4 genotype is associated with particularly malignant progression of disease and poor clinical outcome.

It is likely that the pathogenesis of spontaneous lobar ICH differs from that of nonlobar ICH. A large population-based study in Cincinnati, Ohio, found that possession of either an E2 or an E4 allele was an independent risk factor for lobar (adjusted OR 2.3, 95% CI 1.2–4.4), but not nonlobar, ICH *(8)*. The attributable risk of lobar ICH associated with either allele was 29%.

REFERENCES

1. Elbaz A. Amarenco P. Genetic susceptibility and ischemic stroke. Curr Opin Neurol 1999;12:47–55.
2. Hassan A, Markus HS. Genetics and ischemic stroke. Brain 2000;123:1784–1812.
3. Cardon LR, Bell JI. Association study designs for complex diseases. Nat Rev Genet 2001;2:91–99.
4. Hegele RA. SNP judgments and freedom of association. Arterioscler Thromb Vasc Biol 2002;22:1058–1061.
5. Gretarsdottir S, Sveinbjornsdottir S, Jonsson HH, et al. Localization of a susceptibility gene for common forms of stroke to 5q12. Am J Hum Genet 2002;70:593–603.
6. Martin ER, Lai EH, Gilbert JR, et al. SNPing away at complex diseases: analysis of single-nucleotide polymorphisms around APOE in Alzheimer disease. Am J Hum Genet 2000;67:383–394.
7. Meschia JF. Addressing the heterogeneity of the ischemic stroke phenotype in human genetics research. Stroke 2002;33:2780–32785.

8. Woo D, Sauerbeck LR, Kissela BM, et al. Genetic and environmental risk factors for intracerebral hemorrhage. Stroke 2002;33:1190–1196.
9. Bak S, Gaist D, Sindrup SH, Skytthe A, Christensen K. Genetic liability in stroke. A long-term follow-up study of Danish twins. Stroke 2002;33:769–774.
10. Brass LM, Isaacsohn JL, Merikangas KR, Robinette CD. A study of twins and stroke. Stroke 1992;23:221–223.
11. Tournier-Lasserve E, Joutel A, Melki J, et al. Cerebral autosomal dominant arteriopathy with subcortical infarcts and leucoencephalopathy maps to chromosome 19q12. Nat Genet 1993;3:256–259.
12. Joutel A, Corpechot C, Ducros A, et al. Notch3 mutations in CADASIL, a hereditary adult-onset condition causing stroke and dementia. Nature 1996;383:707–710.
13. Markus HS, Martin RJ, Simpson MA, et al. Diagnostic strategies in CADASIL. Neurology 2002;59:1134–1138.
14. Joutel A, Favrole P, Labauge P, et al. Skin biopsy immunostaining with a Notch3 monoclonal antibody for CADASIL diagnosis. Lancet 2001;358:2049–2051.
15. Joutel A, Dodick DD, Parisi JE, et al. De novo mutation in the Notch3 gene causing CADASIL. Ann Neurol 2000;47:388–391.
16. Dong Y, Hassan A, Zhang Z, et al. Yield for screening for CADASIL mutations in lacunar stroke and leukoariosis. Stroke 2003;34:203–206.
17. Mudd SH, Levy HL, Kraus JP. Disorders of transsulfuration. In: Valle D, ed. The Metabolic and Molecular Basis of Inherited Disease. 8th ed. New York: McGraw Hill, 2001.
18. McCully K. Vascular pathology of homocysteinemia: implications for the pathogenesis of atherosclerosis. Am J Pathol 1969;56:111–128.
19. Kelly PJ, Furie KL, Kistler JP, et al. Stroke in young patients with hyperhomocysteinemia due to cystathionine beta-synthase deficiency. Neurology 2003;60: 275–279.
20. Davi G, Di Minno G, Coppola A, et al. Oxidative stress and platelet activation in homozygous homocystinuria. Circulation 2001;104:1124–1128.
21. Wilcken DE, Wilcken B. The natural history of vascular disease in homocystinuria and the effects of treatment. J Inherit Metab Dis 1997;20:295–300.
22. Yap S, Naughten ER, Wilcken B, Wilcken DE, Boers GH. Vascular complications of severe hyperhomocysteinemia in patients with homocystinuria due to cystathionine β-synthase deficiency: effects of homocysteine-lowering therapy. Semin Thromb Hemost 2000;26:335–340.
23. Pavlakis SG, Phillips PC, DiMauro S, et al. Mitochondrial myopathy, encephalopathy, lactic acidosis, and stroke-like episodes. A distinctive clinical syndrome. Ann Neurol 1984;16:481.
24. Schmiedel J, Jackson S, Schafer J, Reichmann H. Mitochondrial cytopathies. J Neurol 2003;250:267–277.
25. Gretarsdottir S, Thorleifsson G, Reynisdottir ST, et al. The gene encoding phosphodiesterase 4D confers risk of ischemic stroke. Nat Genet 2003;35:131–138.
26. Williams MS, Bray PF. Genetics of arterial prothrombotic risk states. Exp Biol Med 2001;226:409–419.
27. Weiss EJ, Bray PF, Tayback M, et al. A polymorphism of a platelet glycoprotein receptor as an inherited risk factor for coronary thrombosis. N Engl J Med 1996; 334:1090–1094.

28. Wagner KR, Giles WH, Johnson CJ, et al. Platelet glycoprotein receptor IIIa polymorphism P1A2 and ischemic stroke risk: the Stroke Prevention in Young Women Study. Stroke 1998;29:581–585.
29. Reiner AP, Kumar PN, Schwartz SM, et al. Genetic variants of platelet glycoprotein receptors and risk of stroke in young women. Stroke 2000;31:1628–1633.
30. Green FR. Fibrinogen polymorphisms and atherothrombotic disease. Ann N Y Acad Sci 2001;936:549–559.
31. Anwar R, Gallivan L, Edmonds SD, Markham AF. Genotype/phenotype correlations for coagulation factor XIII: specific normal polymorphisms are associated with high or low factor XIII specific activity. Blood 1999;93:897–905.
32. Zee RY, Lou YK, Griffiths LR, Morris BJ. Association of a polymorphism of the angiotensin I-converting gene with essential hypertension. Biochem Biophys Res Commun 1992;184:9–15.
33. Keavney B, McKenzie C, Parish S, et al. Large scale test of hypothesized associations between the angiotensin-converting enzyme insertion/deletion polymorphism and myocardial infarction in about 5000 cases and 6000 controls. Lancet 2000;355: 434–442.
34. Sharma P. Meta-analysis of the ACE gene in ischemic stroke. J Neurol Neurosurg Psychiatry 1998;64:227–230.
35. Akhtar Sethi A, Nordestgaard BG, Tybjaerg-Hansen A. Angiotensinogen gene polymorphism, plasma angiotensinogen, and risk of hypertension and ischemic heart disease. A meta-analysis. Arterioscler Thromb Vasc Biol 2003;23:1269.
36. Sayed-Tabatabaei F, Houwing-Duistermaat JJ, van Duijn CM, Witteman JCM. Angiotensin-converting enzyme gene polymorphism and carotid artery wall thickness. A meta-analysis. Stroke 2003;34:1634–1639.
37. Nakata Y, Katsuya T, Rakugi H, et al. Polymorphism of angiotensin converting enzyme, angiotensinogen, and apolipoprotein E genes in a Japanese population with cerebrovascular disease. Am J Hypertens 1997;10:1391–1395.
38. Barley J, Markus H, Brown M, Carter N. Lack of association between angiotensinogen polymorphism (M235T) and cerebrovascular disease and carotid atheroma. J Hum Hypertens 1995;9:681–683.
39. Takami S, Imai Y, Katsuya T, et al. Gene polymorphism of the renin–angiotensin system associates with risk for lacunar infarction. The Ohasama study. Am J Hypertension 2000;13:121–127.
40. Schmidt R, Schmidt H, Fazekas F, et al. Angiotensinogen polymorphism M235T, carotid atherosclerosis, and small-vessel disease-related cerebral abnormalities. Hypertension 2001;38:110–115.
41. Sierra C, Coca A, Gomez-Angelats E, et al. Renin-angiotensin system genetic polymorphisms and cerebral white matter lesions in essential hypertension. Hypertension 2002;39:343–347.
42. Frosst P, Blom HJ, Milos R, et al. A candidate genetic risk factor for vascular disease: a common mutation in methylenetetrahydrofolate reductase. Nat Genet 1995; 10:111–113.
43. Li Z, Sun L, Zhang H, et al. Elevated plasma homocysteine was associated with hemorrhagic and ischemic stroke, but MTHFR C677T polymorphism was a risk factor for thrombotic stroke. A multicenter case–control study in China. Stroke 2003; 34:2085–2090.

44. Klerk M, Verhoef P, Clarke R, et al. MTHFR 677C→T polymorphism and risk of coronary heart disease: a meta-analysis. JAMA 2002;288:2023–2031.
45. Kelly PJ, Rosand J, Kistler JP, et al. Homocysteine, MTHFR 677C→T polymorphism, and risk of ischemic stroke: results of a meta-analysis. Neurology 2002;59: 529–536.
46. McCarron MO, Delong A, Alberts MJ. APOE genotype as a risk factor for ischemic stroke. A meta-analysis. Neurology 1999;53:2176–2179.
47. Teasdale GM, Nicoll JAR, Murray G, Fiddes M. Association of apolipoprotein E polymorphism with outcome after head injury. Lancet 1997;350:1069–1071.
48. Lichtman SW, Seliger G, Tycko B, Marder K. Apolipoprotein E and functional recovery from brain injury following postacute rehabilitation. Neurology 2000;55: 1536–1539.
49. Alberts MJ, Graffagnino C, McClenny C, et al. ApoE genotype and survival from intracerebral hemorrhage. Lancet 1995;346:575.
50. McCarron MO, Muir KW, Nicoll JA, et al. Prospective study of apolipoprotein E genotype and outcome following ischemic stroke. Arch Neurol 2000;57;1480–1484.
51. McCarron MO, Hoffman KL, DeLong DM, et al. Intracerebral hemorrhage outcome: APOE, hematoma and edema volumes. Neurology 1999;53:2176–2179.
52. Weir CJ, McCarron MO, Muir KW, et al. Apolipoprotein E genotype, coagulation, and survival following acute stroke. Neurology 2001;57:1097–1100.
53. Treger I, Froom P, Ring H, Friedman G. Association between apolipoprotein E4 and rehabilitation outcome in hospitalized ischemic stroke patients. Arch Phys Med Rehabil 2003;84:973–976.
54. McCarron MO, Nicoll JA. Apolipoprotein E genotype and cerebral amyloid angiopathy-related hemorrhage. Ann NY Acad Sci 2000;903:176–179.
55. Greenberg SM. Cerebral amyloid angiopathy and vessel dysfunction. Cerebrovasc Dis 2002;13(Suppl 2):42–47.

Index

A

D